Echography and Doppler of the Brain

Chiara Robba • Giuseppe Citerio
Editors

Echography and Doppler of the Brain

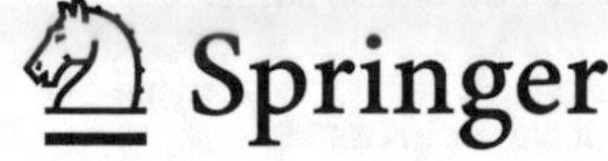
Springer

Editors
Chiara Robba
Anesthesia and Intensive Care
Policlinico San Martino
IRCCS for Oncology and Neuroscience
Genoa
Italy

Giuseppe Citerio
Anesthesia Neurosurgical Intensive Care
ASST Monza School of Medicine
University of Milano
Bicocca
Milano
Italy

ISBN 978-3-030-48204-6 ISBN 978-3-030-48202-2 (eBook)
https://doi.org/10.1007/978-3-030-48202-2

This Springer imprint is published by the registered company Springer Nature Switzerland AG
The registered company address is: Gewerbestrasse 11, 6330 Cham, Switzerland

Foreword

The care of critically ill patients with neurological diseases is challenging, and often involves compromises to select a least-worst rather than a best option. This is particularly true in the case of neuromonitoring. Clinical monitoring of brain function in our patients is often confounded by sedative drugs, and we have to rely to a greater extent on neuroimaging and bedside monitoring devices.

Imaging essentially provide snapshots of disease, rather than representing an approach to ongoing patient monitoring. As a consequence, many neuro-ICUs have had to primarily rely on multimodality physiological monitoring (intracranial pressure monitoring, often combined with brain oximetry and cerebral microdialysis) to understand evolving pathophysiology, select appropriate therapies, and assess their impact. However, the risks involved make their use inappropriate in patients with less severe disease, in the prehospital phase, when patients are being screened before ICU admission, and after patients have left the ICU. Finally, substantial cost of disposable equipment limits their use in resource-limited contexts. There is a clear need for noninvasive monitoring with limited consumable costs, which can be used through the entire disease narrative.

While neurophysiological monitoring does fulfil some of these requirements, it tends to be cumbersome to initiate and often requires specialist expertise for interpretation. Further, while it can detect seizures and may aid in the titration of sedative, it does not provide information about many of the physiological parameters we can influence with ICU interventions.

The case for ultrasound-based investigation of cerebral and cerebrovascular physiology is compelling. These techniques provide key data in several areas where we have potential therapies, including intracranial pressure, cranial compliance, cerebral blood flow, cerebral autoregulation, and vasospasm. The noninvasive nature of the technique allows extension of its application from the prehospital phase to late follow-up, and also to extracranial diseases where secondary neurological compromise is suspected. Finally, the negligible consumable costs facilitate use in resource-limited environments.

Given these clear benefits of ultrasound-based diagnosis and monitoring, this book, edited by Dr. Robba and Professor Citerio, is a welcome contribution. Written by experienced clinicians who have wide knowledge of the literature and use these techniques regularly, the chapters cover all aspects of brain ultrasound and echography—including anatomy and physiology, methodology, clinical evidence, and practical application and interpretation. The information that it provides will support the use of ultrasound in both clinical care and research—either on its own or as a complement to neuroimaging, invasive monitoring, and neurophysiology.

Ultrasound-based diagnosis and monitoring of brain dysfunction have a growing role in the care of patients with brain dysfunction and disease—and this book will contribute to that growth.

Cambridge, UK David Menon

Foreword

"Learning never exhausts the mind"—Leonardo da Vinci

For decades, clinicians have attempted to use monitoring techniques to try to understand the pathophysiology of brain disease. In the early 1980s, Aaslid and colleagues first demonstrated that cerebral arterial flow velocities could be measured by pulsed Doppler ultrasound, heralding a new era of noninvasive monitoring of cerebral hemodynamics.

As technology continued to evolve over recent years, a variety of invasive and noninvasive monitors were developed which introduced the concept of multimodal neuromonitoring. Whilst this has been supplemented by complex imaging methodologies, giving us increasingly detailed information about brain pathophysiology, the principle of bedside monitoring remains the ultimate goal of neuroscientists around the world.

The use of ultrasound moves a long way in achieving this goal, and its application for the brain and other organ systems continues to expand. Whilst clinicians continue to push the boundaries of the use of ultrasound, dissemination of their expertise to the next generation of scientists and clinicians is a responsibility that must not be ignored.

This book, co-edited by leaders in the field of neurosciences and neuromonitoring, establishes a firm foundation to promote knowledge and understanding in this area of neurosciences. It is an excellent educational asset for those interested in the use of ultrasound and Doppler as applied to brain pathophysiology and clinical management of neurological disease. As well as covering a breadth of conditions, readers will find the link to pathology and clinical applications in each section both stimulating and informative. Although the basic technique of ultrasound is not complex, this book will allow readers to refine their understanding of the technique, its application, and interpretation of information that the technique gives them. As with any skill however, continued practice is essential!

I look forward in the coming years that I will see more clinicians using the technique of ultrasound in the management of complex neurological conditions as a result of the learning from this unique book.

I wish you enjoyable and informative reading!

Cambridge, UK Arun Gupta

Acknowledgements

The authors would like to thank Dr Alberto Addis for his help in revieweing the book content.

Contents

List of Videos

Video 4.1 Optic nerve sheath diameter measurement using ocular sonography in the horizontal and vertical axes

Video 17.1 TCCD, transtemporal approach, midbrain plane. In the transtemporal approach, the midbrain plane is recognizable for its typical butterfly-shaped hypoechogenic structure surrounded by the hyperechogenic basal cisterns. By tilting the probe above the midbrain of 10°, the thalamic plane with the third ventricle is visualized

Video 17.2 TCCD, transtemporal approach, midbrain plane. Typical vascular representation in color-mode pattern of the midbrain plane where the ipsilateral MCA M1–M2 segments and ACA-A1 are visualized; also contralateral ACA-A1 and MCA-M1 may be visible. Note the optimal quality of the temporal window. By tilting the probe above the midbrain of 100, the thalamic plane with the third ventricle is visualized. In this plane are typically visible the PCA-P2 segment, the distal part of ACA-A2, and MCA-M2. By lowering the insonation angle by 10° from the midbrain plane, the upper pontine plane is displayed. Here, the distal ICA is recognized as well as the PCA-P1 segment (also partially visible in the midbrain plane)

Electronic Supplementary Material is available in the online version of the related chapter on https://doi.org/10.1007/978-3-030-48202-2_4 and https://doi.org/10.1007/978-3-030-48202-2_17.

Part I

Technology, Views and Normal Echo Anatomy

1 Principles of Transcranial Doppler Ultrasonography

Danilo Cardim and Chiara Robba

Contents

1.1 Introduction

Two basic modalities are currently available in clinical practice for brain ultrasonography: transcranial Doppler (TCD) and brightness (B)-mode transcranial colour-coded duplex (TCCD).

Transcranial Doppler ultrasonography technique is based on the phenomenon called Doppler effect, observed by the physicist Christian Andreas Doppler in the nineteenth century. The Doppler effect states that when a sound wave with a certain frequency strikes a moving object, the reflected wave changes its frequency (the Doppler shift, f_d) directly proportionally to the velocity of the reflector. In other words, when the relative movement results in the wave source and wave observer becoming closer together, the wavelength is decreased giving the perception of a higher frequency; on the other hand, when the relative movement results in the source and observer becoming farther apart, the wavelength is increased giving the perception of a lower frequency (Fig. 1.1). When translated to medical applications, this principle has been applied to monitor erythrocyte motion inside an insonated blood vessel by measuring the difference in ultrasound frequencies between emission and reception [1]. The equation derived from this principle is the basis for calculating the cerebral blood flow velocity (FV, in cm/s), which is a function of the parameters affecting the relative motion (velocity and angle) and parameters determining the

D. Cardim (✉)
Department of Neurology and Neurotherapeutics, University of Texas Southwestern Medical Center, Dallas, TX, USA

Institute for Exercise and Environmental Medicine, Texas Health Presbyterian Hospital Dallas, Dallas, TX, USA

C. Robba
Anesthesia and Intensive Care, Policlinico San Martino, IRCCS for Oncology and Neuroscience, Genoa, Italy

C. Robba, G. Citerio (eds.), *Echography and Doppler of the Brain*,
https://doi.org/10.1007/978-3-030-48202-2_1

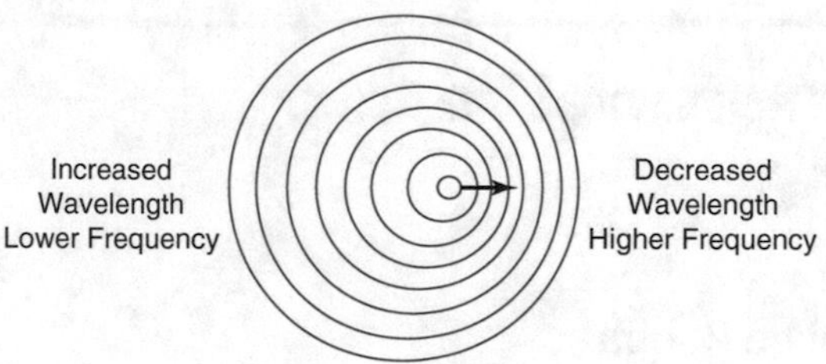

Fig. 1.1 Visual representation of the Doppler effect. As the wave source and wave observer become closer together, the wavelength decreases giving the perception of a higher frequency. In contrast, as the source and observer become farther apart, the wavelength increases giving the perception of a lower frequency

wavelength (operating frequency and propagation velocity):

$$v = \frac{(c \times f_d)}{2 \times f_0 \times \cos\theta}$$

where c is the speed of the incident wave, f_0 is the incident pulse frequency, f_d is the Doppler shift and θ is the angle of the reflector relative to the ultrasound probe [2].

There are two main forms of spectral Doppler, continuous-wave (CW) and pulsed-wave (PW) Doppler. With CW, a transmitter continuously listens for echoes and since the reception and transmission are continuous, echoes reflected from all depths are heard simultaneously without any depth discrimination. Unless there is a reference image indicating the source of specific flow velocity ranges, CW does not provide information relative to the source of the detected signals. On the other hand, with PW Doppler the transmitter and receiver obey a pulse repetition frequency (PRF) mode in which they are alternately turned on and off so signals reflected at a specific time can be received with good range resolution. In this case, the time for the echo signal to return is associated with a specific depth.

Reid and Spencer popularised the Doppler principle applied to imaging of blood vessels in the 1970s [3]. The application of TCD in clinical practice was first described by Rune Aaslid and collaborators in 1982 [1], as a technique applying ultrasound probes for dynamic monitoring of cerebral blood flow and vessel pulsatility in the basal cerebral arteries.

The brightness mode (B-mode) and Doppler ultrasound capabilities, consisting of the transcranial colour-coded duplex (TCCD) technology, were implemented to TCD by Schoning et al. in the late 1980s to overcome some of the TCD limitations [4]. Since then, advancements in the TCCD technology, such as transducer design, implementation of computational capabilities and better sonographic contrast materials, have promoted enhanced image quality and enabled its application in current clinical practice.

1.2 Transcranial Doppler Ultrasonography

TCD relies on pulsed-wave Doppler to insonate vessels at multiple depths. The received echoes generate an electrical impulse in the ultrasound probe and it is processed to calculate f_d and v, yielding a spectral waveform with peak systolic velocity (FV_s) and end diastolic velocity (FV_d) values (Fig. 1.1).

The blind identification of the basal cerebral arteries provided by TCD is based on the ultrasound wave spectral display and certain standard criteria, including appropriate acoustic window, probe angle, target artery depth, blood flow direction (towards or away from the insonation probe) and waveform envelope analysis which allows the monitoring of cerebral blood flow velocity (Fig. 1.2). Acoustic windows represent regions of thin bone in the skull that allow transmission of ultrasound waves to the basal cerebral arteries. There are four feasible acoustic windows for TCD insonation: the transtemporal, suboccipital, transorbital and submandibular. For instance, the transtemporal window, located above the zygomatic ridge between the lateral canthus of the eye and auricular pinna, is the most frequently used for the insonation of the middle cerebral artery (MCA), anterior cerebral artery (ACA), posterior cerebral artery (PCA) and terminal internal carotid artery (ICA) [5].

An ultrasound frequency of $\leq$2 MHz is required to penetrate the skull acoustic windows and reach the basal cerebral arteries. However, inadequate transtemporal windows (e.g. due to thicker skull bone layers impeding the penetra-

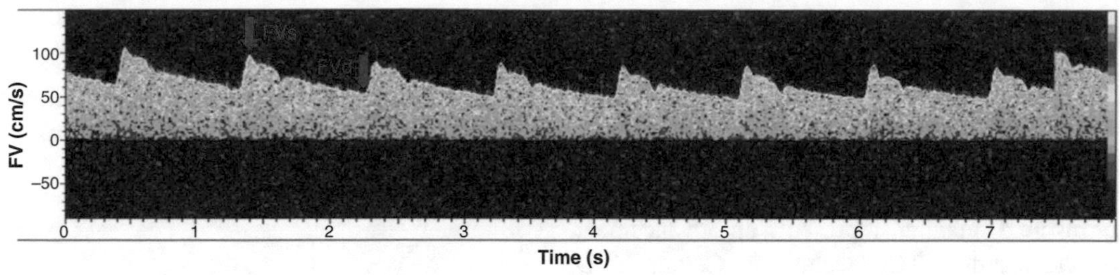

Fig. 1.2 Representation of the systolic (FV_s) and diastolic (FV_d) components of the spectral cerebral blood flow (CBF) velocity (FV) waveform

tion of ultrasound waves) have been reported in 10–20% of patients and represent a limitation of this insonation technique [5]. TCD allows intermittent monitoring of cerebral blood flow velocity by fixating the probe with appropriate headsets (probe holders) at the skull's temporal window. In contrast to other brain monitoring modalities (e.g. intracranial pressure, brain tissue oxygenation), at the current state of development, continuous TCD monitoring is unfeasible since proper and stable insonation is dependent on constant position and angle of insonation which can be easily affected by movement artefacts causing probe misplacement and consequently disrupted data acquisition. However, new state-of-the-art robotic TCD probes with automated correction for angle of insonation are being tested in different clinical settings to overcome the intermittent nature of TCD monitoring [6]. Overall, the exploration of more continuous ways to perform TCD monitoring can improve the reliability of TCD parameters.

In the scientific literature, the TCD technique has been extensively reported for non-invasive multimodal brain monitoring and evaluation of cerebral blood flow using basic and advanced parameters (described in Part II of this book). Basic parameters include mean cerebral blood flow velocity (calculated from the peak systolic and end diastolic cerebral blood flow velocity waveform), Gosling pulsatility index (PI) [7], Pourcelot resistive index (RI) and Lindegaard ratio (LR) [8]:

$$PI = \frac{FV_s - FV_d}{FV_m} (a.u.)$$

$$RI = \frac{FV_s - FV_d}{FV_s} (a.u.)$$

$$LR = \frac{FV_{mMCA}}{FV_{mEICA}} (a.u.)$$

where FV (s, d and m) represents the systolic, diastolic and mean components of the cerebral blood flow velocity waveform; MCA, middle cerebral artery; and EICA, extracranial internal carotid artery.

Advanced parameters include the detection of microembolic signals [9] and measures of cerebral vasomotor reactivity via breath holding (e.g. breath holding index (BHI)) and CO_2-induced hypercapnia [10]. Other advanced parameters such as cerebral blood flow autoregulation, non-invasive assessment of intracranial pressure and cerebral perfusion pressure, critical closing pressure and cerebral arterial compliance can be assessed with TCD and depend on the combined and synchronised assessment of cerebral blood flow velocity and systemic arterial blood pressure [8].

The general indications for TCD are subdivided into ischaemic cerebrovascular disease (e.g. sickle cell disease, right-to-left cardiac shunts, arteriovenous malformations), periprocedural (e.g. coronary artery bypass, carotid angioplasty and stenting surgeries) and neurointensive care categories (e.g. vasospasm, cerebral circulatory arrest, head injury) [11].

1.3 Transcranial Colour-Coded Duplex Ultrasonography

TCCD, an ultrasound modality combining transcranial colour-coded Doppler vessel representation with bi-dimensional pulsed-wave Doppler ultrasound imaging, represents an advancement of the standard TCD technique. Certain TCD limitations such as blind identification of blood vessels, poor spatial resolution, non-visualisation of anatomical landmarks, inaccurate blood velocity metrics and misclassification of specific blood vessels in the presence of normal anatomical variants formed the basis for the development of TCCD [12].

TCCD provides multiple advantages compared with TCD sonography: (I) direct visualisation and easier identification of the cerebral arteries with high resolution in specific intracranial vessel segments; (II) detailed allocation of vessel pathologies; and (III) possibility for software-assisted angle of insonation correction, resulting in more accurate measurement of cerebral blood flow velocities. Regarding the latter feature, the Doppler effect equation demonstrates that the detected Doppler shift is dependent on the cosine of the angle of insonation (formed between the emitted Doppler signal and the vessel flow direction) with maximal Doppler shifts detected at 0° and 180°. Since vascular Doppler rarely affords detections of the maximum Doppler shift due to insufficient imaging views, angle correction is necessary to compensate for the partial frequency shift detection. When the insonation angle is less than 90°, the reflected frequency is higher than the emitted frequency, and a positive Doppler shift is detected (the angle cosine is positive). Similarly, if the angle is greater than 90°, the reflected frequency is lower than the emitted frequency, and a negative Doppler shift is detected (the angle cosine is negative). Most important is that unless the Doppler angle is 0° or 180°, the system cannot detect the full frequency shift. As the insonation angle approaches 90°, the frequency shift approaches 0. For conditions in which the shift is not completely detected the ultrasound system allows for software-assisted angle correction. This can be done by aligning a Doppler flow indicator with the detected direction of the flow. Using basic geometry algorithms, the system software can determine the Doppler angle, calculate the angle cosine and correct the partially detected Doppler frequency shift. The basic differences between TCD and TCCD are listed in Table 1.1.

Table 1.1 Basic differences between TCD and TCCD

	TCD	TCCD
Free-hand assessment	Yes	Yes
Monitoring over time	Yes	No
Imaging of intracranial structures	No	Yes
Correction for angle of insonation	No	Yes
FV data output	Yes	No

Although TCCD provides direct visualisation of the brain parenchyma structures (e.g. ventricular system, midline shift) and vessels through combined ultrasound B-mode, at the current state of development it does not allow prolonged continuous monitoring of cerebral blood flow. In contrast to TCD devices, TCCD is most suitable for free-hand monitoring given the robust characteristics of the probes, which makes their fixation on the patient's head impractical in the absence of probe holders (not currently provided by manufacturers). Another potential limitation in comparison to TCD consists of the fact that most manufacturers do not provide analogic or digital outputs of the cerebral blood flow velocity data, which precludes the assessment of parameters that might require monitoring over time, such as continuous assessment of cerebral blood flow autoregulation or non-invasive intracranial pressure estimation (discussed in Chaps. 7 and 8).

Clinical evaluations with TCCD can be performed using 2–2.5 MHz probes that allow high-resolution visualisation of the main intracranial structures and vessels. At this ultrasound frequency range, probes at different configurations (e.g. phased array, sector or echo probes) can insonate brain structures located at depths of up to 12–15 cm [13, 14]. By applying the duplex imaging mode, the typical insonation through the transtemporal window will reveal the midbrain and individual basal arteries at the circle of Willis. Similarly to TCD, individual arteries can be identified by their depth of insonation and blood flow direction, but in the case of TCCD these arteries can be easily visualised on the device display.

TCCD devices provide basic parameters regarding cerebral blood flow velocity (systolic and diastolic components of the waveform) as well as calculated values such as mean cerebral blood flow velocity and indices based on the envelope of the cerebral blood flow velocity, for instance, PI, RI and LR. Advanced parameters, such as TCD-based cerebral autoregulation indices and critical closing pressure of the cerebrovascular bed that depends on continuous high-resolution data, cannot be obtained using the state-of-the-art TCCD machines due to the impracticality to output the collected data in real time.

Besides the shared indications TCCD has with TCD regarding the assessment of ischaemic cerebrovascular conditions in different clinical settings, its ability to image the intracranial anatomy allows the prompt identification of many critical disorders, such as intracranial haematomas, hydrocephalus and brain midline shift that previously relied mostly on more sophisticated (but less clinically practical) imaging techniques like computed tomography, magnetic resonance imaging and angiography.

1.4 Final Remarks

Notably, TCD and TCCD occupy different niches in brain ultrasonography. Owing to the ability of providing monitoring over time, even if intermittently, TCD has been a remarkable research tool in clinical neurosciences and has supported important scientific findings in cerebral blood flow physiology, not only in neurocritical care but also vastly in other clinical and experimental conditions. TCCD, on the other hand, finds its niche mostly in neurocritical care wards, with emerging applications in general critical care, being utilised for prompt diagnosis of derangements in cerebral blood flow circulation. The different sections of this book will discuss thoroughly the applications and usefulness of TCD and TCCD for research and clinical practice.

References

1. Aaslid R, Markwalder TM, Nornes H. Noninvasive transcranial Doppler ultrasound recording of flow velocity in basal cerebral arteries. J Neurosurg. 1982;57(6):769–74.
2. Aaslid R. In: Vienna RA, editor. Transcranial Doppler sonography. New York, NY: Springer; 1986. p. 22–38.
3. Reid JM, Spencer MP. Ultrasonic Doppler technique for imaging blood vessels. Science. 1972;176(4040):1235–6.
4. Schöning M, Grunert D, Stier B. Transkranielle Real-Time-Sonographie bei Kindern und Jugendlichen, Ultraschallanatomie des Gehirns. Ultraschall der Medizin. 1988;9(06):286–92.
5. Moppett IK, Mahajan RP. Transcranial Doppler ultrasonography in anaesthesia and intensive care. Br J Anaesth. 2004;93(93):710–24.
6. Zeiler FA, Smielewski P. Application of robotic transcranial Doppler for extended duration recording in moderate/severe traumatic brain injury: first experiences. Crit Ultrasound J. 2018;10(1):16.
7. De Riva N, Budohoski KP, Smielewski P, Kasprowicz M, Zweifel C, Steiner LA, et al. Transcranial Doppler pulsatility index: what it is and what it isn't. Neurocrit Care. 2012;17(1):58–66.
8. Robba C, Goffi A, Geeraerts T, Cardim D, Via G, Czosnyka M, et al. Brain ultrasonography: methodology, basic and advanced principles and clinical applications. A narrative review. Intensive Care Med. 2019;45:913.
9. Basic Identification Criteria of Doppler Microembolic Signals. Stroke. 1995;26(6):1123.
10. Nicoletto HA, Boland LS. Transcranial Doppler Series Part V: Specialty Applications. Am J Electroneurodiagnostic Technol. 2011;51(1):31–41.
11. Sloan MA, Alexandrov AV, Tegeler CH, Spencer MP, Caplan LR, Feldmann E, et al. Assessment: transcranial Doppler ultrasonography: report of the Therapeutics and Technology Assessment Subcommittee of the American Academy of Neurology. Neurology. 2004;62(9):1468–81.
12. Bogdahn U, Becker G, Winkler J, Greiner K, Perez J, Meurers B. Transcranial color-coded real-time sonography in adults. Stroke. 1990;21:1680.
13. Baumgartner RW. Transcranial color duplex sonography in cerebrovascular disease: a systematic review. Cerebrovasc Dis. 2003;16:4.
14. Bartels E, Fuchs HH, Flügel KA. Color Doppler imaging of basal cerebral arteries: normal reference values and clinical applications. Angiology. 1995;46:877.

Basic Anatomy with TCCD and Vessels

2

Pierre Bouzat and Thibaud Crespy

Contents

2.1 Introduction

Anatomy of major intracranial arteries has been described as the circle of Willis, which is a vascular anastomotic system at the base of the brain. From an embryologic standpoint, the circle of Willis is an important communicating system for blood supply between the forebrain and the hindbrain. Transcranial color-coded Doppler (TCCD) explores these different arteries through the skull [1]. Since bone blocks ultrasounds, regions with

P. Bouzat (✉)
Department of Anesthesiology and Intensive Care, Univ. Grenoble Alpes, INSERM 1216, Grenoble Institut Neurosciences, Grenoble University Hospital, Grenoble, France
e-mail: pbouzat@chu-grenoble.fr

T. Crespy
Department of Anesthesiology and Intensive Care, Grenoble University Hospital, Grenoble, France
e-mail: tcrespy@chu-grenoble.fr

C. Robba, G. Citerio (eds.), *Echography and Doppler of the Brain*,
https://doi.org/10.1007/978-3-030-48202-2_2

thinner walls, the so-called acoustic windows, generate less distortion for sound waves and provide blood flow velocities in each cerebral artery [2]. Age, sex, and race may affect bone thickness and porosity, resulting in more difficult examinations. Three main cranial windows are used to image major intracranial basal arteries: the orbital window for the ophthalmic and the internal carotid arteries; the temporal window for the anterior, middle, and posterior cerebral arteries; and the occipital window for intracranial segments of vertebral arteries and basilar artery [3]. Finally, the submandibular window has also been described to measure cerebral blood flow velocities on internal carotid arteries and basilar artery [4]. Apart from the arterial vasculature, the description of the cerebral veins and sinuses can also be done using the temporal window. Beyond vascular exploration, TCCD can also provide a comprehensive description of brain anatomy and several brain structures can be observed with ultrasonography [5]. As a result, TCCD has moved from a simple Doppler exam to a more complex description of brain anatomy.

2.2 Vascular Anatomy

2.2.1 The Circle of Willis

Sir Thomas Willis, in 1664, described the anatomy of basal intracranial vessels [6]. The circle of Willis provides an essential communicating system between the anterior (internal carotid arteries, anterior cerebral arteries, middle cerebral arteries) and posterior (posterior, vertebral, and basilar arteries) vessels thanks to the anterior and posterior communicating arteries [7]. The internal carotid arteries (ICA) enter the cranial cavity through the foramen lacerum and divide into anterior cerebral arteries (ACA) and middle cerebral arteries (MCA) on each side. The ACAs are connected to each other by an anterior communicating (ACOM) artery. Posteriorly, the right and left vertebral arteries join to form the basilar artery, which runs along the ventral surface of the pons and terminates by dividing into right and left posterior cerebral arteries (PCA). The ICAs on both sides are connected with the PCAs by posterior communicating arteries, creating the posterior part of the circle of Willis (Fig. 2.1).

The circle of Willis is a natural vascular hub so that blood flow can be diverted in case of proximal vessel occlusion. As a network of cerebral arteries, its role as the main collateral circuit is to compensate for stenosis and occlusions of the carotid or vertebral arteries [8]. However, a complete circle of Willis is present in only 18–20% of the individuals, due to various anatomic variations [9]. With TCCD, vessels are identified with the depth of insonation, direction of blood flow to the transducer, and simple notions of anatomy.

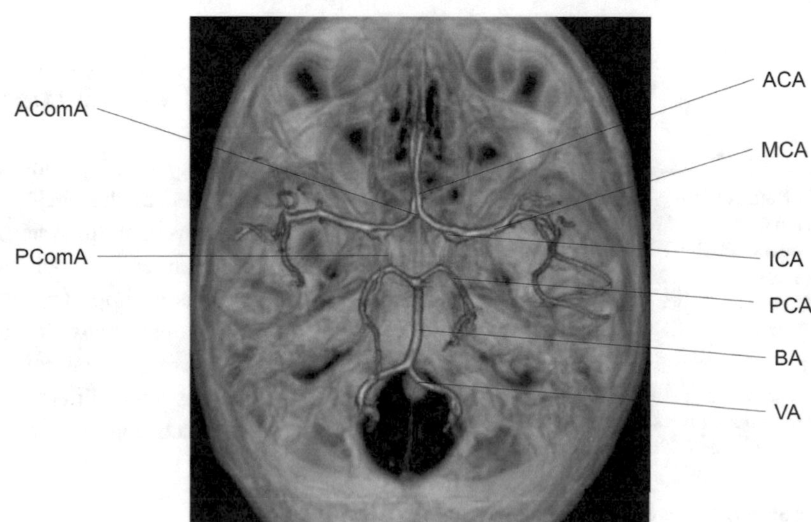

Fig. 2.1 The circle of Willis. *AComA* anterior communicating artery, *PComA* posterior communicating artery, *ACA* anterior cerebral artery, *MCA* middle cerebral artery, *ICA* internal carotid artery, *PCA* posterior cerebral artery, *BA* basilar artery, *VA* vertebral artery

2.2.2 Vascular Anatomy Through the Temporal Window

The temporal window is the main access to basal cerebral arteries since the entire polygon of Willis is imaged through this acoustic window. Bilateral examination is considered as a standard of care for TCCD examination in many clinical situations [10, 11]. The temporal area is located above the zygomatic arch, delineating a line from the tragus to the external canthus, i.e., the outer edge of the orbit. Three different windows have been described: A for anterior, M for middle, and P for posterior, which is often the only one in older people. The middle part of the temporal window is considered as the best acoustic window since it allows a reduction of the insonation angle close to zero. In up to 23% of women, there is no temporal window, especially in older women with hyperostosis or osteoporosis [12].

Using color mode, the entire circle of Willis with ACA and MCA can be visualized, together with PCA, internal carotid, and basilar artery in patients with favorable anatomy. The first part of the MCA (M1) is usually insonated at a depth ranging between 40 and 60 mm. A positive blood flow toward the probe is observed, usually labeled in red. The ACA, between 60 and 70 mm, has negative blood flow velocities since ACA flows away from the probe. The PCA is insonated between 65 and 70 mm. The PCA flow is positive within the first portion of the artery, P1, and becomes negative in its second part, P2. Deeper, the contralateral MCA, ACA, and PCA may be observed (Fig. 2.2).

2.2.3 Vascular Anatomy Through the Transorbital Window

The orbital window explores the ophthalmic artery and the internal carotid syphon. This window relates to the thinness of the orbital plates and bony defects caused by the optic foramina and superior orbital fissures. The probe is placed directly on the eye through the closed eyelid and is angled slightly medial and upward. The operator should not stay too long with the ultrasound probe on the eye to avoid any damage. Theoretically, ultrasounds may induce cataracts if used repeatedly. However, no harmful effect has been reported with the transorbital window providing a reduction in the power output (less than 17 mW/cm^2) in order to minimize the risk of traumatic subluxation of the crystalline lens of the eye.

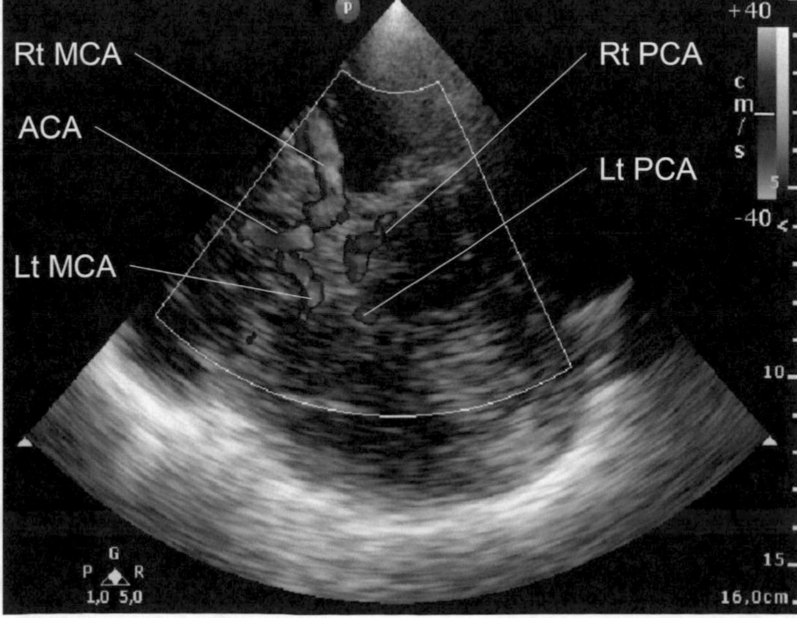

Fig. 2.2 Vascular anatomy through the transtemporal window. The entire circle of Willis is imaged through this acoustic window. *Rt* right, *Lt* left, *ACA* anterior cerebral artery, *MCA* middle cerebral artery, *ICA* internal carotid artery, *PCA* posterior cerebral artery

The ophthalmic artery is imaged at a depth of 45–60 mm, with a positive and resistive signal. The ICA siphon, beyond 60 mm, is a curved artery, whose flow may be directed toward or away from the probe (Fig. 2.3). Bidirectional signals may be obtained when the genu of the ICA siphon is insonated.

2.2.4 Vascular Anatomy Through the Suboccipital Window

The occipital or transforaminal window images the intracranial segment of the vertebral arteries and the basilar artery due to a natural defect between the occipital bone and atlas vertebra. The probe is placed below and medial to the mastoid processes. This window may require turning the patient to one side but is also feasible in a patient seated with the head flexed slightly forward. The probe is directed toward the bridge of the nose or contralateral eye. This orientation permits obtaining flow signals from the ipsilateral VA at a depth ranging from 50 to 70 mm. The basilar artery is imaged with the probe directed medially at a depth higher than 80 mm (Fig. 2.4). Corresponding flows go away from the probe.

2.2.5 Vascular Anatomy Through the Submandibular Window

The transducer is placed in an anatomically defined triangle in the submandibular area.

This triangle is formed by a medial line passing through the sternal notch and the cricoid cartilage, a line parallel to and just below the horizontal branch of the mandible, and a line coming from the mastoid process to the cricoid cartilage [4]. The Doppler probe is slightly angled medially and toward the occipital notch. The direction of the head is always maintained in its normal axis, neither extended nor flexed, while the probe is directed toward the occipital notch. The submandibular window also allows imaging the distal ICA (extradural segment) in the neck at a depth ranging between 40 and 60 mm (Fig. 2.5).

2.2.6 Sonography of Cerebral Veins and Sinus

Through the temporal window, in the axial plane, veins and sinuses can be insonated according to their anatomic location and flow direction. Regarding cerebral veins, the deep middle and basal cerebral

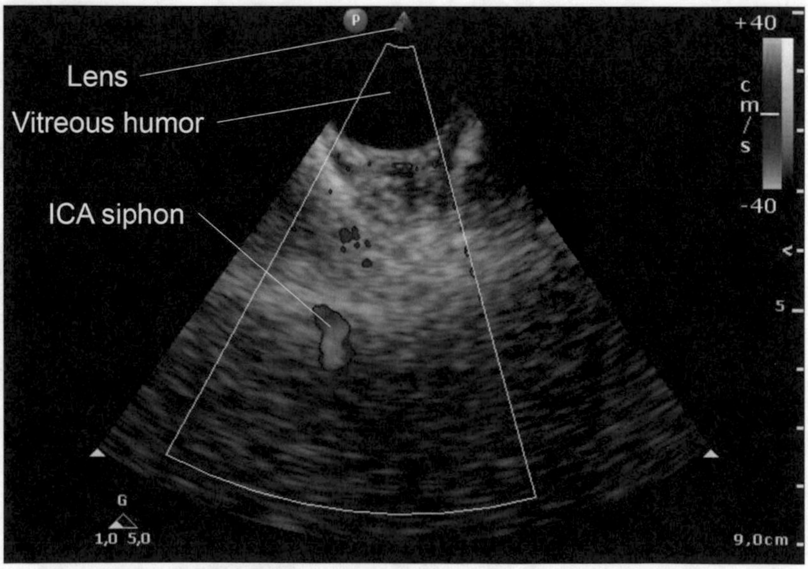

Fig. 2.3 Vascular anatomy through the transorbital window. *ICA* internal carotid artery

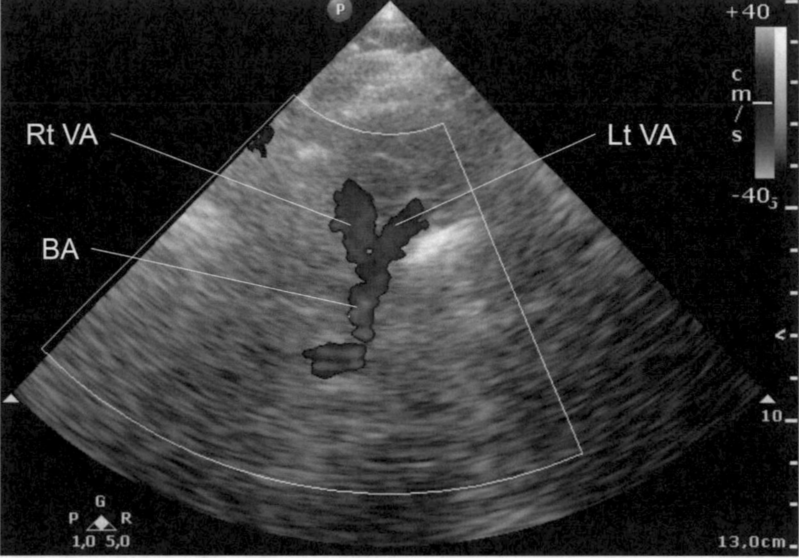

Fig. 2.4 Vascular anatomy through the suboccipital window. *VA* vertebral artery, *BA* basilar artery

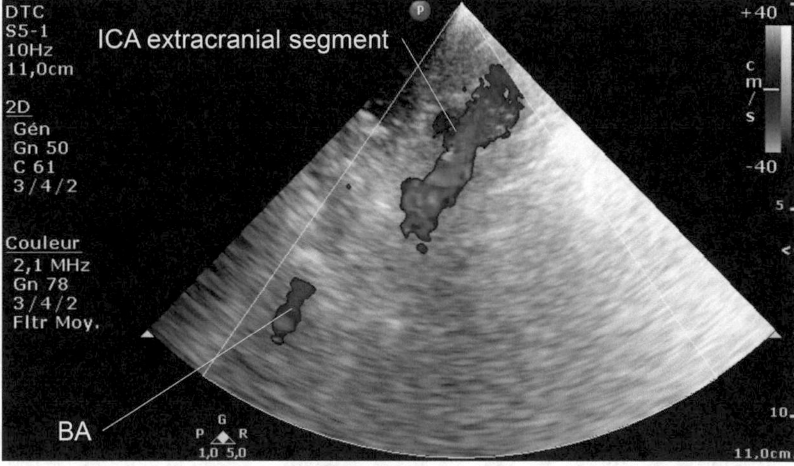

Fig. 2.5 Vascular anatomy through the submandibular window. The internal carotid artery (ICA) is imaged as well as the basilar artery (BA)

veins can be explored through the temporal bone window as well as the straight, transverse, inferior, and superior sagittal sinuses [13].

The deep middle cerebral vein (Fig. 2.6) is located above and posterior to the middle cerebral artery, with a flow direction opposite to the middle cerebral artery [14]. The basal vein originates by union of the deep middle cerebral vein and the anterior and inferior striate veins [15]. Since the anterior and inferior striate veins are not imaged by TCCD and their modes of confluence are diverse, the transition from the deep middle cerebral vein to the basal vein cannot be visualized by sonography. According to anatomic data, the origin of the basal vein may theoretically reach insonation depths of 49–55 mm. To minimize the possibility of confusing the deep middle cerebral vein for the basal vein, the depth used for insonation of the deep middle cerebral vein should be less than 50 mm. The basal vein (Fig. 2.7) is imaged in its peduncular segment, where it is located parallel and above the posterior cerebral artery [14]. Direction of blood flow in this basal vein

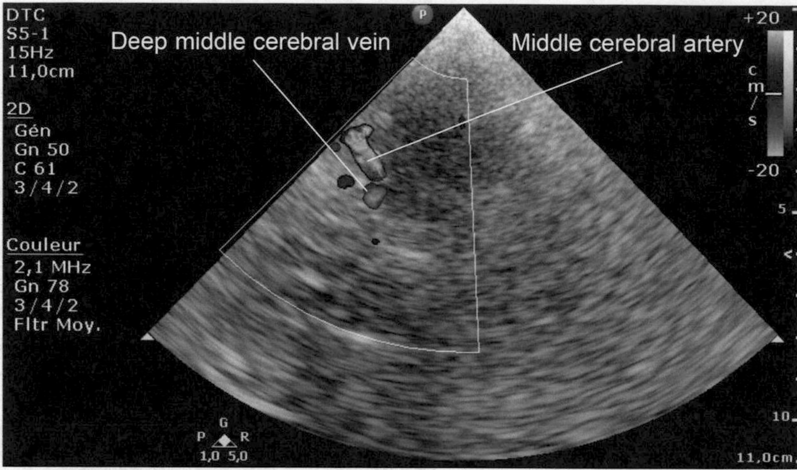

Fig. 2.6 Deep middle cerebral vein through the temporal window. The deep middle cerebral vein is located above and posterior to the middle cerebral artery, with a flow direction opposite to the middle cerebral artery

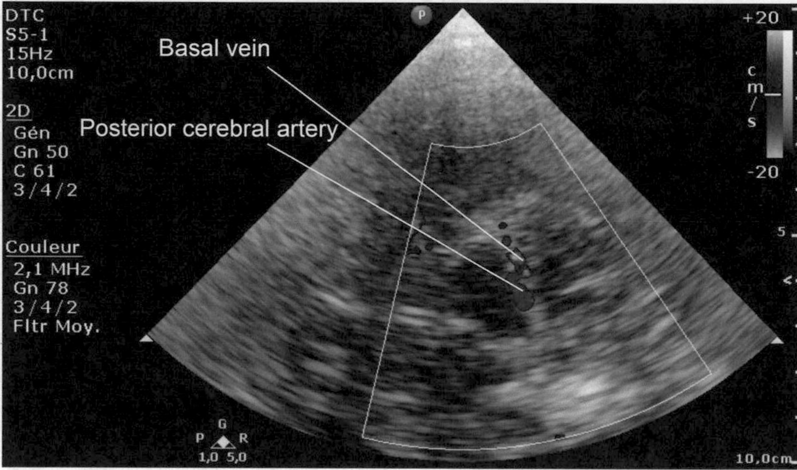

Fig. 2.7 Basal vein through the temporal window. The basal vein is imaged in its peduncular segment, where it is located parallel and above the posterior cerebral artery

segment is identical to that of the posterior cerebral artery [14].

The straight sinus has an oblique course in the sagittal plane with an angle ranging from 40° to 71° [16]. Therefore, the transducer is rotated in the sagittal plane to obtain parallel insonation of the straight sinus. The straight sinus can be insonated in the middle of its course to distinguish it from the great cerebral vein and the inferior sagittal sinus proximally, and to distinguish it from the torcular Herophili (confluens sinuum), transverse sinus, and superior sagittal sinus distally (Fig. 2.8). The transverse sinus is insonated where it courses horizontally along the occipital bone. To avoid confusion with the straight sinus, torcular Herophili, and superior sagittal sinus, the Doppler sample volume is placed in the lateral part of the horizontal section of the contralateral transverse sinus, just before it curves anteriorly and downward. The inferior sagittal sinus is imaged in its middle and distal thirds, and the superior sagittal sinus in its distal part before it enters the torcular Herophili.

2.3 Brain Anatomy with Ultrasonography

In patients with skull integrity, the acoustic window that is used for brain exploration is the temporal one. Otherwise, patients with craniectomy offer a unique opportunity to image intracranial structures. In this chapter we only focus on patients with no craniectomy to further describe brain sono-anatomy through the transtemporal window.

2.3.1 Anatomic Landmarks

The hyperechoic lesser sphenoid wing and superior margin of the petrous pyramid are usual bony landmarks that are imaged through the temporal window in the mesencephalic plane (Fig. 2.9). The hyperechoic posterior part of the sagittal sinus allows anterior-to-posterior orientation of the intracranial structures. Usually, the examination starts with the identification of a classic brain structure: the mesencephalic brainstem, which is the central structure for orientation in the axial sonographic plane [17]. The brainstem is visualized as a hypoechoic butterfly-shaped image, surrounded by hyperechoic subarachnoid cisterns (Fig. 2.9). Tilting the probe about 10° upwards, the diencephalic plane is imaged. The anechoic lumen of the third ventricle is framed by two

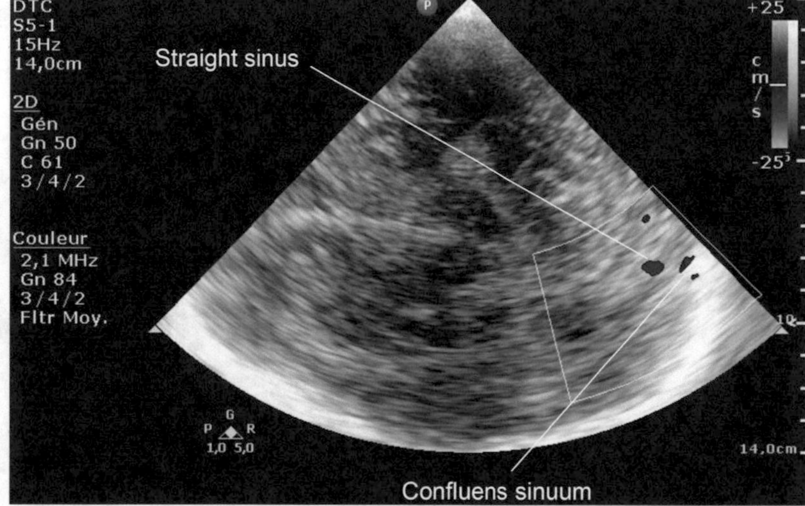

Fig. 2.8 Straight sinus through the temporal window. The transducer is rotated in the sagittal plane to obtain parallel insonation of the straight sinus. The straight sinus can be insonated in the middle of its course to distinguish it from the great cerebral vein and the inferior sagittal sinus proximally, and to distinguish it from the torcular Herophili (confluens sinuum), transverse sinus, and superior sagittal sinus distally

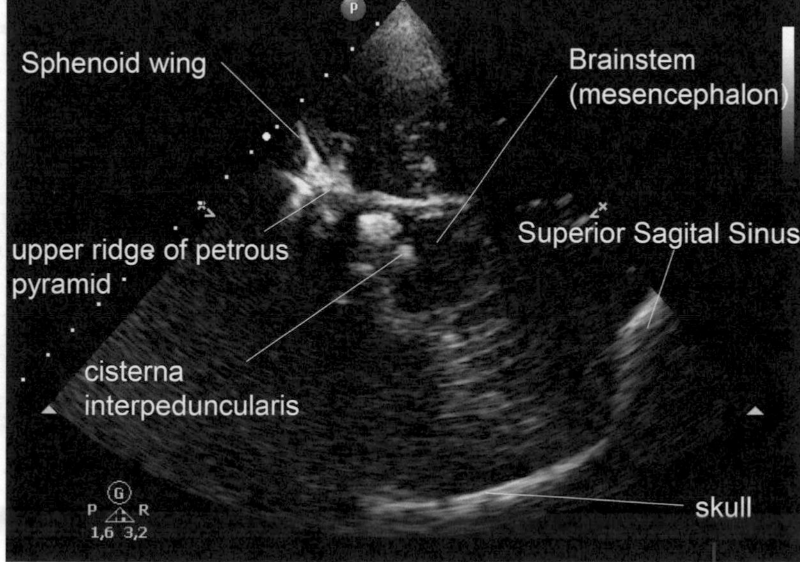

Fig. 2.9 Brain anatomy through the temporal window: typical oblique axial plane showing main cerebral landmarks such as brainstem, surrounding cisterna, and sphenoid wing

hyperechoic ependymal linings (Fig. 2.10). Just posteriorly, thalami are depicted as hypoechogen/isoechogen structures surrounding the third ventricle. Lateral ventricle can also be imaged by directing ultrasound beam slightly cranially (Fig. 2.11) [5]. At this ventricular plane, the largest transverse diameters of the third ventricle may be measured as well as lateral ventricles [18].

2.3.2 Clinical Implications

2.3.2.1 Intracranial Hemorrhage

The progression of intracranial hemorrhage (ICH) is one of the most important prognostic factors after spontaneous or post-traumatic ICH [19]. Follow-up can be done with repeated CT scanning but requires transferring patient from the ICU to a CT scan facility. TCCD may provide a noninvasive follow-up of brain hematomas at the bedside since ICH is imaged as a hyperechoic sharply demarcated mass within the brain parenchyma [17]. However, this follow-up is limited to the first 7 days, when brain hematomas appear more echogenic than the surrounding brain tissue. TCCD was also used to differentiate ischemic and hemorrhagic stroke in 151 stroke patients [20]. Early monitoring of ICH was also done by Perez et al. [21], showing a good correlation between TCCD and CT scan measurements of hematoma volume. TCD only missed eight ICH patients with a small hemorrhage (five

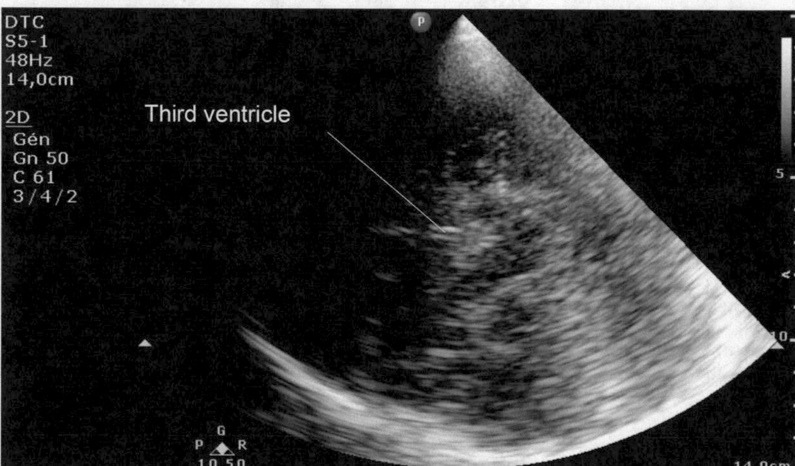

Fig. 2.10 Brain anatomy through the temporal window: the anechoic lumen of the third ventricle is framed by two hyperechoic ependymal linings

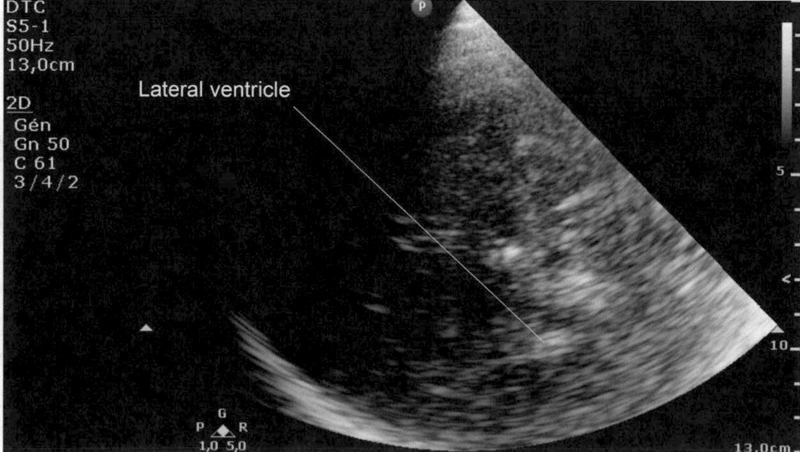

Fig. 2.11 Brain anatomy through the temporal window: lateral ventricles are imaged by directing ultrasound beam cranially

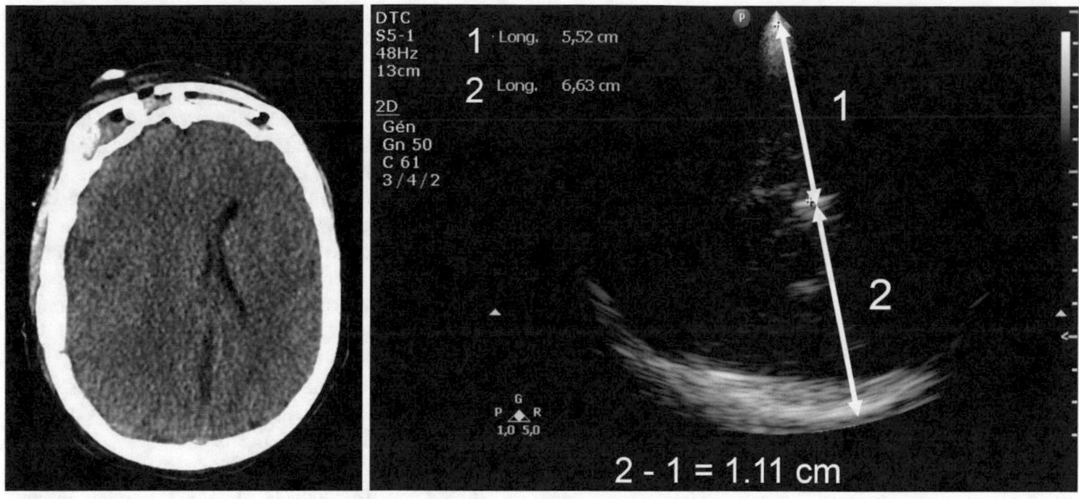

Fig. 2.12 Midline shift in a patient with a cerebral empyema. Ultrasonography found same value (right image) as that of CT scan (left image)

patients) or an infratentorial hemorrhage (three patients). TCCD was also used to detect hemorrhagic transformation of ischemic strokes [22]. The follow-up of brain hematomas is even easier in patients with decompressive craniectomy. Brain hematomas can be imaged and their volumes may be accurately estimated with ultrasonography [23].

2.3.2.2 Epidural/Subdural Hematomas

Epidural and subdural hematomas are surgical lesions that should be promptly diagnosed to evaluate their surgical removal. CT scan is the gold standard for their diagnosis but TCCD detection of these hematomas has been described [24]. Using the classic midbrain plan, the contralateral skull is visualized. Epidural hematoma is observed as a hyperechogenic image inside the skull. Subdural hematoma has also been quantified by measuring the distance between the skull and the dural border of the arachnoid, described as a highly echogenic membrane [25].

2.3.2.3 Brain Midline Shift

Brain midline shift is an emergency that requires prompt treatment. The diagnosis is based on cerebral CT scan, which is the gold standard for brain imaging [26]. Brain ultrasonography may also provide useful information regarding midline shift by measuring the distance between the skull and the third ventricle on both sides (clinical case in Fig. 2.12, midline shift equal to A – B/2). First description of this method was performed in stroke patients after malignant ischemic stroke [27, 28]. More recently, an observational study mixing TBI and ICH patients found a good correlation between this noninvasive method and CT scanning values, suggesting the use of TCCD as a bedside tool to diagnose midline shift in diverse clinical situations [29].

2.3.2.4 Hydrocephalus

Another clinical implication is the diagnosis of brain ventricle enlargement. Indeed, the visualization of brain ventricles allows a comparison of their sizes across patient's stay in intensive care unit [30]. Several authors found a good correlation between TCCD and CT scan measurements of third and lateral ventricles [18, 31]. This diagnosis is even easier in patients with decompressive craniectomy [23]. The follow-up of brain ventricle enlargement after external ventricular drain (EVD) clamping trial has also been described, showing a good sensitivity of TCCD when ventricle enlargement was greater than 5.5 mm [32]. Finally, the location of EVD tip can also be imaged with TCCD particularly in patients with decompressive craniectomy [33].

2.3.2.5 Stroke

TCCD can be used at the early phase of stroke for different purposes. TCCD may visualize arterial occlusion and potential collateral circulation. It can also assess arterial recanalization after thrombolysis and may detect early complication such as hemorrhagic transformation. After malignant ischemic stroke, TCCD may be helpful to measure midline shift, detect high intracranial pressure [34], and assess brain autoregulation. As a consequence, TCCD is a complementary method to standard imaging techniques for the bedside management of stroke patients.

2.4 Conclusion

TCCD has become a standard of care in many neuro-ICU. Its role goes beyond a simple measurement of blood flow velocities since TCCD also explores brain anatomy. With adequate training, TCCD helps clinicians in different situations such as CBF estimation, vasospasm diagnosis, and brain structure exploration. These clinical implications define TCCD as the new stethoscope of the brain in daily ICU practice.

References

1. Aaslid R, Markwalder TM, Nornes H. Noninvasive transcranial Doppler ultrasound recording of flow velocity in basal cerebral arteries. J Neurosurg. 1982;57(6):769–74.
2. Tsivgoulis G, Alexandrov AV, Sloan MA. Advances in transcranial Doppler ultrasonography. Curr Neurol Neurosci Rep. 2009;9(1):46–54.
3. Robba C, Cardim D, Sekhon M, Budohoski K, Czosnyka M. Transcranial Doppler: a stethoscope for the brain-neurocritical care use. J Neurosci Res. 2018;96(4):720–30.
4. Geeraerts T, Thome W, Tanaka S, Leblanc PE, Duranteau J, Vigue B. An alternative ultrasonographic approach to assess basilar artery flow. Neurosurgery. 2011;68(2 Suppl Operative):276–81. discussion 81
5. Krejza J, Mariak Z, Melhem ER, Bert RJ. A guide to the identification of major cerebral arteries with transcranial color Doppler sonography. AJR Am J Roentgenol. 2000;174(5):1297–303.
6. Wragge-Morley A. Imagining the soul: Thomas Willis (1621-1675) on the anatomy of the brain and nerves. Prog Brain Res. 2018;243:55–73.
7. Grand W. The anatomy of the brain, by Thomas Willis. Neurosurgery. 1999;45(5):1234–6. discussion 6-7
8. Mukherjee D, Jani ND, Narvid J, Shadden SC. The role of circle of Willis anatomy variations in cardio-embolic stroke: a patient-specific simulation based study. Ann Biomed Eng. 2018;46(8):1128–45.
9. Machasio RM, Nyabanda R, Mutala TM. Proportion of variant anatomy of the circle of Willis and association with vascular anomalies on cerebral CT angiography. Radiol Res Pract. 2019;2019:6380801.
10. White H, Venkatesh B. Applications of transcranial Doppler in the ICU: a review. Intensive Care Med. 2006;32(7):981–94.
11. Bouzat P, Oddo M, Payen JF. Transcranial Doppler after traumatic brain injury: is there a role? Curr Opin Crit Care. 2014;20(2):153–60.
12. Babikian VL, Feldmann E, Wechsler LR, Newell DW, Gomez CR, Bogdahn U, et al. Transcranial Doppler ultrasonography: year 2000 update. J Neuroimaging. 2000;10(2):101–15.
13. Baumgartner RW, Gonner F, Arnold M, Muri RM. Transtemporal power- and frequency-based color-coded duplex sonography of cerebral veins and sinuses. AJNR Am J Neuroradiol. 1997;18(9):1771–81.
14. Chung JI, Weon YC. Anatomic variations of the deep cerebral veins, tributaries of basal vein of Rosenthal: embryologic aspects of the regressed embryonic tentorial sinus. Interv Neuroradiol. 2005;11(2):123–30.
15. Ono M, Rhoton AL Jr, Peace D, Rodriguez RJ. Microsurgical anatomy of the deep venous system of the brain. Neurosurgery. 1984;15(5):621–57.
16. Mattle H, Edelman RR, Reis MA, Atkinson DJ. Flow quantification in the superior sagittal sinus using magnetic resonance. Neurology. 1990;40(5):813–5.
17. Caricato A, Pitoni S, Montini L, Bocci MG, Annetta P, Antonelli M. Echography in brain imaging in intensive care unit: state of the art. World J Radiol. 2014;6(9):636–42.
18. Seidel G, Kaps M, Gerriets T, Hutzelmann A. Evaluation of the ventricular system in adults by transcranial duplex sonography. J Neuroimaging. 1995;5(2):105–8.
19. Dowlatshahi D, Demchuk AM, Flaherty ML, Ali M, Lyden PL, Smith EE, et al. Defining hematoma expansion in intracerebral hemorrhage: relationship with patient outcomes. Neurology. 2011;76(14):1238–44.
20. Maurer M, Shambal S, Berg D, Woydt M, Hofmann E, Georgiadis D, et al. Differentiation between intracerebral hemorrhage and ischemic stroke by transcranial color-coded duplex-sonography. Stroke. 1998;29(12):2563–7.
21. Perez ES, Delgado-Mederos R, Rubiera M, Delgado P, Ribo M, Maisterra O, et al. Transcranial duplex sonography for monitoring hyperacute intracerebral hemorrhage. Stroke. 2009;40(3):987–90.
22. Seidel G, Cangur H, Albers T, Burgemeister A, Meyer-Wiethe K. Sonographic evaluation of hemorrhagic transformation and arterial recanaliza-

tion in acute hemispheric ischemic stroke. Stroke. 2009;40(1):119–23.
23. Caricato A, Mignani V, Bocci MG, Pennisi MA, Sandroni C, Tersali A, et al. Usefulness of transcranial echography in patients with decompressive craniectomy: a comparison with computed tomography scan. Crit Care Med. 2012;40(6):1745–52.
24. Caricato A, Mignani V, Sandroni C, Pietrini D. Bedside detection of acute epidural hematoma by transcranial sonography in a head-injured patient. Intensive Care Med. 2010;36(6):1091–2.
25. Niesen WD, Burkhardt D, Hoeltje J, Rosenkranz M, Weiller C, Sliwka U. Transcranial grey-scale sonography of subdural haematoma in adults. Ultraschall Med. 2006;27(3):251–5.
26. Srairi M, Hoarau L, Fourcade O, Geeraerts T. What is the gold standard method for midline structures shift assessment using computed tomography? Crit Care Med. 2012;40(12):3332–3.
27. Gerriets T, Stolz E, Konig S, Babacan S, Fiss I, Jauss M, et al. Sonographic monitoring of midline shift in space-occupying stroke: an early outcome predictor. Stroke. 2001;32(2):442–7.
28. Gerriets T, Stolz E, Modrau B, Fiss I, Seidel G, Kaps M. Sonographic monitoring of midline shift in hemispheric infarctions. Neurology. 1999;52(1):45–9.
29. Motuel J, Biette I, Srairi M, Mrozek S, Kurrek MM, Chaynes P, et al. Assessment of brain midline shift using sonography in neurosurgical ICU patients. Crit Care. 2014;18(6):676.
30. Berg D, Becker G. Perspectives of B-mode transcranial ultrasound. NeuroImage. 2002;15(3):463–73.
31. Becker G, Bogdahn U, Strassburg HM, Lindner A, Hassel W, Meixensberger J, et al. Identification of ventricular enlargement and estimation of intracranial pressure by transcranial color-coded real-time sonography. J Neuroimaging. 1994;4(1):17–22.
32. Kiphuth IC, Huttner HB, Struffert T, Schwab S, Kohrmann M. Sonographic monitoring of ventricle enlargement in posthemorrhagic hydrocephalus. Neurology. 2011;76(10):858–62.
33. Robba C, Simonassi F, Ball L, Pelosi P. Transcranial color-coded duplex sonography for bedside monitoring of central nervous system infection as a consequence of decompressive craniectomy after traumatic brain injury. Intensive Care Med. 2019;45(8):1143–4.
34. Poca MA, Benejam B, Sahuquillo J, Riveiro M, Frascheri L, Merino MA, et al. Monitoring intracranial pressure in patients with malignant middle cerebral artery infarction: is it useful? J Neurosurg. 2010;112(3):648–57.

Windows and the Practical Approach: The MOTOr

3

Aoife Quinn and Andrea Rigamonti

Contents

3.1 Introduction

Ultrasound examination of the brain is an evolving tool in our armamentarium for the provision of real-time individualized patient care. The absence of spicules in skull bones allows for ultrasonographic assessment. Data obtained complements information already gleaned from history, clinical examination, and imaging. Satisfactory intra- and interobserver reliability has been demonstrated [1, 2]. Brain ultrasound is not a replacement for current gold standard brain imaging modalities nor direct intracranial pressure measurements should these be required. However, ultrasound of the brain provides many advantages. Results obtained from ultrasound examination of the brain have been shown to correlate with CT and MRI examination findings [3–5]. It is a portable, bedside, easily repeatable, real-time investigation. The avoidance of the

A. Quinn
Cambridge University Hospitals, Cambridge, UK
e-mail: aoife.quinn@addenbrookes.nhs.uk

A. Rigamonti (✉)
St Michael's, Unity Health Toronto,
University of Toronto, Toronto, ON, Canada
e-mail: rigamontia@smh.ca

C. Robba, G. Citerio (eds.), *Echography and Doppler of the Brain*,
https://doi.org/10.1007/978-3-030-48202-2_3

need to transfer or expose the patient to contrast and radiation minimizes any biological cost to the patient.

Ultrasound of the brain has a role to play in the evaluation of both structural and vascular issues, notably assessment of hematoma expansion [6], midline shift, hydrocephalus [7], elevations of intracranial pressure (ICP) [8], demonstration of flow status [9], vasospasm [10], and autoregulation [11–13]. Measurements of these indices are particularly relevant for the management of a variety of neurological conditions including stroke, subarachnoid hemorrhage, traumatic brain injury, and intracerebral hemorrhage [14–18]. There is an emerging role for transcranial ultrasound as part of a point-of-care examination in the emergency department [19]. The value obtained from transcranial ultrasound in outpatient, ward, and all intensive care unit settings continues to expand and become more substantial as technical expertise evolves [20]. Its portable nature is of particular benefit for patients on extracorporeal circuits and as a means of assessing the impact of lung-protective ventilator strategies on the brain [21, 22]. The ability to obtain noninvasive intracranial pressure estimations is a potentially useful tool in the management of coagulopathic patients [23–25] or in situations where standard invasive ICP monitoring is unavailable.

Ultrasound of the brain is performed by examining the brain via four windows. A systematic approach to the examination is presented in this chapter. The approach utilized is the MOTOr approach—mandibular, occipital, transtemporal, orbital. In many cases the transtemporal window yields the most fruitful information. However, a complete examination mandates interrogation of the brain structures via all four windows. Visualizing vessels in different windows allows for tracking of the vessels and changes in the flow and facilitates identification of vascular anomalies.

3.2 Anatomy Abnormalities

Abnormalities of the circle of Willis are common and occur in up to 80% of the population. Anatomical abnormalities are more frequent in the posterior circulation. The most common abnormality is a hypoplastic vessel, which is found to occur in 24–35% of patients. Hypoplasia of the first portion of the anterior cerebral artery (A1 segment) may occur in 10–20% of patients. Fetal origin of the posterior cerebral artery (PCA) describes the arrangement when the origin of the PCA is from the internal carotid artery and not the basilar artery. This occurs in 15–25% of patients. A further 6% of patients may have an absent PCA. Accessory vessels also occur with some series reporting 12% of patients having duplications or triplications of the anterior communicating artery [26–28].

3.3 Measurements and Basic Calculations

Structural landmarks are identified using B-mode imaging. The combination of color- and pulsed-wave (PW) Doppler allows demonstration of the vessel and measurements to be made which give information regarding velocity [29]. Following location of a vessel, depth, and flow direction in relation to the probe, parenchyma and other vessels may be ascertained using color Doppler. After obtaining an optimal view of the vessel PW Doppler can be used to sample the vessel. Once the waveform has been recorded, values for peak systolic (PSV), peak diastolic (PDV), and mean flow velocities (MFV) can be measured. Comparison of measurements in sequential segments at 5 mm intervals allows inferences to be drawn to diagnose pathology [30]. Factors that cause an increase in blood flow velocity and therefore impact data interpretation include female gender, pregnancy, lower hematocrit, higher PCO2, increasing MAP, and mental or motor activity. Age has a variable effect with increased velocities until 10 years of age and then a decrease as shown in Table 3.1 (flow velocities in cm/s).

These measurements allow calculation of pulsatility and resistivity indices and an assessment of vasospasm, intact autoregulation, and intracranial pressure [31, 32]. Key velocity indices to perform a basic investigation are outlined in Table 3.2.

Table 3.1 Typical flow velocities in intracranial vessels

Artery	20–40 years of age	40–60 years of age	>60 years of age
ACA	56–60	53–61	44–51
MCA	74–81	72–73	58–59
PCA			
P1	48–57	41–56	37–47
P2	43–51	40–57	37–47
Vertebral artery	37–51	29–50	30–37
Basilar artery	39–58	27–56	29–47

ACA anterior cerebral artery, *MCA* middle cerebral artery, *PCA* posterior cerebral artery, P1: first component of PCA, P2: second component of PCA, values are in cm/s

Table 3.2 Key velocity indices to perform a basic TCCS investigation

Peak systolic velocity (PSV)	This is the maximum value of flow velocity in systole at the apex of the waveform
End diastolic velocity (EDV)	This is measured at the end of diastole and is usually the lowest point before a new waveform begins
Mean flow velocity (MFV)	(PSV + 2*EDV)/3
Gosling's Pulsatility Index (PI)	(PSV – EDV)/MFV
Pourcelot Resistivity Index (RI)	(PSV – EDV)/PSV

Pulsatility of blood flow reflects the resistance to blood flow. Normal pulsatility index (PI) values range from 0.8 to 1.2. Deviations from the normal range can provide clues as to pathology [33]. Values greater than 1.2 suggest a downstream stenosis as a narrowing will increase the mean flow velocity. Increased values over 1.2 may also reflect an increased peripheral resistance secondary to an elevated intracranial pressure [34]. ICP affects PI in a linear fashion. Hypocapnia, aortic insufficiency, or bradycardia may all increase the PI. Causes of a PI lower than 0.8 include an arteriovenous malformation which causes decreased peripheral resistance, or the fact that the point of the vessel being examined is vasodilated and is positioned downstream to a proximal obstruction or stenosis. The resistivity index (RI) measures resistance to blood flow distal to the site of measurement. A measurement of greater than 0.8 implies increased downstream resistance.

Lindegaard ratio (LR) compares the MFV in intracranial to extracranial arteries by calculating the ratio between the MFV in the artery under examination and the MFV in the extracranial portion of the internal carotid artery (ICA) [18]. It differentiates hyperdynamic flow from vasospasm. Intracranial increased flow velocities without a concomitant increase in flow velocity in the supplying extracranial component imply vasospasm [10]. A LR >3 implies vasospasm, and an abnormally low LR implies hyperdynamic flow (for instance caused by an AVM). A modified LR ratio has been developed for the posterior circulation [15, 35].

3.4 Setup

Ideally the sonographer would be positioned behind the patient's head, with the ultrasound machine on one side within easy reach. This facilitates performing the examination in a systematic manner, and for the sequential evaluation of both sides of the patient's brain. Practically speaking a patient in an intensive care unit poses several challenges to this setup. The ventilator, multiple infusion pumps, external ventricular drainage devices, and ICP monitors may obfuscate access to the head of the bed. Movement of the patient may be prohibited by spinal injuries. Patients with poorly compliant brains postinjury may not tolerate changing position and only a limited examination may be possible. It is therefore vital to be flexible in the approach to examination. Dressings and operation sites in neurosurgical patients do not pose insurmountable challenges. Probe position may have to be adjusted slightly to avoid staple lines. Decompressive craniectomy sites do not negatively impact image acquisition, although care must be taken with regard to the amount of pressure applied to the probe. As a matter of fact, the lack of bone makes the acquisition of imaging easier, provided that the anatomy is not excessively distorted by brain swelling. Changes in systemic physiology impact intracerebral physiology. ECG and blood pressure measurements are mandatory as part of the assessment. Patient factors and a pretest probability of a particular diagnosis must be taken into account in the assimilation of data. Patient factors to be considered include diagnosis, operations performed, and intensity of ICU therapies.

3.5 The MOTOr Approach

3.5.1 Mandibular

This window allows the sonographer to identify and examine the extracranial component of the internal carotid artery. Ideally the patient is positioned supine with the head slightly extended. Further extension of the neck may be necessary if the patient has a particularly short neck. Patients in cervical spine collars are precluded from this examination. The probe is placed slightly lateral to the angle of the jaw, and aimed upwards and medially. The probe is placed on a soft-tissue surface rather than a bony window and therefore additional coupling gel may be necessary to obtain reasonable views (Fig. 3.1a). There is great variability in the views of the vessels visualized using this approach. Flow in the extracranial component of the ICA should be away

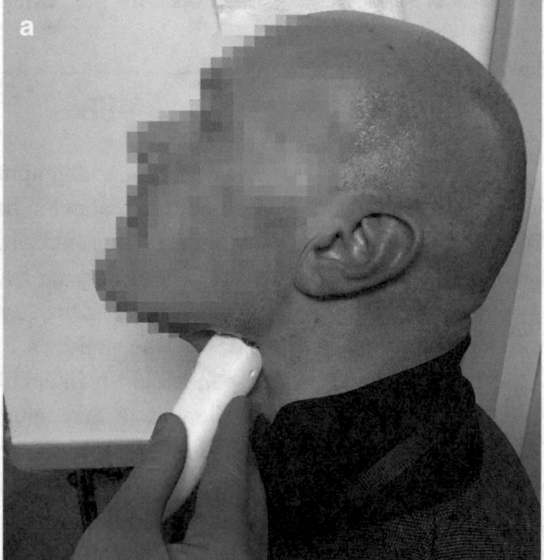

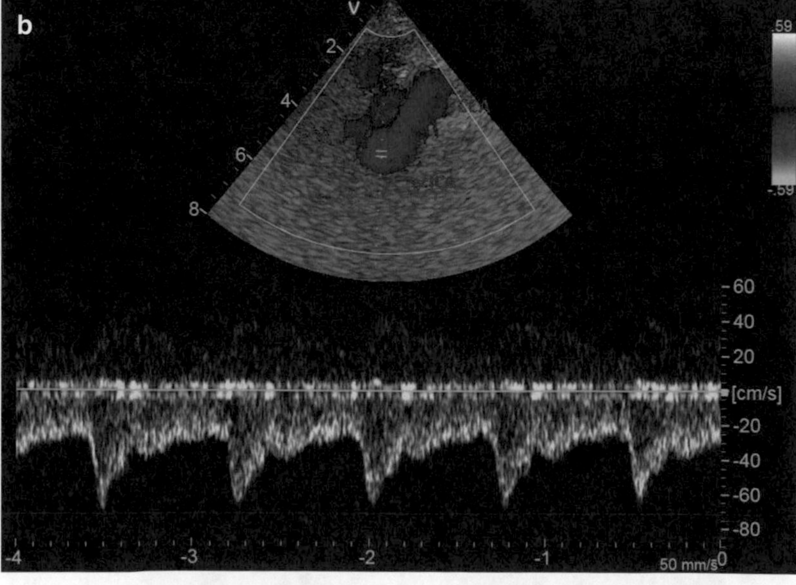

Fig. 3.1 (**a**) Mandibular window. (**b**) *CCA* common carotid artery, *ECA* external carotid artery, ecICA: extracranial internal carotid artery

from the probe. Normal velocity of the artery should be 24–28 cm/s. The distal ICA is found at a depth of 40–60 mm (Fig. 3.1b). The external carotid artery is found more medially in the neck, and has a higher resistance and numerous branches [36, 37]. TCCS can identify changes in the ICA in children with sickle cell disease and serve as a marker of stroke risk secondary to infarction in watershed areas [38]. Carotid trauma has the potential to cause an intimal flap with consequent problems of dissection, thrombosis, stenosis, or occlusion. Unilateral changes in flow velocity in a trauma patient may indicate an intimal flap, and help direct further investigation and management [39]. The information regarding flow dynamics in the extracranial vessels compared to the intracranial vessels is central to making a determination as to the potential for vasospasm to be present.

3.5.2 Occipital

The interface of the occipital bone and the atlas vertebrae creates a natural gap [40]. This is the window for the suboccipital view (Fig. 3.2a). It provides a view of the vertebral and basilar artery (Fig. 3.2b). Optimal images are obtained with the neck flexed forward [41]. This is not particularly feasible for the majority of intensive care patients. For the supine ICU patient, it may be possible to obtain views by tilting the head to contralateral side of interrogation [42]. The two key orientation landmarks of this window are the foramen magnum, which is hypoechoic, and the hyperechoic clivus. Positioning the probe below and medial to the mastoid and angling towards the contralateral eye may give a view of the ipsilateral vertebral artery. Identifying features include a depth of 50–75 mm, and flow that is directed away from the probe. When attempting to insonate the vertebral artery, flow directed towards the probe may be detected. This suggests that the extradural portion of the vertebral artery is being interrogated. This can be corrected by making the angulation more superior [43]. The basilar artery is visualized by placing the probe just below the occipital protuberance. The probe should be angled towards the nasal bridge, and angled slightly more superiorly than when visualizing the vertebral artery. Scanning more medially may improve the view of the basilar artery if not immediately apparent. The basilar artery is typically found at depths of 60–70 mm, but sometimes may be present at up to 100 mm. Flow in the basilar artery is away from the probe [44]. By optimizing the view for an individual patient the Y-shaped confluence of the two vertebral arteries as they converge into the basilar may be demonstrated. Flow velocities in the vertebral arteries and basilar artery are in the range of 39–60 cm/s [45]. The Lindegaard ratio has a modification for assessing vasospasm in the posterior circulation [46, 47].

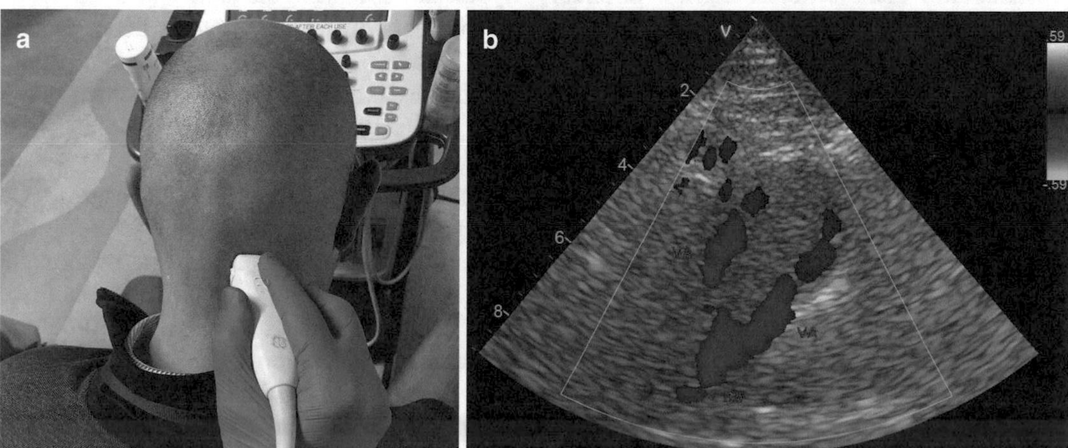

Fig. 3.2 (**a**) Occipital window. (**b**) *BA* basilar artery, *VA* vertebral artery

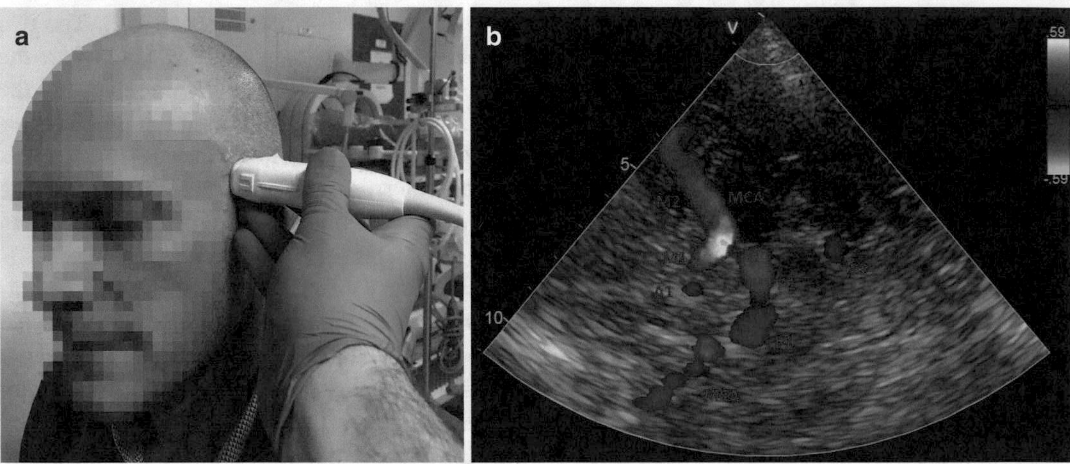

Fig. 3.3 (**a**) Temporal window. (**b**) *MCA* middle cerebral artery (M1: first portion; M2 second portion); A1: first portion of the anterior cerebral artery; P1: first portion of the posterior cerebral artery; P2: second portion of the posterior cerebral artery. With this window you can see both ipsilateral and contralateral circulation

Visualization of the basilar artery can be challenging. Using a combination of occipital and transtemporal windows the basilar artery and posterior cerebellar artery can be identified in 84–94% of patients [48, 49]. The distal segments of the basilar artery are visualized in only 45% of patients. TCCS shows some promise as a diagnostic tool in the evaluation of acute posterior circulation pathology [50] but it cannot be considered reliable enough to exclude serious pathology [51] when compared to angiography techniques. It is particularly difficult to determine if there are impendences to flow. A proximal stenosis or occlusion may be suggested by highly pulsatile blow in the vertebral arteries. Vertebral artery flow may be normal if the occlusion is more distal. The interpretation of indirect signals leads to problems with drawing inferences from the data.

3.5.3 Transtemporal

The transtemporal approach is the high-yield window when performing TCCS. It allows evaluation of the parenchyma [5] and the vasculature of the Circle of Willis [52]. The window is through the pterion—the confluence of the great wing of the sphenoid, the squamous part of the temporal bone, the frontal and the parietal bones. The probe should be orientated with the index mark towards the anterior aspect of the patient. This should correlate with the index mark being on the left of the ultrasound screen. If the patient is in a sitting position the probe should initially be held parallel to the floor and placed just superior to the zygomatic arch (Fig. 3.3a). Slight adjustments in angulation will be needed to obtain adequate views. Initially the probe should be placed 1 cm anterior to the ear, but this distance may need to be adjusted for each individual [53]. Up to 20% of people [54] will have poor transtemporal windows impeding examination. Hyperostosis impacts the ability to examine, as the thickness of the bone impairs image quality [55]. This is particularly pronounced in certain populations like African American women, Asian men, Taiwanese people [56], and women irrespective of race as they age.

The first step in acquiring an image in the transtemporal window is to identify the contralateral temporal bone. The temporal bone is the curved bright white line visualized in the far field. Initially the depth should be set to 10–15 cm to facilitate recognition of the temporal bone (Fig. 3.4). The sphenoid bone with its typical butterfly wing appearance can be seen as a white line in the near field; angling the tail of the probe

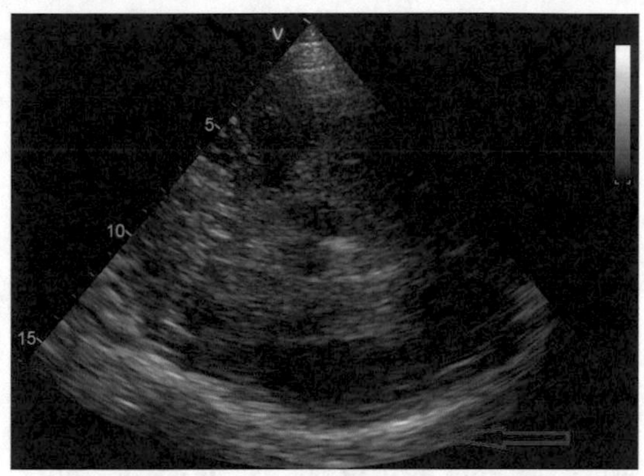

Fig. 3.4 Visualization of the contralateral bone (red arrow) through the transtemporal window

helps bring this into view. The cerebral peduncles are hypoechoic and heart shaped and surrounded by the highly echogenic basal cisterns. It is worth noting that signal brightness is low within the ventricles, but that the perimesencephalic basal cisterns appear bright. The third ventricle is recognized as a slit-like hypoechoic structure with two horizontal hyperechoic lines, which represents the CSF-filled space and the ventricle walls. The third ventricle should be a midline structure in the absence of pathology.

Identification of the contralateral temporal bone, cerebral peduncles, and third ventricle is a critical step. Visualization of these structures confirms that the window is adequate and that the vessels can be investigated with confidence. The depth can be reduced so that the cerebral peduncles are in the far field of the ultrasound image, allowing for easier visualization of vessels with the application of color.

Manipulation of the probe at the transtemporal window allows visualization of numerous key cerebral structures. If there are satisfactory bony windows the mesencephalon, pons, third ventricle, anterior and posterior horns of the lateral ventricles, falx cerebri, thalamus, basal ganglia, pineal gland, and temporal lobe can be identified greater than 75% of the time [5].

By angling the transducer 30° superiorly towards the skull vault the thalamic plane can be visualized. Anatomical landmarks in this plane include the pineal gland, which is typically calcified and therefore hyperechoic. The thalami are hypoechoic. The third ventricle lies in front of the pineal gland, surrounded by the two oval-shaped thalami. The frontal horns of the lateral ventricles are hypoechoic and run into the third ventricle. Enlargement of the third ventricle is one of the ultrasonographic markers of brain atrophy [57]. The width of the third ventricle is typically 3–4 mm, though a range from 2.76 to 7.31 mm has been reported [58]. The caudate and lenticular nucleus are situated between the frontal horns and the thalamus [59].

By angling the probe a further 10° superiorly the cella media plane comes into view. At this point the hypoechoic lateral ventricles can be recognized. Tilting the probe inferiorly from the axial mesencephalic plane allows visualization of the middle temporal fossa. This is comprised of the greater wing of the sphenoid bone anteriorly and the petrosal part of the temporal bone posteriorly. The cerebellum is apparent as a hypoechoic structure.

The transtemporal window can be further evaluated by angling the probe anteriorly and posteriorly. This examines the anterior middle and posterior portions of the window. The posterior window is just anterior to the ear. This window provides the best separation of the anterior and posterior cerebral circulations, which helps with the identification of vessels [45]. The middle window is approx. 1.5 cm anterior to the posterior window and the anterior window is 1.5 cm anterior to the middle window. All windows should be examined to ascertain the optimal views for the individual patient.

Recognition of parenchymal structures and bony landmarks allows for ascertaining if midline shift, hydrocephalus, or masses are present. Measuring from the third ventricle to the temporal bone allows for determination of any midline shift by the following calculation.

TCCS allows demonstration of both vessel proximity to fixed structures and flow direction. In contrast to TCD it does not rely on accurate evaluation of vessel depth to aid identification. Knowledge of anticipated depth is a useful adjunct to facilitate identification and normal anatomy. The vessels of the circle of Willis are located adjacent to the cerebral peduncles. Scanning in the orbitomeatal axial plane demonstrates the mesencephalic brainstem. The cerebral peduncles can then be located. The area immediately lateral to the peduncles can then be interrogated with the color function of the Doppler to delineate the vessels. Once the flow is determined the probe can slowly be angled and tilted to obtain optimal images.

The ICA typically bifurcates at 55–65 mm, into the anterior and middle cerebral arteries. There is simultaneous bidirectional flow at the bifurcation facilitating identification, as both red and blue color flow is apparent. The anterior cerebral artery flows away from the probe and the middle cerebral artery flows towards the probe (Fig. 3.3b).

The MCA lies anterior and lateral to the basal cisterns. It is typically found at depths of 55–60 mm. In a healthy patient the MCA is a low-resistance vessel. Flow runs anteriorly and laterally towards the probe, until the trifurcation of the vessel is reached. The MCA should be interrogated in 2–5 mm increments, from its origin from the ICA to the M1 segment.

The ACA is located by scanning MCA progressively deeper until flow signal in opposite direction is obtained; the proximal ACA can be quite short and can only be sampled over short distances [53]. The ACA is usually found at a depth of approximately 60 mm and it flows medially and away from the probe (Fig. 3.3b). If flow at a deeper distance of 80 mm is detected towards the probe this is probably the contralateral A1 ACA [40]. It is only possible to visualize the A1 segment of the anterior cerebral artery. The 90-degree curve at A2 precludes its visualization using brain ultrasound.

In some patients the PCA may be visible as part of a complete circle of Willis when the MCA is first identified. If not, maneuvers will need to be introduced to visualize the posterior cerebellar arteries. Having first visualized the MCA, the probe can then be aimed posterior and slightly caudal. Typically the PCA is 1–2 cm posterior to the ICA bifurcation in the same plane as the circle of Willis. P1 flows towards the probe and is red and P2 flows away from the probe and hence is blue (Fig. 3.3b). PCAs exhibit lower velocities than the MCAs. P1 is difficult to identify in the fetal PCA configuration. In this arrangement the PCA derives most of its flow through a large posterior communicating artery and the PCA may be hypoplastic [21].

3.5.4 Orbital

The orbital approach can be used to visualize both vascular structures and optic nerve. Measurements of the optic nerve provide information that can be used to deduce if intracranial pressure is raised. Thus TCCS has potentially a substantial role to play in the management of neurocritical care patients in the absence of standard ICP monitors.

When examining the transorbital window time should be minimized as much as possible and power output of the machine should be reduced to 10% to avoid damage to the delicate orbital contents [40]. The probe required is a high-frequency linear transducer probe [60]. The depth should initially be set to 0.5–2 cm. The eyelids should be gently opposed and covered with a clear dressing to prevent damage from the gel. The transducer should be angled upwards and medially to visualize the structures.

3.5.4.1 Optic Nerve Sheath

The optic nerve sheath is continuous with the meninges and therefore continuous with the subarachnoid space. It has previously been demonstrated that elevations in ICP correlate with an increase in the optic nerve sheath diameter (ONSD) [61, 62]. It is possible to use ONSD to determine that ICP is elevated but not to determine the extent to which it is elevated. ONSD assessment is not a replacement for formal continuous ICP monitoring. It does provide an alternate means of assessment for patients in whom LP or cranial probe placement might be contraindicated, e.g., the encephalopathic liver failure patient [63], prior to an ICP probe insertion, or where external ventricular drainage devices or intraparenchymal monitors are unavailable.

The globe of the eye is anechoic. The retrobulbar fat is echogenic. The optic nerve and its surrounding sheath extend from the posterior aspect of the globe through the retrobulbar fat. The optic nerve is anechoic and the sheath is a thin hypoechoic line lying on the outer aspect of each side of the nerve. Measurements of the sheath are made 3 mm posterior to the origin of the nerve. The horizontal distance from each hypoechoic line running along the nerve is measured. The upper limit of normal in adults is considered to be 5 mm. The optic nerve sheath diameter should be ascertained. Bilateral increase is consistent with an increase in intracranial pressure [64]. It is important to ensure that there is a crisp outline of the optic nerve sheath. Turning on color function to ensure that no vessels are running parallel to the sheath and thus inducing inaccuracies in the measurement is prudent.

The optic canal is typically situated medially and contains the carotid syphon. The usual depth is in the range of 55–70 mm. The various portions have different flow directions with the supraclinoid portion flowing away from the probe, and the parasellar portion flowing towards the probe. Signals detected both forward and away indicate the genu portion of the carotid siphon. The ophthalmic artery is typically at a depth of 60 mm, has flow towards the probe, and demonstrates a high-resistance flow pattern.

3.6 Troubleshooting

Oscillation maneuvers may help identify certain vessels [36]. An oscillation may be generated by gently tapping a feeding vessel and observing for changes in the vessel being examined. The terminal ICA and the PCA both lie at posterior angles and occasionally it may be difficult to differentiate between the two. Generating oscillations in the vertebral artery by tapping on the skull base will cause reverberations in the PCA (provided that the PCA is not of fetal origin). Tapping on the carotid at the clavicular level will cause oscillations in vessels of the anterior circulation. The ICA is the supply vessel for the anterior circulation. Briefly occluding the carotid artery (provided that there are no contraindications to doing so) can help differentiate the vessels. If the flow is reduced or reversed this implies that the vessel is originating from the ICA and hence part of the anterior circulation. If no flow changes are produced it implies that the vessel is part of the posterior circulation.

3.7 Summary

Ultrasonography of the brain is a minimally invasive means of examining the brain and its vasculature. It can be used in a variety of pathological states, gives real-time data, and is easily repeatable after therapeutic interventions have been made. It provides reliable data to guide management of isolated intracranial issues, and also provides information about intracranial complications subsequent to systemic pathology. A stepwise methodical approach such as the MOTOr approach outlined in this chapter yields the most information.

References

1. Kaczynski J, Home R, Shields K, Walters M, Whiteley W, Wardlaw J, et al. Reproducibility of transcranial Doppler ultrasound in the middle cerebral artery. Cardiovasc Ultrasound. 2018;16(1):15.
2. Baumgartner RW, Mathis J, Sturzenegger M, Mattle HP. A validation study on the intraobserver reproducibility of transcranial color-coded duplex sonography velocity measurements. Ultrasound Med Biol. 1994;20(3):233–7.
3. Cattalani A, Grasso VM, Vitali M, Gallesio I, Magrassi L, Barbanera A. Transcranial color-coded duplex sonography for evaluation of midline-shift after chronic-subdural hematoma evacuation (TEMASE): a prospective study. Clin Neurol Neurosurg. 2017;162:101–7.
4. Niesen W-D, Rosenkranz M, Weiller C. Bedside transcranial sonographic monitoring for expansion and progression of subdural hematoma compared to computed tomography. Front Neurol. 2018;9:374.
5. Kern R, Perren F, Kreisel S, Szabo K, Hennerici M, Meairs S. Multiplanar transcranial ultrasound imaging: standards, landmarks and correlation with magnetic resonance imaging. Ultrasound Med Biol. 2005;31(3):311–5.
6. Seidel G, Kaps M, Dorndorf W. Transcranial color-coded duplex sonography of intracerebral hematomas in adults. Stroke. 1993;24(10):1519–27.

7. Blanco P, Blaivas M. Applications of transcranial color-coded sonography in the emergency department: transcranial Doppler in the ED. J Ultrasound Med. 2017;36(6):1251–66.
8. Rasulo FA, Bertuetti R, Robba C, Lusenti F, Cantoni A, Bernini M, et al. The accuracy of transcranial Doppler in excluding intracranial hypertension following acute brain injury: a multicenter prospective pilot study. Crit Care. 2017;21(1). [Internet] [cited 2019 Jun 13] http://ccforum.biomedcentral.com/articles/10.1186/s13054-017-1632-2
9. Müller M, Hermes M, Brückmann H, Schimrigk K. Transcranial Doppler ultrasound in the evaluation of collateral blood flow in patients with internal carotid artery occlusion: correlation with cerebral angiography. AJNR Am J Neuroradiol. 1995;16(1):195–202.
10. Schebesch K-M, Woertgen C, Schlaier J, Brawanski A, Rothoerl RD. Doppler ultrasound measurement of blood flow volume in the extracranial internal carotid artery for evaluation of brain perfusion after aneurysmal subarachnoid hemorrhage. Neurol Res. 2007;29(2):210–4.
11. Sorrentino E, Budohoski KP, Kasprowicz M, Smielewski P, Matta B, Pickard JD, et al. Critical thresholds for transcranial Doppler indices of cerebral autoregulation in traumatic brain injury. Neurocrit Care. 2011;14(2):188–93.
12. Panerai RB. Transcranial Doppler for evaluation of cerebral autoregulation. Clin Auton Res. 2009;19(4):197–211.
13. Bellapart J, Fraser JF. Transcranial Doppler assessment of cerebral autoregulation. Ultrasound Med Biol. 2009;35(6):883–93.
14. Lupetin AR, Davis DA, Beckman I, Dash N. Transcranial Doppler sonography. Part 2. Evaluation of intracranial and extracranial abnormalities and procedural monitoring. Radiographics. 1995;15(1):193–209.
15. Moppett IK, Mahajan RP. Transcranial Doppler ultrasonography in anaesthesia and intensive care. Br J Anaesth. 2004;93(5):710–24.
16. Brunser AM, Mansilla E, Hoppe A, Olavarría V, Sujima E, Lavados PM. The role of TCD in the evaluation of acute stroke: TCD in acute stroke. J Neuroimaging. 2016;26(4):420–5.
17. Gerriets T, Stolz E, König S, Babacan S, Fiss I, Jauss M, et al. Sonographic monitoring of midline shift in space-occupying stroke: an early outcome predictor. Stroke. 2001;32(2):442–7.
18. Kirsch JD, Mathur M, Johnson MH, Gowthaman G, Scoutt LM. Advances in transcranial Doppler US: imaging ahead. Radiographics. 2013;33(1):E1–14.
19. Ketelaars R, Reijnders G, van Geffen G-J, Scheffer GJ, Hoogerwerf N. ABCDE of prehospital ultrasonography: a narrative review. Crit Ultrasound J. 2018;10(1). [Internet] [cited 2019 Apr 29] https://criticalultrasoundjournal.springeropen.com/articles/10.1186/s13089-018-0099-y
20. Robba C, Goffi A, Geeraerts T, Cardim D, Via G, Czosnyka M, et al. Brain ultrasonography: methodology, basic and advanced principles and clinical applications. A narrative review. Intensive Care Med. 2019;. [Internet] [cited 2019 Apr 29]; http://link.springer.com/10.1007/s00134-019-05610-4
21. Corradi F, Robba C, Tavazzi G, Via G. Combined lung and brain ultrasonography for an individualized "brain-protective ventilation strategy" in neurocritical care patients with challenging ventilation needs. Crit Ultrasound J. 2018;10(1). [Internet] [cited 2019 Apr 29] https://criticalultrasoundjournal.springeropen.com/articles/10.1186/s13089-018-0105-4
22. Young N, Rhodes JKJ, Mascia L, Andrews PJD. Ventilatory strategies for patients with acute brain injury. Curr Opin Crit Care. 2010;16(1):45–52.
23. Robba C, Cardim D, Tajsic T, Pietersen J, Bulman M, Donnelly J, et al. Ultrasound non-invasive measurement of intracranial pressure in neurointensive care: a prospective observational study. Schreiber M, editor. PLoS Med. 2017;14(7):e1002356.
24. Vaquero J, Fontana RJ, Larson AM, Bass NMT, Davern TJ, Shakil AO, et al. Complications and use of intracranial pressure monitoring in patients with acute liver failure and severe encephalopathy. Liver Transpl. 2005;11(12):1581–9.
25. Karvellas CJ, Fix OK, Battenhouse H, Durkalski V, Sanders C, Lee WM, et al. Outcomes and complications of intracranial pressure monitoring in acute liver failure: a retrospective cohort study. Crit Care Med. 2014;42(5):1157–67.
26. Nicoletto HA, Burkman MH. Transcranial Doppler series. Part I: understanding neurovascular anatomy. Am J Electroneurodiagnostic Technol. 2008;48(4):249–57.
27. Iqbal S. A comprehensive study of the anatomical variations of the circle of Willis in adult human brains. J Clin Diagn Res. 2013;7(11):2423–7.
28. Pascalau R, Padurean VA, Bartoş D, Bartoş A, Szabo BA. The geometry of the circle of Willis anatomical variants as a potential cerebrovascular risk factor. Turk Neurosurg. 2019;29(2):151–8.
29. Puls I, Berg D, Mäurer M, Schliesser M, Hetzel G, Becker G. Transcranial sonography of the brain parenchyma: comparison of B-mode imaging and tissue harmonic imaging. Ultrasound Med Biol. 2000;26(2):189–94.
30. Robba C, Cardim D, Sekhon M, Budohoski K, Czosnyka M. Transcranial Doppler: a stethoscope for the brain-neurocritical care use. J Neurosci Res. 2018;96(4):720–30.
31. Lavinio A, Schmidt EA, Haubrich C, Smielewski P, Pickard JD, Czosnyka M. Noninvasive evaluation of dynamic cerebrovascular autoregulation using Finapres Plethysmograph and Transcranial Doppler. Stroke. 2007;38(2):402–4.
32. Cardim D, Robba C, Bohdanowicz M, Donnelly J, Cabella B, Liu X, et al. Non-invasive monitoring of intracranial pressure using transcranial Doppler ultrasonography: is it possible? Neurocrit Care. 2016;25(3):473–91.

33. Michel E, Zernikow B. Gosling's Doppler pulsatility index revisited. Ultrasound Med Biol. 1998;24(4):597–9.
34. Kassab MY, Majid A, Farooq MU, Azhary H, Hershey LA, Bednarczyk EM, et al. Transcranial Doppler: an introduction for primary care physicians. J Am Board Fam Med. 2007;20(1):65–71.
35. Vinciguerra L, Lanza G, Puglisi V, Pennisi M, Cantone M, Bramanti A, et al. Transcranial Doppler ultrasound in vascular cognitive impairment-no dementia. Ginsberg SD, editor. PLoS One. 2019;14(4):e0216162.
36. Nicoletto HA, Burkman MH. Transcranial Doppler series part III: interpretation. Am J Electroneurodiagnostic Technol. 2009;49(3):244–59.
37. Nicoletto HA, Burkman MH. Transcranial Doppler series part II: performing a transcranial Doppler. Am J Electroneurodiagnostic Technol. 2009;49(1):14–27.
38. Bogdahn U, Becker G, Winkler J, Greiner K, Perez J, Meurers B. Transcranial color-coded real-time sonography in adults. Stroke. 1990;21(12):1680–8.
39. Gorman MJ, Nyström K, Carbonella J, Pearson H. Submandibular TCD approach detects post-bulb ICA stenosis in children with sickle cell anemia. Neurology. 2009;73(5):362–5.
40. Lee TS, Ducic Y, Gordin E, Stroman D. Management of carotid artery trauma. Craniomaxillofac Trauma Reconstr. 2014;7(3):175–89.
41. Bathala L, Mehndiratta MM, Sharma VK. Transcranial Doppler: technique and common findings (part 1). Ann Indian Acad Neurol. 2013;16(2):174–9.
42. Arnolds BJ, Kunz D, von Reutern GM. Spatial resolution of transcranial pulsed Doppler technique in vitro evaluation of the sensitivity distribution of the sample volume. Ultrasound Med Biol. 1989;15(8):729–35.
43. Hennerici M, Rautenberg W, Sitzer G, Schwartz A. Transcranial Doppler ultrasound for the assessment of intracranial arterial flow velocity--part 1. Examination technique and normal values. Surg Neurol. 1987;27(5):439–48.
44. Hennerici M, Rautenberg W, Schwartz A. Transcranial Doppler ultrasound for the assessment of intracranial arterial flow velocity–part 2. Evaluation of intracranial arterial disease. Surg Neurol. 1987;27(6):523–32.
45. Purkayastha S, Sorond F. Transcranial Doppler ultrasound: technique and application. Semin Neurol. 2013;32(04):411–20.
46. Lupetin AR, Davis DA, Beckman I, Dash N. Transcranial Doppler sonography. Part 1. Principles, technique, and normal appearances. Radiographics. 1995;15(1):179–91.
47. Soustiel JF, Shik V, Shreiber R, Tavor Y, Goldsher D. Basilar vasospasm diagnosis: investigation of a modified "Lindegaard index" based on imaging studies and blood velocity measurements of the basilar artery. Stroke. 2002;33(1):72–7.
48. Sviri GE, Ghodke B, Britz GW, Douville CM, Haynor DR, Mesiwala AH, et al. Transcranial Doppler grading criteria for basilar artery vasospasm. Neurosurgery. 2006;59(2):360–6. discussion 360-366
49. Becker G, Lindner A, Bogdahn U. Imaging of the vertebrobasilar system by transcranial color-coded real-time sonography. J Ultrasound Med. 1993;12(7):395–401.
50. Pade O, Eggers J, Schreiber S, Valdueza J. Complete basilar artery assessment by Transcranial color-coded duplex sonography using the combined transforaminal and transtemporal approach. Ultraschall Med – Eur J Ultrasound. 2011;32(S 02):E63–8.
51. Kermer P, Wellmer A, Crome O, Mohr A, Knauth M, Bähr M. Transcranial color-coded duplex sonography in suspected acute basilar artery occlusion. Ultrasound Med Biol. 2006;32(3):315–20.
52. Brandt T, Knauth M, Wildermuth S, Winter R, von Kummer R, Sartor K, et al. CT angiography and Doppler sonography for emergency assessment in acute basilar artery ischemia. Stroke. 1999;30(3):606–12.
53. Aaslid R, Markwalder TM, Nornes H. Noninvasive transcranial Doppler ultrasound recording of flow velocity in basal cerebral arteries. J Neurosurg. 1982;57(6):769–74.
54. Bazzocchi M, Quaia E, Zuiani C, Moroldo M. Transcranial Doppler: state of the art. Eur J Radiol. 1998;27(Suppl 2):S141–8.
55. Naqvi J, Yap KH, Ahmad G, Ghosh J. Transcranial Doppler ultrasound: a review of the physical principles and major applications in critical care. Int J Vasc Med. 2013;2013:1–13.
56. Kollár J, Schulte-Altedorneburg G, Sikula J, Fülesdi B, Ringelstein EB, Mehta V, et al. Image quality of the temporal bone window examined by transcranial Doppler sonography and correlation with postmortem computed tomography measurements. Cerebrovasc Dis. 2004;17(1):61–5.
57. Lin Y-P, Fu M-H, Tan T-Y. Factors associated with no or insufficient temporal bone window using transcranial color-coded sonography. J Med Ultrasound. 2015;23(3):129–32.
58. Müller M, Esser R, Kötter K, Voss J, Müller A, Stellmes P. Width of 3. Ventricle: reference values and clinical relevance in a cohort of patients with relapsing remitting multiple sclerosis. Open Neurol J. 2013;7:11–6.
59. Puz P, Lasek-Bal A, Radecka P. Transcranial sonography of subcortical structures in patients with multiple sclerosis. Acta Neurol Scand. 2017;136(1):24–30.
60. Llompart Pou JA, Abadal Centellas JM, Palmer Sans M, Pérez Bárcena J, Casares Vivas M, Homar Ramírez J, et al. Monitoring midline shift by transcranial color-coded sonography in traumatic brain injury. A comparison with cranial computerized tomography. Intensive Care Med. 2004;30(8):1672–5.
61. Soldatos T, Chatzimichail K, Papathanasiou M, Gouliamos A. Optic nerve sonography: a new window for the non-invasive evaluation of intracranial pressure in brain injury. Emerg Med J. 2009;26(9):630–4.
62. Hansen HC, Helmke K. The subarachnoid space surrounding the optic nerves. An ultrasound study of the optic nerve sheath. Surg Radiol Anat. 1996;18(4):323–8.

63. Liu D, Kahn M. Measurement and relationship of subarachnoid pressure of the optic nerve to intracranial pressures in fresh cadavers. Am J Ophthalmol. 1993;116(5):548–56.
64. Liu D, Li Z, Zhang X, Zhao L, Jia J, Sun F, et al. Assessment of intracranial pressure with ultrasonographic retrobulbar optic nerve sheath diameter measurement. BMC Neurol. 2017;17(1). [Internet] [cited 2019 Mar 26] http://bmcneurol.biomedcentral.com/articles/10.1186/s12883-017-0964-5

4 Optic Nerve Sheath Diameter

Thomas Geeraerts, Louis Delamarre, and Charles-Henri Houze-Cerfon

Contents

4.1 Introduction

Ocular ultrasound has recently emerged as a promising tool to assess noninvasive intracranial pressure (ICP). The optic nerve, as a part of the central nervous system, is surrounded by a subarachnoid

Electronic Supplementary Material The online version of this chapter (https://doi.org/10.1007/978-3-030-48202-2_4) contains supplementary material, which is available to authorized users.

T. Geeraerts (✉)
Anesthesiology and Critical Care Department, University Hospital of Toulouse, University Toulouse 3-Paul Sabatier, Toulouse, France

Coordination d'Anesthésie, CHU Toulouse, Hôpital Pierre Paul Riquet, Toulouse, France
e-mail: geeraerts.t@chu-toulouse.fr

L. Delamarre
Anesthesiology and Critical Care Department, University Hospital of Toulouse, University Toulouse 3-Paul Sabatier, Toulouse, France
e-mail: delamarre.l@chu-toulouse.fr

C.-H. Houze-Cerfon
Emergency Medicine Department, SAMU 31, University Hospital of Toulouse, University Toulouse 3-Paul Sabatier, Toulouse, France
e-mail: houze-cerfon.ch@chu-toulouse.fr

C. Robba, G. Citerio (eds.), *Echography and Doppler of the Brain*, https://doi.org/10.1007/978-3-030-48202-2_4

space containing cerebrospinal fluid (CSF). The subarachnoid space surrounding the optic nerve communicates with intracranial cavity and changes in intracranial CSF pressure can be transmitted along the optic nerve sheath. The retrobulbar optic nerve sheath is distensible and can inflate in case of CSF accumulation in the retrobulbar space due to raised pressure in the cerebrospinal fluid. Ocular sonography can be used to precisely measure the optic nerve sheath diameter.

4.2 Anatomical Background

In 1806, Tenon described the optic nerve sheath and the optic sclera as continuous to the dura mater. The optic nerve, as a part of the central nervous system, is surrounded by a dural sheath. In vivo, the CSF circulates in this space, from the posterior to the anterior part. In the absence of obstruction in CSF circulation, the intraorbital CSF is subject to similar pressure changes as those in the intracranial and lumbar compartments [1]. In 1964, Hayreh showed in monkeys that the cranial cavity communicated with the optic nerve sheath and that a rise in CSF pressure in subarachnoid space was transmitted along the optic nerve sheath [2]. Hayreh also demonstrated that a rise in pressure in the optic nerve sheath is essential for the development of edema of the optic disk. Papilledema is probably a delayed consequence of chronic CSF accumulation in the retrobulbar area [3]. In case of raised ICP, and in accordance with Monro-Kellie doctrine [4], CSF can be redistributed toward the caudal compartment, and due to the cul-de-sac anatomy of the optic nerve, CSF can accumulate in the retrobulbar compartment. Direct measurement of such CSF accumulation by measuring optic nerve sheath diameter may provide an early and reactive measure of intracranial hypertension.

Dense adhesions between the optic nerve and its sheath are observed in the posterior part of the nerve, in the optic canal. However, in the anterior part of the optic nerve and particularly in the retrobulbar segment, the sheath has fewer adherences to the nerve, and is only surrounded by orbital fat. The retrobulbar optic nerve sheath is therefore distensible and can inflate in case of raised pressure in the CSF. In cadavers, the ONSD displays predominantly anterior enlargement following injection into the orbital perineural subarachnoid space [5]. In humans, following an intrathecal lumbar infusion of Ringer's solution, ONSD dilation reaches a maximum at peak CSF pressure, strongly suggesting a close relationship between CSF pressure and dilation of the orbital perineural subarachnoid space [5]. This dilation occurs within seconds after rise in CSF pressure. This dynamic property appears to be clinically relevant to detect acute changes in ICP.

4.3 Technology and Methods

4.3.1 Technology

To allow precise measurements, a high-frequency probe of at least 7.5 MHz must be used. Multipurpose ultrasound units with high-frequency transducers (more than 7.5 MHz, usually a 7.5–10 MHz probe), now available in most ultrasound systems, have high lateral and axial precision [6]. Complex and specialized probes for ONSD measurement are probably not needed [7]. Linear high-frequency probes, corresponding to the probes used for vascular ultrasound, can be used. Depth should be set at 4 cm and the two-dimensional mode should be used.

4.3.2 Methods

Patients must be placed in supine position, at 20–30° to the horizontal. A thick layer of gel must be applied over the closed upper eyelid (Movie 4.1). Attention must be paid to avoid generating pressure on the eye with the probe. The probe must be placed on the gel in the temporal area of the eyelid, and not on the eye itself, to prevent pressure being exerted on the eye. The placement of the probe must be adjusted to give a suitable angle for displaying the entry of the optic nerve into the globe.

4.3.3 Normal Views

The normal sonographic aspect of the optic nerve is from center to peripheral: hypoechogenic nerve fibers are closely surrounded by the echogenic pia mater; the subarachnoid space appears anechogenic or hypoechogenic and is surrounded by hyperechogenic dura mater and periorbital fat [6].

The 2D mode is generally used and ONSD must be measured in its retrobulbar segment, 3 mm behind the ocular globe, corresponding to the anterior part of the ONSD that can dilate in case of raised pressure (Fig. 4.1, Movie 4.1). This identification is carried out using an electronic caliper and perpendicularly to the optic nerve axis. The ONSD corresponds to the distance between the external part of the subarachnoid space, in other words to the distance corresponding to hypoechogenic CSF inside the hyperechogenic orbital fat.

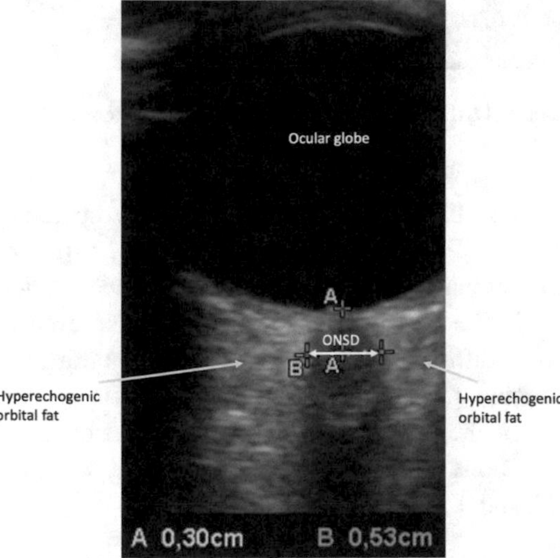

Fig. 4.1 Normal view of ocular ultrasound and optic nerve sheath diameter (ONSD) measurement. The 2D mode is used. A first caliper is placed in the posterior part of the retina, and 3 mm behind the ocular globe in the optic nerve axis (distance between both A). A second caliper is placed to measure ONSD, perpendicularly to the nerve axis. The ONSD corresponds to the distance between the external part of the subarachnoid space, in other words to the distance corresponding to hypoechogenic CSF inside the hyperechogenic orbital fat. The ONSD is 5.3 mm

ONSD measurement should be performed bilaterally. Some authors measured ONSD in several axes by rotating the probe. ONSD is usually measured in the horizontal and vertical axes, for both eyes, the final ONSD reading corresponding to the mean of these four values (Fig. 4.2). Blehar et al. showed that measurements in the horizontal axis are consistently larger than those in the vertical axis [8]. This could be related to a nonspherical ONSD, but also in some cases to a shadow image, resulting from an acoustic artifact rising from the lamina cribrosa, or from unintended reconstruction when using outdated ultrasound systems. In our experience, measurements in the horizontal axis alone are sufficient to discriminate patients with or without raised ICP.

To avoid posterior artifacts, ONSD measurement should not be made through the lens. A correct image should be able to allow a clear differentiation between the nerve and the arachnoid, with the outer border of the subarachnoid being identifiable. The visualization of the entry of the optic nerve into the globe should be without interposition of hyperechogenic layer of the sclera, with the nerve and the globe being hypoechogenic. The placement of probe must be adjusted so that the optic nerve axis is aligned with the middle of the posterior part of the image. A summary of quality criteria is proposed in Table 4.1.

There is a growing body of evidence in the clinical setting suggesting that millimetric increases in sonographic optic nerve sheath diameter (ONSD) are related to raised ICP. Optic nerve diameter (OND, i.e., not taking into consideration the sheath but only the nerve itself) has a poor relationship with ICP, and changes in ICP cannot be detected by changes in OND [9]. The variation of ONSD during raised ICP cannot therefore be related to optic nerve dilatation (as during nerve edema) but to its sheath distension, probably due to the increase in CSF pressure surrounding the optic nerve.

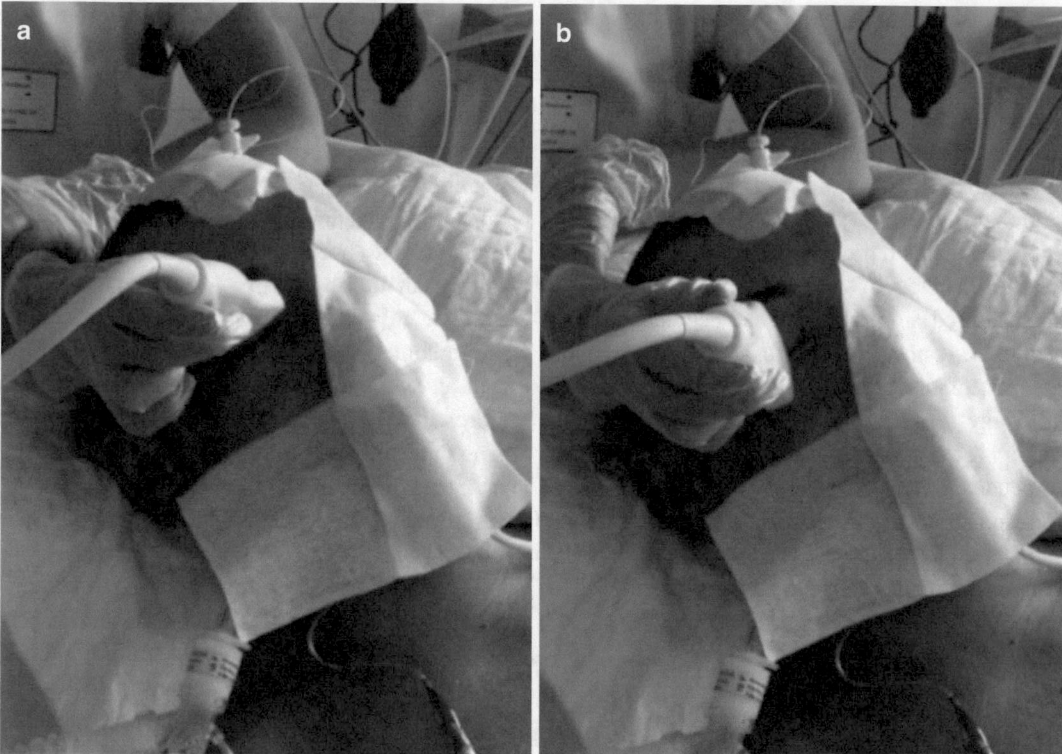

Fig. 4.2 Placement of the probe for optic nerve sheath diameter (ONSD) measurement. A 7.5 MHz linear probe is used, in the horizontal axis (**a**) and in the vertical axis (**b**)

Table 4.1 Quality criteria for optic nerve sheath measurement

1. ONSD measurement should *not* be made through the lens
2. Visualization of the entry of the hypoechogenic optic nerve into the hypoechogenic globe without interposition of hyperechogenic layer of the sclera
3. Optic nerve axis aligned with the middle of the posterior part of the image
4. Differentiation between the nerve and the arachnoid should be obvious
5. The outer border of the subarachnoid must be identifiable
6. Absence of posterior artifact (hypoechogenic line, without attenuation with depth)
7. Standardized ONSD measurement: 4 mm behind the retina, perpendicularly to the nerve axis
8. Bilateral measurements: Both eye: Horizontal + vertical axis or horizontal axis alone

4.3.4 Feasibility and Reproducibility

ONSD measurement has been shown to be feasible in difficult conditions, such as prehospital setting, in high altitude [10, 11], in the operating room [12], or even during microgravity exposure in astronauts in the International Space Station [13]. The overall quality was acceptable even in such difficult settings. Variability in ultrasonographic measurement of ONSD seems to be limited, as the median intra-observer and inter-observer variations were shown to be, respectively, less than 0.2 and 0.3 mm [9, 14–16].

4.4 Limits and Safety Issues

4.4.1 Limits

There are some limitations to the use of ocular sonography. These limits should be known to avoid misinterpretations of ONSD.

Inexperience with sonography may be an important limitation for the use of this method. The learning curve seems however to be rapid: an experienced sonologist needs as few as ten measurements and three abnormal scans to obtain adequate results, while for novice sonologists, 20–25 scans may be needed [17, 18].

Sonography allows only sequential measures while ICP is a dynamic parameter which can change very rapidly. Significant episodes of raised ICP can therefore remain unrecognized by sonographic examination. Precise ICP prediction remains difficult with sonography as an ICP range of more than 10 mmHg can be observed for a given ONSD value.

Hansen et al. [19] have shown in isolated human optic nerve preparations that following submission to pressure, the diameter of the nerve sheath increased up to 140% of its baseline value. However, when the applied pressure was very high (up to 45–55 mmHg or more) the ONSD did not reach its baseline during decompression, suggesting a loss in ONSD elasticity. This could be of importance in patients who have experienced a very high increase in ICP with subsequent treatment (osmotherapy or decompression), and who will have a sustained enlarged ONSD despite normal ICP. Moreover, the relationship between ONSD and ICP is not linear. The maximum distension of ONSD is around 7.5–8 mm, as measured in brain-dead patients [20].

In adults, ONSD does not vary with age [21]. In children however, ONSD has been described to decrease with age before 1 year [22]. Hence, the upper limit of normal ONSD value is considered to be 4.5 mm in children over 1 year of age, and 4 mm under 1 year of age.

4.4.2 Safety

Ocular sonography has been used for more than 25 years in ophthalmology [23]. Ocular ultrasound is regarded as safe, when Doppler frequency analysis is not used for prolonged duration [24]. B (or 2D) mode, most commonly used, is safe regarding the production of harmful temperature [25]. Nevertheless, prolonged exposition to high-frequency Doppler may be harmful by causing heating to the retina. Safety issues should be considered when using ocular ultrasound. The British Medical Ultrasound Society produced in 2010 helpful guidelines for the safe use of diagnostic ultrasound equipment [26]. For eye sonography it is recommended to monitor thermal and mechanical indexes. The thermal index should be less than 1. If the thermal index is more than 1, scanning of the eye is not recommended. The mechanical index should be less than 0.3. In case of mechanical index over 0.7, there is a risk of cavitation.

4.5 Recent Innovation and Future Perspectives

Very recently, the ratio of ONSD to eyeball transverse diameter has been described to better estimate ICP than ONSD alone [27]. This could be an elegant way for normalizing ONSD for patient's size.

Recent advances in sonographic allow promising 3D measurements. Volumetric measurements of the optic nerve sheath may improve the accuracy of the prediction of the risk of raised ICP [28, 29].

Automatic estimation of the ONSD has also been recently described, using an algorithm allowing extraction of the optic nerve region below the eye using the eye location and size estimates, smoothing, and scaling of intensities to alleviate attenuation effects [30].

These advances could help clinicians to use ONSD in their daily practice and better estimate the risk of raised ICP.

4.6 Conclusion

The distension of the optic nerve sheath reflects CSF redistribution during rise in ICP. Ocular sonography, when respecting simple rules for quality measurements, is a valid measurement of the distension of the dural sheath surrounding the optic nerve. Ocular sonography with optic nerve sheath diameter (ONSD) measurement does not require specialized skills. This simple and rapid method may offer opportunities to estimate the risk of raised ICP, and maybe to better individualized treatment in the very early management of brain-injured patients.

References

1. Helmke K, Hansen HC. Fundamentals of transorbital sonographic evaluation of optic nerve sheath expansion under intracranial hypertension II. Patient study. Pediatr Radiol. 1996;26:706–10.
2. Hayreh SS. Pathogenesis of oedema of the optic disc (papilloedema) a preliminary report. Br J Ophthalmol. 1964;48:522–43.
3. Hayreh SS. Optic disc edema in raised intracranial pressure: V. pathogenesis. Arch Ophthalmol. 1977;95:1553–65.
4. Cross ME, Plunkett EVE. The Monro–Kellie doctrine. In: Physics, Pharmacol. Physiol. Anaesth. 2014; 310–312.
5. Hansen H-C, Helmke K. Validation of the optic nerve sheath response to changing cerebrospinal fluid pressure: ultrasound findings during intrathecal infusion tests. J Neurosurg. 2009;87:34–40.
6. Bergès O, Koskas P, Lafitte F, Piekarski JD. Sonography of the eye and orbit with a multipurpose ultrasound unit. J Radiol. 2006;87:345–53.
7. Shah S, Kimberly H, Marill K, Noble VE. Ultrasound techniques to measure the optic nerve sheath: is a specialized probe necessary? Med Sci Monit. 2009;15:MT63-8.
8. Blehar DJ, Gaspari RJ, Montoya A, Calderon R. Correlation of visual axis and coronal axis measurements of the optic nerve sheath diameter. J Ultrasound Med. 2008;27:407–11.
9. Geeraerts T, Merceron S, Benhamou D, Vigué B, Duranteau J. Non-invasive assessment of intracranial pressure using ocular sonography in neurocritical care patients. Intensive Care Med. 2008;34:2062–7.
10. Houzé-Cerfon CH, Bounes V, Guemon J, Le Gourrierec T, Geeraerts T. Quality and feasibility of sonographic measurement of the optic nerve sheath diameter to estimate the risk of raised intracranial pressure after traumatic brain injury in prehospital setting. Prehosp Emerg Care. 2019;23:277–83.
11. Canepa CA, Harris NS. Ultrasound in austere environments. High Alt Med Biol. 2019;20:103–11.
12. Verdonck P, Kalmar AF, Suy K, Geeraerts T, Vercauteren M, Mottrie A, De Wolf AM, Hendrickx JFA. Optic nerve sheath diameter remains constant during robot assisted laparoscopic radical prostatectomy. PLoS One. 2014;9:e111916.
13. Sirek AS, Garcia K, Foy M, Ebert D, Sargsyan A, Wu JH, Dulchavsky SA. Doppler ultrasound of the central retinal artery in microgravity. Aviat Space Environ Med. 2014;85:3–8.
14. Ballantyne J, Hollman AS, Hamilton R, Bradnam MS, Carachi R, Young DG, Dutton GN. Transorbital optic nerve sheath ultrasonography in normal children. Clin Radiol. 1999;54:740–2.
15. Soldatos T, Karakitsos D, Chatzimichail K, Papathanasiou M, Gouliamos A, Karabinis A. Optic nerve sonography in the diagnostic evaluation of adult brain injury. Crit Care. 2008;12:R67.
16. Lochner P, Coppo L, Cantello R, Nardone R, Naldi A, Leone MA, Brigo F. Intra- and interobserver reliability of transorbital sonographic assessment of the optic nerve sheath diameter and optic nerve diameter in healthy adults. J Ultrasound. 2016;19:41–5.
17. Tayal VS, Neulander M, Norton HJ, Foster T, Saunders T, Blaivas M. Emergency department sonographic measurement of optic nerve sheath diameter to detect findings of increased intracranial pressure in adult head injury patients. Ann Emerg Med. 2007;49:508–14.
18. Shrestha GS, Upadhyay B, Shahi A, Jaya Ram KC, Joshi P, Poudyal BS. Sonographic measurement of optic nerve sheath diameter: how steep is the learning curve for a novice operator? Indian J Crit Care Med. 2018;22:646–9.
19. Hansen HC, Lagrèze W, Krueger O, Helmke K. Dependence of the optic nerve sheath diameter on acutely applied subarachnoidal pressure—an experimental ultrasound study. Acta Ophthalmol. 2011;89:e528–32.
20. Topcuoglu MA, Arsava EM, Bas DF, Kozak HH. Transorbital ultrasonographic measurement of optic nerve sheath diameter in brain death. J Neuroimaging. 2015;25:906–9.
21. Chan PYN, Mok KL. Transorbital sonographic evaluation of optic nerve sheath diameter in normal Hong Kong Chinese adults. Hong Kong J Emerg Med. 2008;15:197–204.
22. Newman WD, Hollman AS, Dutton GN, Carachi R. Measurement of optic nerve sheath diameter by ultrasound: a means of detecting acute raised intracranial pressure in hydrocephalus. Br J Ophthalmol. 2002;86:1109–13.
23. Bedi DG, Gombos DS, Ng CS, Singh S. Sonography of the eye. Am J Roentgenol. 2006;187:1061–72.
24. Williamson TH, Harris A. Color Doppler ultrasound imaging of the eye and orbit. Surv Ophthalmol. 1996;40:255–67.
25. Barnett SB, Ter Haar GR, Ziskin MC, Rott HD, Duck FA, Maeda K. International recommendations and guidelines for the safe use of diagnostic ultrasound in medicine. Ultrasound Med Biol. 2000;26:355–66.
26. Safety Group of the British Medical Ultrasound Society. Guidelines for the safe use of diagnostic ultrasound equipment. Ultrasound. 2010;18:52–9.
27. Du J, Deng Y, Li H, Qiao S, Yu M, Xu Q, Wang C. Ratio of optic nerve sheath diameter to eyeball transverse diameter by ultrasound can predict intracranial hypertension in traumatic brain injury patients: a prospective study. Neurocrit Care. 2019; https://doi.org/10.1007/s12028-019-00762-z.

28. Hoffmann J, Schmidt C, Kunte H, Klingebiel R, Harms L, Huppertz HJ, Lüdemann L, Wiener E. Volumetric assessment of optic nerve sheath and hypophysis in idiopathic intracranial hypertension. Am J Neuroradiol. 2014;35:513–8.
29. Dentinger A, MacDonald M, Ebert D, Garcia K, Sargsyan A. Volumetric ophthalmic ultrasound for inflight monitoring of visual impairment and intracranial pressure. Acta Neurochir Suppl. 2018;126:97–101.
30. Gerber S, Jallais M, Greer H, McCormick M, Montgomery S, Freeman B, Kane D, Chittajallu D, Siekierski N, Aylward S. Automatic estimation of the optic nerve sheath diameter from ultrasound images. Imaging Patient Cust Simul Syst Point Care Ultrasound. 2017;10549:113–20.

Limitations and Pitfalls

5

Aarti Sarwal

Contents

5.1 Introduction

Cranial ultrasound imaging utilizes the B mode of ultrasound to visualize the brain parenchyma and ventricles. Pulse Doppler imaging of the cerebral vasculature supported by color-mode and B-mode imaging is called transcranial color-coded duplex sonography (TCCS) or imaging transcranial Doppler (TCD). Non-imaging machines displaying only pulse Doppler spectral waveforms obtained without B-mode imaging guidance are conventionally termed transcranial Doppler or non-imaging TCD. Each of these modalities can be used to study the cerebral circulation through temporal windows, suboccipital windows, or transorbital windows, depending on the placement of the probe. Each Doppler modality can be used for multiple clinical indications in sickle cell disease, cerebral ischemia, detection of right-to-left shunts, subarachnoid hemorrhage, brain death, and periprocedural or surgical monitoring. Many emerging applications in critical care have enlightened cerebrovascular changes in systemic diseases and expanded clinical applications of TCCS, TCD, and cranial ultrasound [1].

A. Sarwal (✉)
Neurology, Wake Forest School of Medicine, Winston Salem, NC, USA
e-mail: asarwal@wakehealth.edu

C. Robba, G. Citerio (eds.), *Echography and Doppler of the Brain*,
https://doi.org/10.1007/978-3-030-48202-2_5

This chapter discusses the limitations of the cranial ultrasound, non-imaging pulse Doppler, and color duplex imaging in various windows. Also reviewed are technical pitfalls of these studies, anatomical nuances, as well as drawbacks to consider in major clinical applications. *Pitfalls in the technical use and clinical applications of these imaging modalities are also discussed* (*see* Table 5.1).

5.2 Technical Considerations

5.2.1 Acquisition of Images

Studies comparing acquisition of intracranial signals through TCCS and TCD have not found any difference, but individual sonographers may find steeper learning curves on one modality compared to the other [2]. Non-imaging TCD can be

Table 5.1 Limitations and pitfalls of transcranial ultrasound and Doppler imaging

	Limitations	Pitfalls
B-mode ultrasound Imaging of the intracranial anatomy	• Lack of temporal windows • Ultrasound has not been sensitive enough to replace head CT for volumetric measurements of midline shift, ventricular size, ischemic stroke, intracranial hemorrhage	• Quantitative measurements need experienced operators for reliability • Measurements are difficult to reproduce due to inability to replicate standardized insonation planes and may be better for trends than absolute values • Focal lesions may not produce a shift measured by ultrasound; hence absence of midline shift does not exclude intracranial pathology
Non-imaging transcranial Doppler of circle of Willis	• Lack of temporal windows and suboccipital windows in a small proportion of patients • Identifies the cerebral arteries "blindly," on the basis of the spectral display and standard criteria including arterial depth, arterial blood flow direction, and waveform analysis. May need power motion mode Doppler to increase the efficiency of insonation by providing multi-depth insonation • The rate of complete exam is lower for cerebral circulation due to relatively laborious process	• Identification of vessels in the presence of anatomical variations and without a visual guidance of the course of the vessel may be difficult • Waveform analysis itself may not reveal the nature of anatomic variants in circle of Willis • Identifying of each vessel segment at successive depths is guided by hit-and-trial "angling and inching" and may miss segments when focal pathology is present • Possibility of missing highest velocity in focal stenosis or tandem stenosis
Transcranial color-coded duplex imaging or imaging transcranial Doppler of circle of Willis	• Lack of temporal windows and suboccipital windows in a small proportion of patients • Difficult to perform prolonged continuous monitoring due to the manual holding of probe • Distal basilar artery through the suboccipital window (posterior coronal plane) may not be easy to insonate in patients with unfavorable neck anatomy	• Color signals may not be obtainable in all patients • Higher gain, power Doppler, or B-mode-guided placement of pulse Doppler gate may be needed
Transorbital windows for optic nerve sheath diameter	• Needs high-frequency probe for reliable insonation • Requires a low mechanical index in preset to avoid ultrasound-mediated strain on lens capsule	• Important to measure optic nerve sheath diameter in cross sections with "target" view • Measurements in longitudinal view may be erroneous
Transorbital windows with TCD or TCCS for ophthalmic artery	• Requires a low mechanical index in preset to avoid ultrasound-mediated strain on lens capsule	• Important to distinguish ophthalmic artery insonation from internal carotid artery siphon

used for prolonged studies and continuous imaging due to a smaller probe easily tethered on a headband. Imaging TCD or TCCS, on the other hand, suffers from limitations for prolonged continuous monitoring, due to the need to use a phased-array probe that requires manual holding throughout the study.

Cranial ultrasound requires a preset that allows high-intensity ultrasound to penetrate through the layers of the skull. 5–40% of patients may have thick skull that may not allow insonation through the temporal bone [3, 4].

On TCCS, the lack of adequate acoustic temporal bone window may allow some B-mode imaging and visualization of midbrain but may not allow capture of any Doppler shifts, making it impossible for color Doppler and pulse Doppler signals to be obtained during insonation (Fig. 5.1a). Some patients though may have only one temporal window, thus allowing visualization of ipsilateral vessels; hence both sides should be insonated prior to declaring the examination not possible. Furthermore, depth can be increased within the same window to attempt visualization of contralateral blood vessels. Some patients may have enough output to allow B-mode and pulse Doppler signals to be displayed, but may not produce a color spectrum due to the default low gain settings in color mode. In such patients, power Doppler mode may be used to detect flow and

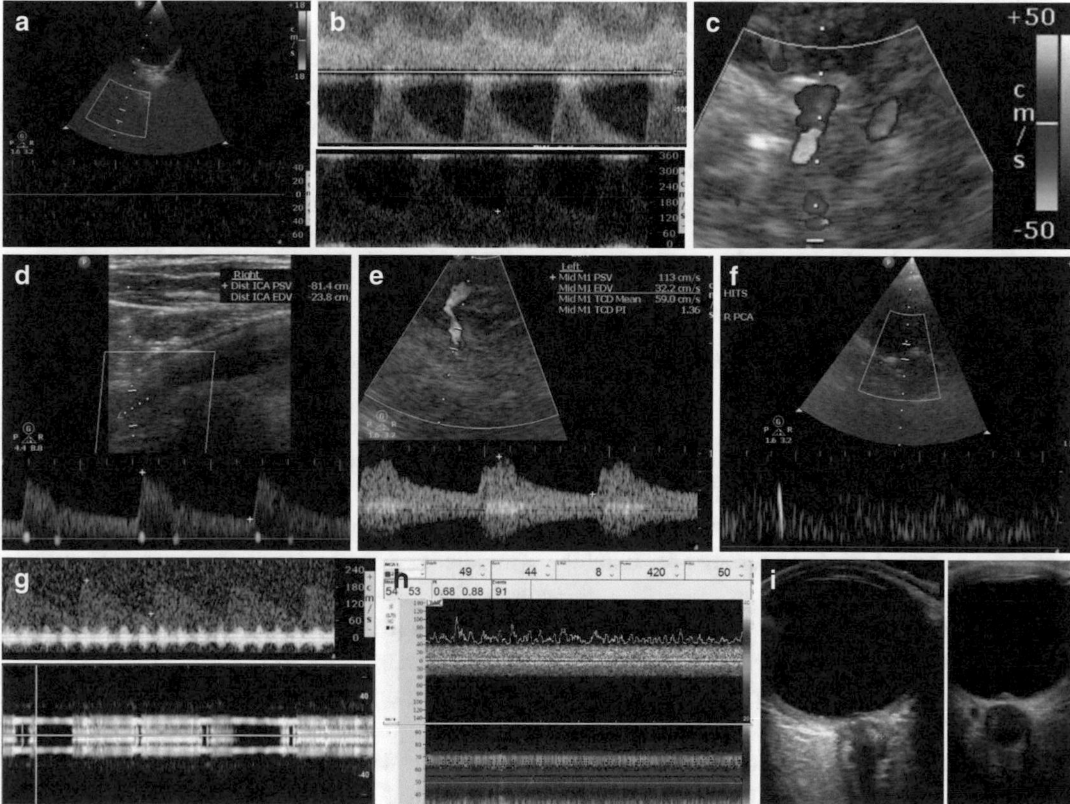

Fig. 5.1 Technical consideration in transcranial ultrasound and Doppler. (**a**) Lack of temporal windows. (**b**) Aliasing (upper panel) and correction to appropriate scale to remove it (lower panel). (**c**). Aliasing seen in color Doppler as colors from extremes of scale present within the vessel as yellow and aqua. (**d**). Systolic clicks vs. a systolic bruit (**e**) which is a sign of turbulence. (**f**) High-intensity thromboembolic signals (HITS). (**g**) Harmonic artifacts produced by high-frequency oscillator ventilation. (**h**) Power M-mode Doppler may help in insonating when using a non-imaging TCD. (**i**) Orbital ultrasound to measure optic nerve sheath diameter should focus on the optic nerve 3 mm behind the retina (left panel) but measurements should be done in axial section after obtaining "target" view as in right panel [1]

guide the placement of the pulse Doppler gate. Alternatively, a wide gate (10–15 mm) can be used to search for Doppler signals in anatomically expected locations on the B-mode image, and then adjusted to standard 5 mm once signals are localized [4]. Non-imaging TCD identifies the cerebral arteries "blindly" on the basis of spectral display, standard criteria of assessing arterial depth, arterial blood flow direction, and waveform analysis [1]. Identifying each segment of the vessel at successive depths is guided by hit-and-trial "angling and inching" method. Power motion (M) mode of Doppler may also be used to increase the efficiency of insonation by providing a visual array of signals from multi-depth insonation (Fig. 5.1h) when using this modality.

Suboccipital insonation on either modality can be difficult due to unfavorable bone windows, a tortuous course of vertebrobasilar system, or patient factors like cervical syndrome or obesity [5]. Orbital windows to assess optic nerve sheath can be challenging in patients with orbitofacial trauma. Careful technique or use of a hypoallergenic gel during eye insonation may help prevent complications related to corneal exposure.

5.2.2 Accuracy of Quantitative Measurements

Like most ultrasound modalities, quantitative measurements on cranial ultrasound, TCD, and TCCS need standardized and thorough insonation protocols and experienced operators for reliability [6].

Cranial ultrasound measurements for midline shift and ventricular size have shown reasonable accuracy in comparison to computed tomography (CT) and good inter-operator reliability in published studies [1, 7, 8]. Reproducibility for these quantitative measurements needs close attention to standardized protocol and experience. Studies have reported midline shift and ventricular width in different planes. For better accuracy when assessing midline shift, both sides of the brain may be measured in the same plane using the same temporal window, instead of insonating each side separately. However, harmonic imaging-related errors at deeper insonation in significantly wide skulls may limit this approach. Challenges in replicating standardized planes on ultrasound imaging and limitations of concordance with CT axial planes due to inherent angulation when insonating through the temporal bone window have limited the widespread use of this clinical application. Furthermore, focal lesions below the temporal level may not result in a shift measurable by ultrasound; hence absence of midline shift does not exclude intracranial pathology. Although ultrasound has not been able to replace head CT for volumetric measurement of intracranial lesions, midline shift, or ventricular size, serial studies in patients too unstable for transport to obtain a head CT may help inform trends that may be more useful than absolute values [1].

Optic nerve sheath diameter measurements using transorbital windows also face the challenge of reproducibility of the most representative axial section being insonated. Guiding insonation to create a "target" pattern for measurements may allow for reproducible measurements, thus improving the accuracy for predicting intracranial pressure (Fig. 5.1i) [9]. Inconsistent data on reproducibility, wide variance in normative values, and cutoffs for predicting raised intracranial pressure have limited the widespread translation of this modality in clinical practice [10, 11].

Multiple studies have reported high sensitivity and specificity of TCCS and TCD in the assessment of intracranial stenoses (sensitivity 94–100%, specificity 99–100%), occlusions (middle cerebral artery: sensitivity 93–100%, specificity 98–100%), and cross-flow through the anterior (sensitivity 98%, specificity 100%) and posterior (sensitivity 84%, specificity 94%) communicating arteries. The lack of complete sensitivity and specificity comes from the absence of physiological windows and the ability to get complete spectral Doppler shifts from some individuals [12]. High correlation coefficient values have been reported in all quantitative assessments of spectral Doppler waveforms, but the challenges of insonating a long segment of a vessel to correct the angle of insonation due to the inherent anatomy of circle of Willis make it prone to errors with change in technique. Many published guidelines hence recommend no correction for angle of insonation for intracranial circulation [4]. Care must still be taken in the identification of vessel segments and tracings, with repeated measures taken, if necessary, to ensure reproducibility, especially when pathological patterns are noted. Lack of vessel lumen visibility on intracranial imaging requires using a standard gate, recommended at 5 mm for most quantitative measurements. However, in low-flow states or when color signals cannot be appropriately identified, larger gates may be used for detecting the most appropriate segment to sample.

When estimating intracranial pressure (ICP) using TCDs, the available formulas tend to overestimate it due to autoregulatory effects and compartmentalization of pressures and its differential effect along the vessel length. Most predictive models for noninvasive ICP measurements are based on initial studies in traumatic brain injury and assume normal caliber of vessels; hence their applicability in focal compartmentalized intracranial pathologies like ischemic or hemorrhagic stroke or in pathologies involving vasospasm, as in subarachnoid hemorrhage, is unclear [1]. Accuracy and normative values for cerebral autoregulation testing using TCDs have been validated only for middle cerebral arteries. The use of mean flow velocities on TCD to predict vasospasm has high sensitivity but low specificity with dissociation between occurrence of sonographic vasospasm and delayed cerebral ischemia. Despite these limitations, TCD continues to be the only diagnostic modality available for routine noninvasive screening of patients at risk [13].

Epidemiological factors must also be considered in using normative values when assessing for pathology, though detailed data on population-based normative need to be investigated for each pathology [14, 15].

5.2.3 Ultrasound-Related Artifacts

Clinicians should make themselves aware of common ultrasound and Doppler artifacts like mirror image artifact, aliasing (Fig. 5.1b), vibration (Fig. 5.1d), and bruits (Fig. 5.1e) when using cranial ultrasound and spectral Doppler for transcranial insonation [16, 17]. While insonating cranial structures, tissue harmonic imaging (THI) is used to enhance the differentiation of brain parenchyma, but this may produce stripe/streak artifacts, especially in Doppler imaging [3, 16, 18–20]. This problem can be negated by using specific transcranial presets in portable machines, or ensuring that harmonic imaging is off when alternate presets are used for Doppler studies [3, 18, 21]. Intracranial coils in aneurysms may serve as powerful reflectors and produce twinkling artifacts in color Doppler mode, with visible color signals making a false-positive impression of flow within a coiled aneurysm. This can usually be confirmed by a no-flow spectrum on pulse Doppler [20].

Small echogenic structures on the lateral sides of the sector image may be enlarged, especially ventricular borders. This artifact should be considered when assessing for an unexpected pathological finding in any visualized echogenic structure. This artifact can also affect measurements of the width of the frontal or temporal horns of the lateral ventricles when assessing for hydrocephalus. A hyperechoic falx cerebri in the midline may rarely produce a mirror artifact in the color insonation of the circle of Willis.

Aliasing (Fig. 5.1b) during Doppler imaging must be addressed by decreasing the baseline or increasing the scale. This increases the pulse repetition frequency and hence the Nyquist limit to obviate the artifact. On color Doppler, aliasing may be visible as extremes of color scale adjacent to each other and can be distinguished from true reversal of flow by the fact that the color changes jump the baseline (Fig. 5.1c) [16].

When diagnosing embolic high-intensity thromboembolic signals (HITS), care must be taken to avoid artifacts produced by motion and voice that can cause highly audible signals in the spectral waveforms. Figure 5.1d, e, f illustrates systolic clicks compared to systolic bruits and HITS. Low-intensity and -amplitude systolic click produced by dynamic valves or hyperdynamic heartbeats marked by its periodicity to cardiac cycle can be distinguished from the high-intensity signals that represent embolizing particles to the intracranial circulation phenomena. Systolic bruits are distinguishable from click artifacts as well as HITS as signals lasting most of the cardiac systole and producing low-amplitude waveforms within the envelope of the spectral waveform of the vessel [22].

5.3 Anatomical Considerations

Anatomical variability of the circle of Willis should be recognized, especially while insonating vessels using pulse Doppler. Up to 50% of brains may show anomalies with 1/4th brains having some vessel hypoplasia. Fetal PCA may be present in 10% of the insonated brains [5, 23]. Additional variations in anatomy like anomalous origins, attenuated vessels, accessory vessels like persistent trigeminal artery, fenestrations, trifurcations, dissections, and vascular malformations may be present. Some of these may be recognized from the color spectrum in TCCS and the insonation using non-imaging TCD may not reveal the nature of variation.

The distal posterior cerebral artery (PCA) and basal vein of Rosenthal can sometimes create a mixed signal with an arterial and venous component (Fig. 5.2a) [24]. Identification of venous waveforms is key to differentiating between post-stenotic waveforms especially when insonating PCA in a region where it is not uncommon to insonate deep cerebral veins (Fig. 5.2b) [24]. A post-stenotic waveform of PCA may be mistaken for a venous waveform. Insonating multiple segments of the vessel and its anatomical relationship to diencephalon may help the distinction.

On suboccipital insonation, only a fraction (25–30%) of patients have codominant vertebral arteries; hence the majority show asymmetry in the color and Doppler flow signals of intracranial vertebral artery segments [5]. Flow reversal in the vertebral artery in the suboccipital window should be explored carefully, to ensure that ipsi-

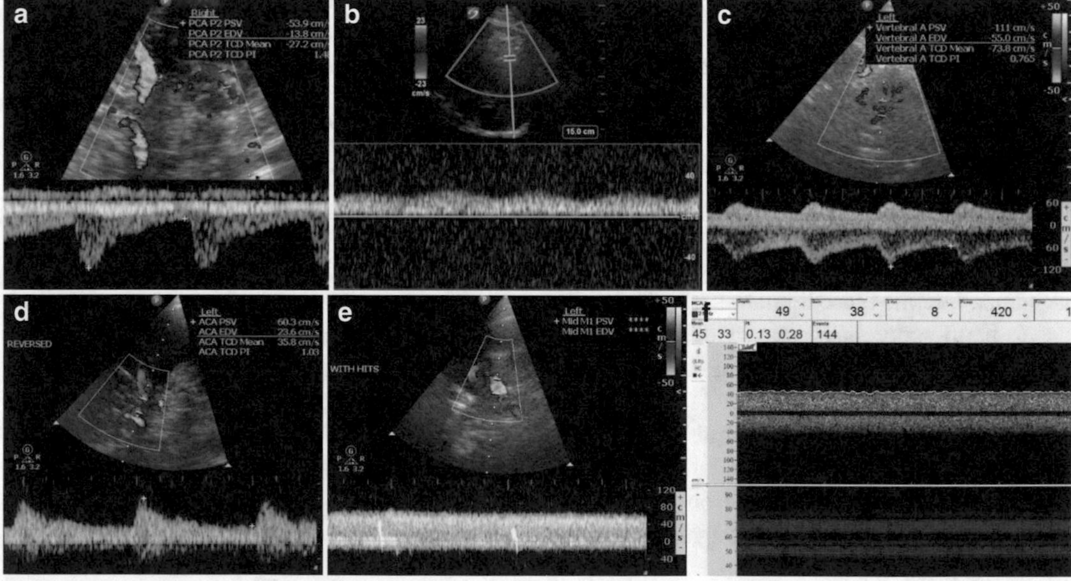

Fig. 5.2 Anatomical considerations in performing transcranial Doppler. (**a**) Identification of venous waveforms is key to differentiating between post-stenotic waveforms while insonating PCA where concomitant insonation of deep cerebral veins is possible. (**b**) Posterior circulation waveforms may commonly appear post-stenotic due to tight posterior cranial fossa and should be distinguished from venous waveforms. (**c**) Care must be taken if vertebral artery appears reversed that PICA is not the source of waveforms. In this figure both PICA at its origin and vertebral are being insonated. (**d**) Reversed ACA must be distinguished from proximal MCA especially when using non-imaging Doppler as it represents a pathological pattern of collateralization related to proximal ICA occlusion. (**e**) Nonpulsatile arterial waveforms in patient with VA-ECMO on imaging TCCS (**e**) and non-imaging TCD (**f**)

lateral posterior inferior cerebellar artery is not being mistaken for a reversed vertebral artery before a diagnosis of subclavian steal is made based on this finding. Bidirectional signals at the cerebellar vessel origin can help discern waveforms from each vessel (Fig. 5.2c) [5]. Similarly reversed ACA must be distinguished clearly from proximal MCA, especially when using standardized depths for vessel identification in non-imaging TCD, as this finding would represent a pathological pattern signifying collateralization from a proximal ICA occlusion (Fig. 5.2d) [25].

5.4 Clinical Considerations

5.4.1 Harmful Effects of Ultrasound Exposure

Though transcranial insonation for brain ultrasound and Doppler is a relatively safe examination, the ALARA (as low as reasonably achievable) principle should be followed when adjusting settings that affect acoustic output and ultrasound insonation times. TCD usually has high intensity to overcome the rapid attenuation of ultrasound by the skull and complete studies may take 30–60 min to insonate all windows and blood vessels [4]. The thermal effects of ultrasound can lead to significant heating of the skull bone and potentially secondary heating of brain tissue. For all prolonged or continuous studies, local heating effect should be closely monitored. For orbital windows, insonation should be performed at a lowest power with mechanical index (MI) set at <0.3 to avoid any risk of injury to the eye due to mechanical strain produced by the ultrasound waves [4].

5.4.2 Systemic Factors Related to Patients' Cardiopulmonary State

Cerebral blood flow velocities and pulsatility indices may be affected by patient factors like systemic blood pressure, carbon dioxide levels, body temperature, cardiac arrhythmias, anemia, or presence of significant cardiac disease. Systemic diseases like sepsis and renal and liver failure may also cause changes in cerebral waveforms due to alteration of cerebral hemodynamics [1]. These factors should be accounted for when reporting pathological findings, especially when present diffusely in spectral analysis of arterial waveforms. Presence of left ventricular assist devices or extracorporeal venoarterial circuits may produce a nonpulsatile waveform in Doppler (Fig. 5.2e,f).

5.4.3 Waveform Analysis in Acute Cerebrovascular Pathology

Cerebral hemodynamic waveform assessment should be done within the global context of findings in other segments of the same vessel as well as findings in other vessels. Interpretation of isolated finding in one vessel may lead to diagnostic errors. TCD insonation of a vessel should be thorough to include insonation along the vessel length to find the highest velocity. Limited sampling may cause the highest velocity segment to be missed in a vessel with vasospasm or tandem stenosis. Similar caution should be exercised in sampling pulse Doppler waveforms for duplex-guided insonation, especially where each segment can be visually identified and gated for measurements.

Hemodynamically significant focal stenosis will cause resistive waveforms proximal to the lesion and is usually followed by post-stenotic waveforms on more distal insonation (Fig. 5.3d, e). If the segment distal to suspected stenosis does show relatively normal waveforms rather than post-stenotic waveforms, then a tandem lesion should be suspected. Diffusely present post-stenotic waveforms across both anterior and posterior circulation should raise the suspicion of a proximal extracerebral pathology, like significant aortic stenosis causing a global parvus et tardus phenomenon [25, 26]. Similarly, diffusely elevated mean flow velocities with resistive waveforms may represent global pathology like cerebral edema causing increased distal resistance, multifocal vasospasm, or an autoregulatory

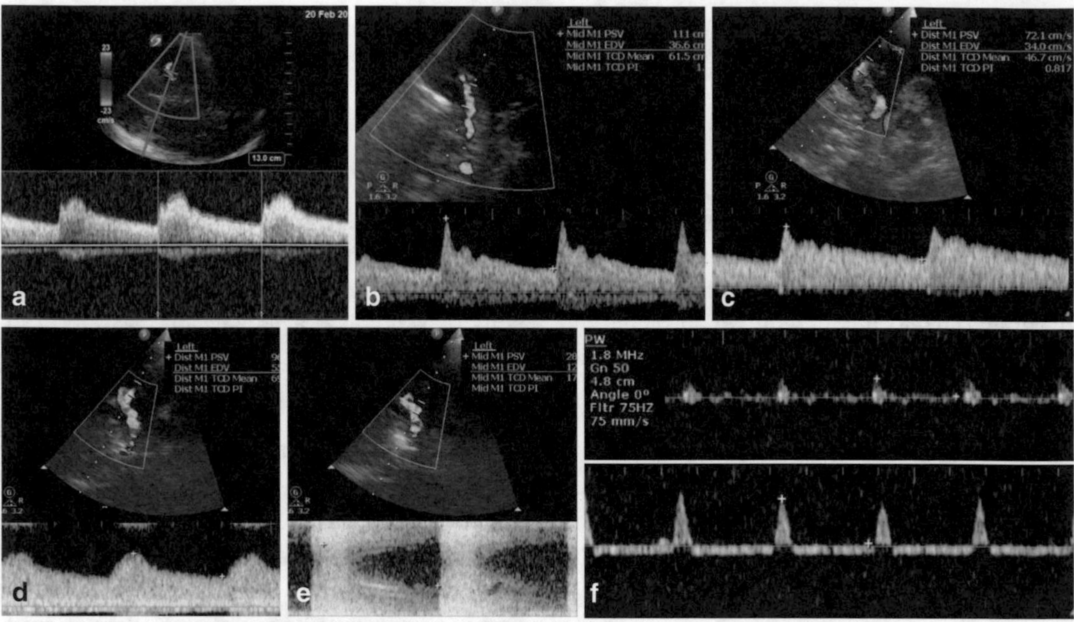

Fig. 5.3 Clinical considerations in transcranial ultrasound and Doppler. (**a**) Windkessel notch is produced by decreasing compliance in the brain and should be distinguished from post-stenotic waveforms. Left image shows the Windkessel notch preceded by a clear systolic upstroke and higher in amplitude compared to the systolic upstroke. Right image shows the waveform where systolic upstroke had the highest amplitude and all succeeding systolic notches are lower in a stepwise decelerating pattern characteristic of normal compliant brain. Abnormal Doppler waveforms can be produced by intracranial stenosis (**b**) and hyperemia (**c**) or from increased distal resistance. Intracranial stenosis will typically have post-stenotic segment (**d**) with resistive waveforms (**e**) insonated more proximally. (**f**) Diagnosis of cerebral circulatory arrest requires demonstration of irreversible waveforms which may manifest as systolic spikes (upper panel) or oscillatory waveforms (lower panel)

response to systemic hypertension. Extracranial internal carotid insonation can allow the assessment for systemic hypertension by calculating the Lindegaard ratio. When elevated velocities are present in an isolated vessel, a differential diagnosis of focal vasospasm, mild stenosis, as well as hyperemia exists. Distinguishing between these pathologies may require a more thorough evaluation of the whole vessel and correlation with findings in other vessels [26]. Hyperemic vessels may have higher diastolic velocities and lower PIs, though collateralization-related hyperemia in autoregulating vessels may only manifest with elevated mean velocities (Fig. 5.3c).

Noncompliant brain affected by intracranial pathology may show the Windkessel notch effect (Fig. 5.3a) compared to the stepwise deceleration seen in compliant brains (Fig. 5.3b). This should be distinguished from post-stenotic waveforms (Fig. 5.3d) [27]. Posterior circulation vessels, specifically PCA and the basilar artery, may show post-stenotic waveforms throughout their course in older patients with distal intracranial atherosclerosis or in younger patients with tight posterior cranial fossa [5]. These can be distinguished from pathological states for their being present throughout the length of PCA bilaterally and basilar course without proximal resistive changes.

High pulsatility index typically represents increased distal resistance but is not specific enough to differentiate between increased resistance produced by a rise in intracranial pressure, intracranial atherosclerosis, or advanced age [25].

5.4.4 Cerebral Circulatory Arrest

A special mention is being made in familiarizing with pitfalls of using TCD or TCCS in brain death evaluation. Transcranial Doppler or TCCS is an accurate test to assess for cerebral circulatory arrest with some caveats. A meta-analysis of 12 studies revealed a pooled sensitivity and specificity of 0.90 (95% CI, 0.87–0.92) and 0.98 (95% CI, 0.96–0.99), respectively, in supporting the diagnosis of cerebral circulatory arrest. The area under the curve with the corresponding standard error (SE) was 0.964 ± 0.018, while index Q test ±SE was estimated at 0.910 ± 0.028 [28].

Presence of temporal windows must be demonstrated prior to using transcranial Doppler or duplex imaging for confirming cerebral circulatory arrest. Complete absence of blood flow on Doppler studies cannot be used as sufficient evidence for ancillary testing since a proportion of physiologically normal patients may have no temporal windows. Transcranial Doppler evaluates cerebral circulatory arrest rather than brainstem function; hence it should not replace the clinical evaluation of brainstem reflexes and apnea test. All anterior and posterior circulation vessels on both sides should be insonated. Extracranial circulation (internal carotid insonation in the neck) should demonstrate physiological forward flow bilaterally. When present across all intracranial vessels in anterior and posterior circulation, oscillatory patterns with equivalent forward and backward flow components or systolic spikes <50 m/s and <200 ms over two studies at least 30 min apart are consistent with cerebral circulatory arrest [29]. Care must be taken to distinguish these systolic spikes from systolic click artifacts (Fig. 5.1d). Attempts must be made to achieve insonation of low flow patterns by reducing pulse repetition frequency, deactivating filters, enlarging Doppler sampling gates (10–15 mm), and increasing Doppler power and gain when feasible [29].

5.5 Summary

Cranial ultrasound, transcranial Doppler, and color-coded duplex imaging are useful noninvasive tools for rapid assessment of acute brain pathologies and cerebrovascular hemodynamics. Appropriate training, experience, and competencies in image acquisition, waveform interpretations, and familiarity with clinical context can help reduce the pitfalls associated with this promising tool.

References

1. Robba C, Goffi A, Geeraerts T, et al. Brain ultrasonography: methodology, basic and advanced principles and clinical applications. A narrative review. Intensive Care Med. 2019;45:913–27.
2. Krejza J, Swiat M, Pawlak MA, et al. Suitability of temporal bone acoustic window: conventional TCD versus transcranial color-coded duplex sonography. J Neuroimaging. 2007;17:311–4.
3. Vignon F, Shi WT, Yin X, Hoelscher T, Powers JE. The stripe artifact in transcranial ultrasound imaging. J Ultrasound Med. 2010;29:1779–86.
4. Alexandrov AV, Sloan MA, Wong LK, et al. Practice standards for transcranial Doppler ultrasound: part I—test performance. J Neuroimaging. 2007;17:11–8.
5. Kaps M, Seidel G, Bauer T, Behrmann B. Imaging of the intracranial vertebrobasilar system using color-coded ultrasound. Stroke. 1992;23:1577–82.
6. Robba C, Poole D, Citerio G, Taccone FS, Rasulo FA. Brain ultrasonography consensus on skill recommendations and competence levels within the critical care setting. Neurocrit Care. 2019;32:502.
7. Motuel J, Biette I, Srairi M, et al. Assessment of brain midline shift using sonography in neurosurgical ICU patients. Crit Care. 2014;18:676.
8. Robba C, Cardim D, Sekhon M, Budohoski K, Czosnyka M. Transcranial Doppler: a stethoscope for the brain-neurocritical care use. J Neurosci Res. 2018;96:720–30.
9. Robba C, Cardim D, Tajsic T, et al. Non-invasive intracranial pressure assessment in brain injured patients using ultrasound-based methods. Acta Neurochir Suppl. 2018;126:69–73.
10. Lochner P, Czosnyka M, Naldi A, et al. Optic nerve sheath diameter: present and future perspectives for neurologists and critical care physicians. Neurol Sci. 2019;40:2447.
11. Robba C, Santori G, Czosnyka M, et al. Optic nerve sheath diameter measured sonographically as non-invasive estimator of intracranial pressure: a systematic review and meta-analysis. Intensive Care Med. 2018;44:1284–94.
12. Baumgartner RW. Transcranial color duplex sonography in cerebrovascular disease: a systematic review. Cerebrovasc Dis. 2003;16:4–13.
13. Kumar G, Alexandrov AV. Vasospasm surveillance with transcranial Doppler sonography in subarachnoid hemorrhage. J Ultrasound Med. 2015;34:1345–50.
14. Bavarsad Shahripour R, Mortazavi MM, Barlinn K, et al. Can STOP trial velocity criteria be applied to Iranian children with sickle cell disease? J Stroke. 2014;16:97–101.

15. Tegeler CH, Crutchfield K, Katsnelson M, et al. Transcranial Doppler velocities in a large, healthy population. J Neuroimaging. 2013;23:466–72.
16. Rubens DJ, Bhatt S, Nedelka S, Cullinan J. Doppler artifacts and pitfalls. Radiol Clin N Am. 2006;44:805–35.
17. Ratanakorn D, Kremkau FW, Myers LG, Meads DB, Tegeler CH. Mirror-image artifact can affect transcranial Doppler interpretation. J Neuroimaging. 1998;8:175–7.
18. Puls I, Berg D, Maurer M, Schliesser M, Hetzel G, Becker G. Transcranial sonography of the brain parenchyma: comparison of B-mode imaging and tissue harmonic imaging. Ultrasound Med Biol. 2000;26:189–94.
19. Srinivasan V, Smith M, Bonomo J. Bedside cranial ultrasonography in patients with hemicraniectomies: a novel window into pathology. Neurocrit Care. 2019;31:432–3.
20. Khan HG, Gailloud P, Martin JB, et al. Twinkling artifact on intracerebral color Doppler sonography. AJNR Am J Neuroradiol. 1999;20:246–7.
21. Maciak A, Kier C, Seidel G, Meyer-Wiethe K, Hofmann UG. Detecting stripe artifacts in ultrasound images. J Digit Imaging. 2009;22:548–57.
22. Guepie BK, Sciolla B, Millioz F, Almar M, Delachartre P. Discrimination between emboli and artifacts for outpatient transcranial Doppler ultrasound data. Med Biol Eng Comput. 2017;55:1787–97.
23. Iqbal S. A comprehensive study of the anatomical variations of the circle of Willis in adult human brains. J Clin Diagn Res. 2013;7:2423–7.
24. Schreiber SJ, Stolz E, Valdueza JM. Transcranial ultrasonography of cerebral veins and sinuses. Eur J Ultrasound. 2002;16:59–72.
25. Alexandrov AV, Sloan MA, Tegeler CH, et al. Practice standards for transcranial Doppler (TCD) ultrasound. Part II. Clinical indications and expected outcomes. J Neuroimaging. 2012;22:215–24.
26. Alexandrov AV. Extra- and intracranial waveform analysis algorithm, descriptions, classifications, and differential diagnosis. J Vasc Ultrasound. 2015;39:192–202.
27. Aggarwal S, Brooks DM, Kang Y, Linden PK, Patzer JF II. Noninvasive monitoring of cerebral perfusion pressure in patients with acute liver failure using transcranial doppler ultrasonography. Liver Transpl. 2008;14:1048–57.
28. Chang JJ, Tsivgoulis G, Katsanos AH, Malkoff MD, Alexandrov AV. Diagnostic accuracy of transcranial Doppler for brain death confirmation: systematic review and meta-analysis. AJNR Am J Neuroradiol. 2016;37:408–14.
29. Ducrocq X, Hassler W, Moritake K, et al. Consensus opinion on diagnosis of cerebral circulatory arrest using Doppler-sonography: task force group on cerebral death of the Neurosonology Research Group of the World Federation of Neurology. J Neurol Sci. 1998;159:145–50.

6 The Minimal, Intermediate, and Advanced Skills: How to Boost Your Competencies

Frank A. Rasulo and Nicola Zugni

Contents

6.1 Introduction

As for most techniques dealing with complicated and sophisticated technology, the path should lead through a training process in order to first apprehend the technique itself, and second to apply it correctly. Hence, when medical instruments are involved, this advice becomes paramount.

The neo-sonographer should take advantage of the numerous certified theoretical and hands-on courses available which are organized by many societies, managed by expert teachers within this field [1].

Although BUS is a relatively simple technique, in order to apply it correctly a great deal of knowledge regarding cerebral anatomy and parameters is required, also necessary in order to perform sophisticated diagnostic tests which will ultimately lead to clinical decision-making. Consequently, the apprehension of BUS and its application become quicker and more efficient when learned from an expert neuro-sonologist. As demonstrated by Klinzing et al. in their study published in 2015 [2], despite being associated with a steep and favorable learning curve, ultrasound identification of the middle cerebral

F. A. Rasulo (✉)
Anesthesiology and Intensive Care, Division of Anesthesiology, Intensive Care & Emergency Medicine, University of Brescia at Spedali Civili Hospital, Brescia, Italy

Residency Program and School in Anesthesiology and Intensive Care, University of Brescia at Spedali Civili Hospital, Brescia, Italy

Neuroanesthesia and Neuro Critical Care section of the SIAARTI Society, Rome, Italy

N. Zugni
Department of Anesthesia, Critical Care and Emergency, Spedali Civili University Hospital, Piazzale Ospedali Civili, Brescia, Italy

C. Robba, G. Citerio (eds.), *Echography and Doppler of the Brain*,
https://doi.org/10.1007/978-3-030-48202-2_6

artery by inexperienced operators after a short theoretical-practical course presented a faster and steeper curve if the operators were supervised by expert tutors.

Few monitoring systems are accompanied by high levels of evidence associated with significant clinical improvements when these tools are adopted into practice. The latest recommendations of the American Society of Echocardiography describe how to perform a complete echocardiographic examination in adult patients and identify accreditation guidelines for advanced echocardiography [3]. For transcranial Doppler (TCD), the lack of unified guidelines has led to the creation of performance standards for conducting TCD examinations, based on available evidence, clinical expertise, and consensus.

It is necessary to define two methods based on the technology involved: TCD (Doppler) and TCCD (B-mode and echo-color functions).

6.2 TCD and TCCD

The term brain ultrasound comprises all types of methods which utilize ultrasonography, including Doppler based. Therefore, ultrasound machines may consist mainly of two types:

- TCD, which evaluates the blood flow velocities within the main cerebral vessels by using the Doppler principle (Fig. 6.1)
- Transcranial color-coded duplex Doppler sonography (TCCD), which combines B-mode (color Doppler imaging, brain parenchyma, and bone) (Fig. 6.2)

The probes differ based on the method utilized. It is suggested that the neo-sonographer becomes familiar with both types of ultrasound methods, since the reliability of some of the diagnostic test may vary based on the technique applied [4, 5].

TCCD has multiple advantages compared to TCD [6]:

- Reliability in recognizing the blood flow of each individual cerebral artery
- More accurate identification of vascular pathology
- Correction of the angle of insonation with consequent greater accuracy in measuring flow velocity
- Evaluation and study of the cerebral parenchyma, vessels, and bone structure

TCCD is accompanied by the same limits as traditional TCD ultrasound, such as the need of a good acoustic window and operator dependence.

These limits, and others, give emphasis to the importance of defining the training necessary for the acquisition of specific skills in order to progress from being an inexperienced operator to an expert in brain ultrasound.

Clinical applications of TCCD include [7–12]:

- Diagnosis of cerebral pathologies: intracranial hemorrhages, hydrocephalus, cerebral edema, etc. (Fig. 6.3)
- Evaluations of the flow velocity waveform: diagnosis of cerebral circulation arrest, estimation of intracranial pressure, performance of self-regulation tests, and diagnosis of vasospasm (Fig. 6.4)

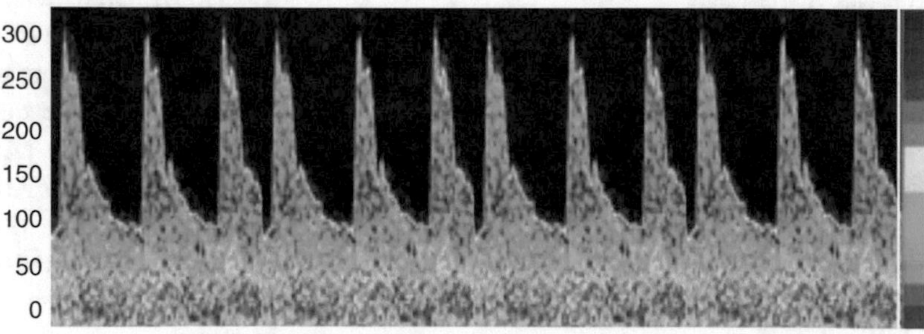

Fig. 6.1 Transcranial Doppler (blood flow velocities)

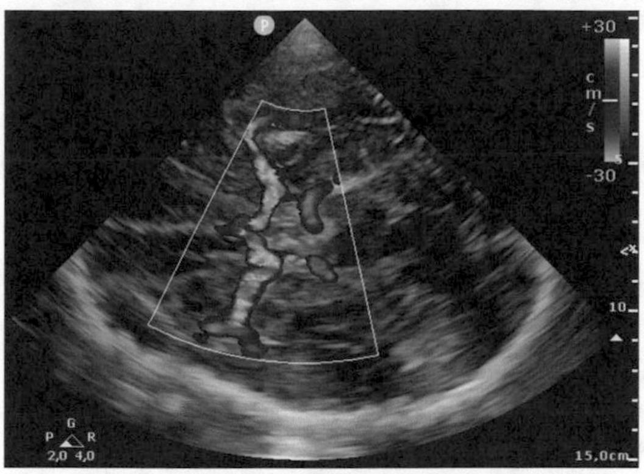

Fig. 6.2 Transcranial color-coded duplex Doppler sonography (circle of Willis)

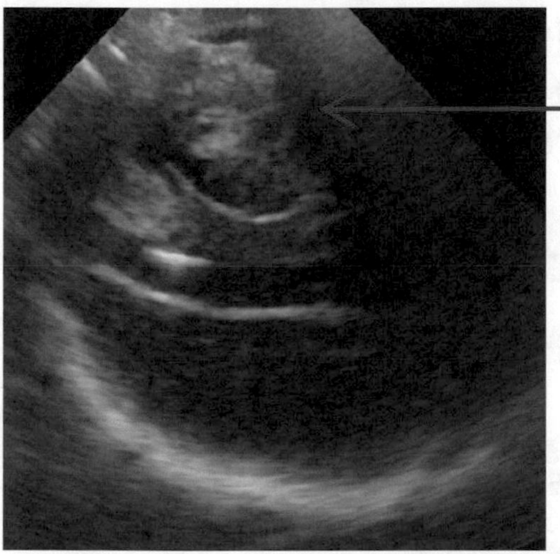

Fig. 6.3 Intracranial hemorrhages (arrow)

6.3 Training Strategies

A recent consensus on cerebral ultrasonography sought to evaluate the experts' opinion regarding the identification of the skills necessary to master to pass from the basic level to the advanced level [13]. They present a staircase approach where the first step represents the basic level from which the neo-sonologist would start training. From there on, in order to pass to the next levels of competence, it is essential to complete the skills of each single previous level.

From the BUS consensus three skill levels were identified based on the experts' responses: minimal, intermediate, and advanced (Fig. 6.5).

It is advisable that the neo-sonographer be familiar with the basic knowledge of brain anatomy, ultrasound technology, and benchmark insonation parameters, followed by the ability to insonate the basic and most easily accessible vessels and anatomical structures (Table 6.1).

It is more difficult, and the exam is less reliable, if the sonographer were to bypass the structures necessary to identify in order to insonate the target vessel.

A few examples:

- When using the temporal acoustic window and the probe is positioned, if the contralateral bone is not visible in B-mode, then it would be unlikely that other structures or vessels be located since the skull bone is hyperintense.

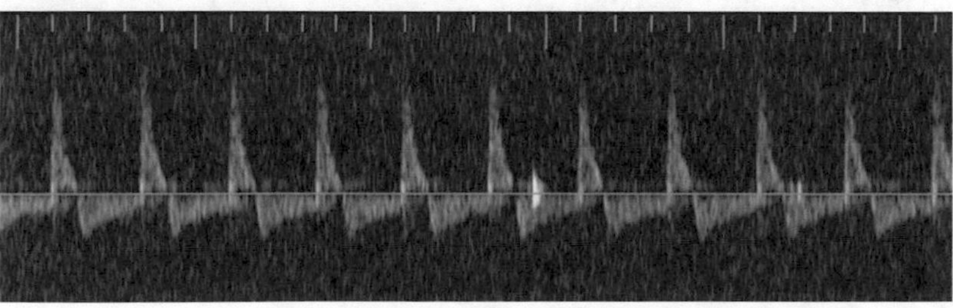

Fig. 6.4 Cerebral circulation arrest (reverberant flow)

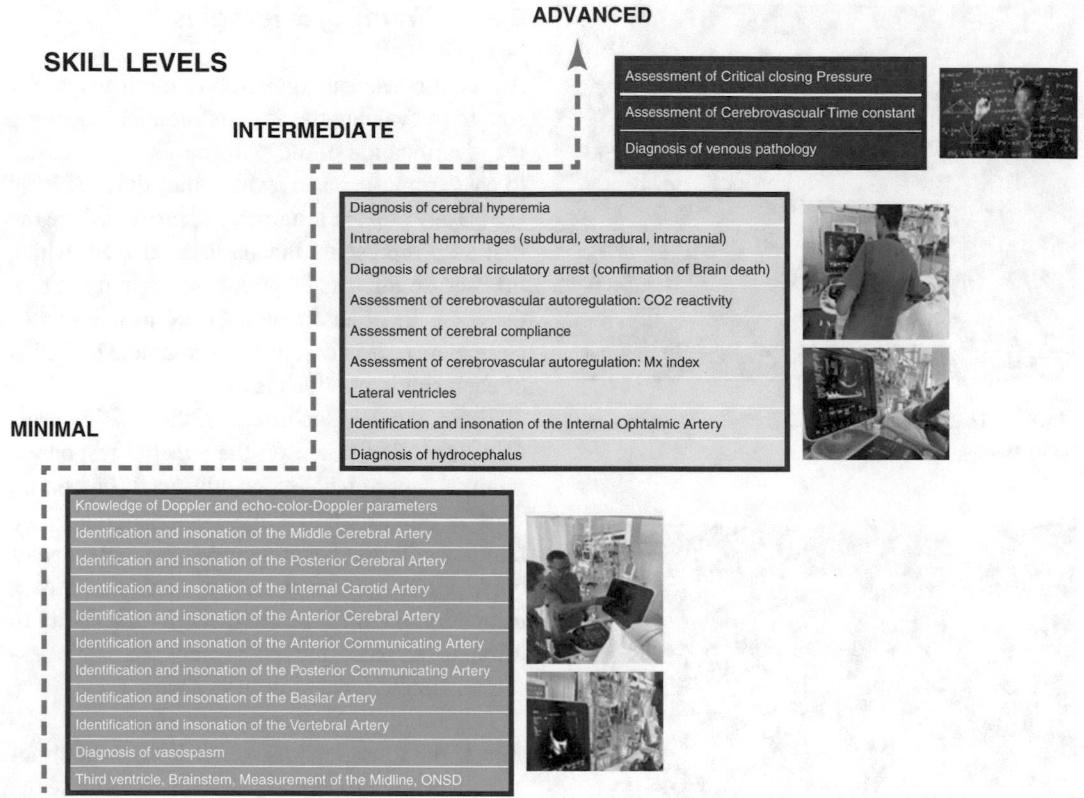

ADVANCED
SKILL LEVELS
INTERMEDIATE
MINIMAL
Assessment of Critical closing Pressure
Assessment of Cerebrovascualr Time constant
Diagnosis of venous pathology
Diagnosis of cerebral hyperemia
Intracerebral hemorrhages (subdural, extradural, intracranial)
Diagnosis of cerebral circulatory arrest (confirmation of Brain death)
Assessment of cerebrovascular autoregulation: CO2 reactivity
Assessment of cerebral compliance
Assessment of cerebrovascular autoregulation: Mx index
Lateral ventricles
Identification and insonation of the Internal Ophtalmic Artery
Diagnosis of hydrocephalus
Knowledge of Doppler and echo-color-Doppler parameters
Identification and insonation of the Middle Cerebral Artery
Identification and insonation of the Posterior Cerebral Artery
Identification and insonation of the Internal Carotid Artery
Identification and insonation of the Anterior Cerebral Artery
Identification and insonation of the Anterior Communicating Artery
Identification and insonation of the Posterior Communicating Artery
Identification and insonation of the Basilar Artery
Identification and insonation of the Vertebral Artery
Diagnosis of vasospasm
Third ventricle, Brainstem, Measurement of the Midline, ONSD

Fig. 6.5 Skill levels for gaining competency in performing BUS

- Without the contralateral bone landmark, it would be impossible to calculate the midline shift.
- By first visualizing the brain peduncles in B-mode it is much easier to locate the cerebral posterior artery (P1 and P2), since this later passes directly on top of the brain stem.
- By locating the sphenoidal wings and petrous arc the middle and anterior cerebral arteries, as for other vessels of the Willis circle, can be identified.

The presence of a tutor during this first phase is preferable in order to guide the student and teach the tips and tricks of performing a correct and efficient BUS exam: for example, correct head position of the patient, finding the anatomical landmarks, correct hand position when holding the probe, correct choice of probe based on the type of exam required, learning the basic machine settings, and safety tips. These and other valuable recommendations when performing BUS are best taught in the presence of a tutor who would correct any faults in executing the exam or simply answer questions regarding the technique itself.

During this level all the skills gained in performing the exam will be put to use in using BUS as a clinical diagnostic tool. Again, although the sonographer is no longer a neophyte, the presence of a tutor, or at least the possibility to contact the tutor when required, is suggested. In this level, along with disease diagnosis through direct visualization of abnormal flow velocities and anatomical structures, the sonographer should be capable of performing certain diagnostic tests and calculations which can aid in the diagnosis but also in therapeutic decision-making. The experts in the consensus previously mentioned stratified within this level certain monitoring parameters and calculations which utilize ultrasound, such as cerebral autoregulation testing, which can be extemporaneous or continuous, while remaining not excessively complicated to execute (Table 6.2).

Table 6.1 Minimal skills

Minimal skill		
Identification and insonation of arteries	Identification and insonation of the middle cerebral artery and anterior cerebral artery	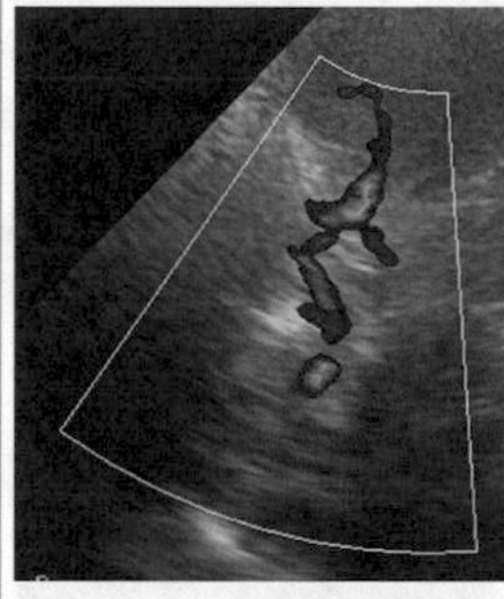
	Identification and insonation of the internal carotid artery	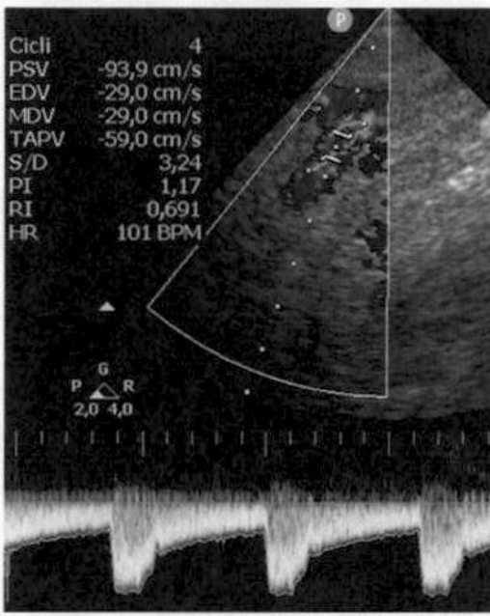
	Identification and insonation of the posterior cerebral artery (P1 in red, P2 in blue)	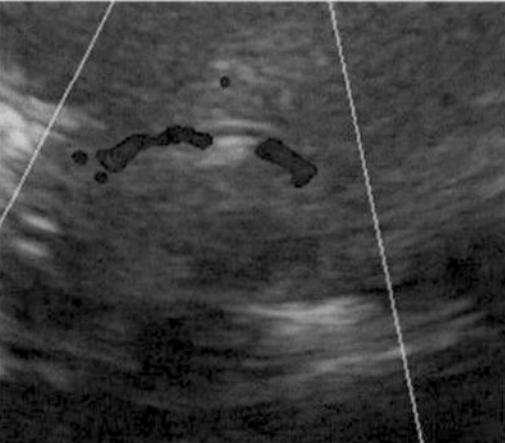
	Identification and insonation of the basilar artery (red line)	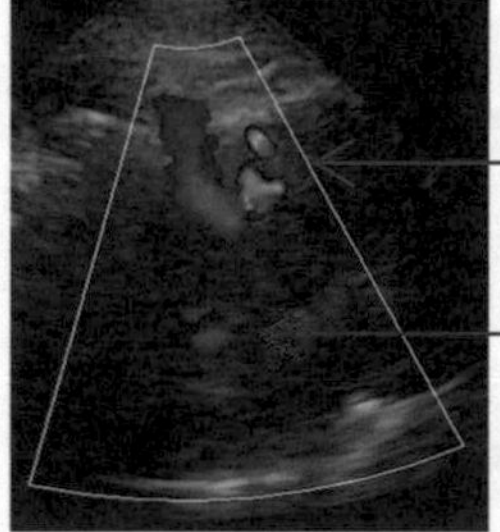
	Identification and insonation of the vertebral artery (blue line)	

(continued)

Table 6.1 (contiued)

Minimal skill		
Identification of other anatomical structures	Optic nerve sheath diameter	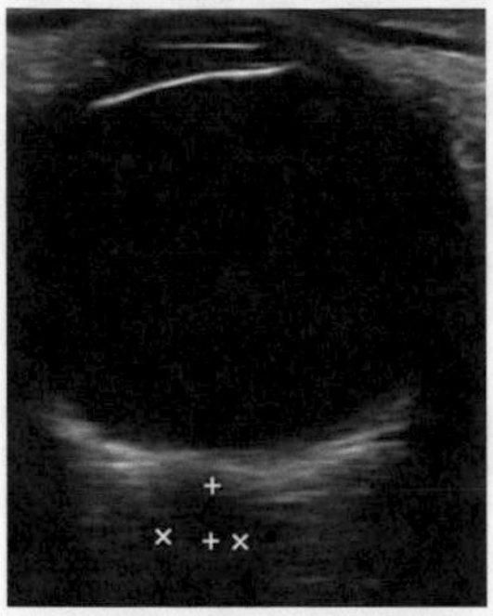
	Third ventricle (blue line)	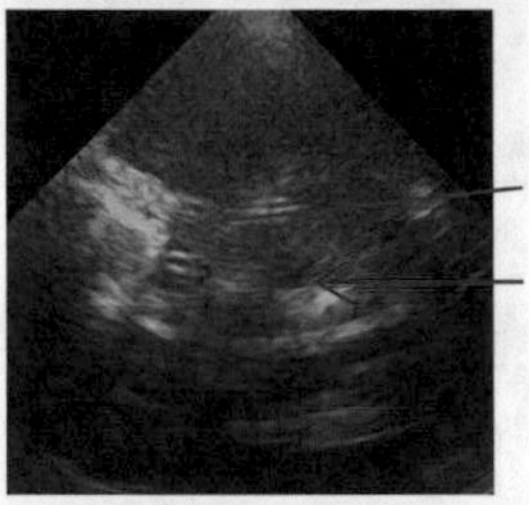
	Brainstem (red line)	
	Measurement of the midline shift	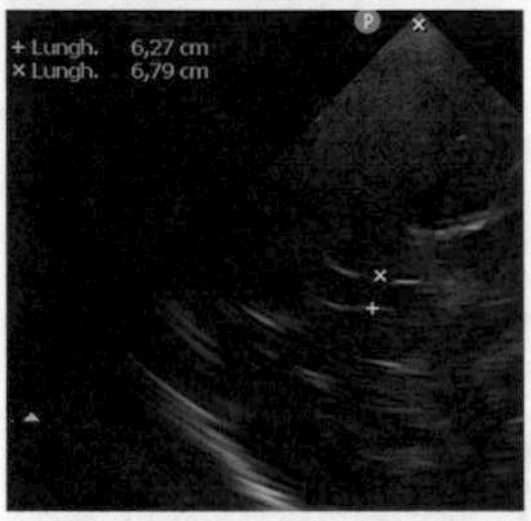
	Contralateral temporal skull bone	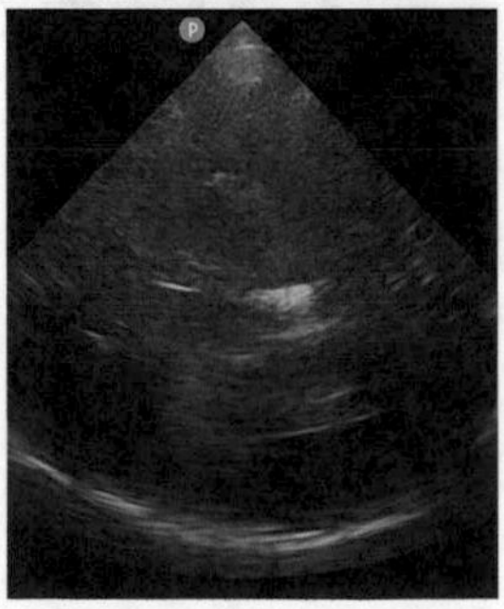

Table 6.1 (contiuned)

Minimal skill			
Diagnosis of brain pathologies	Diagnosis of vasospasm Lindegaard Index (L.I.)	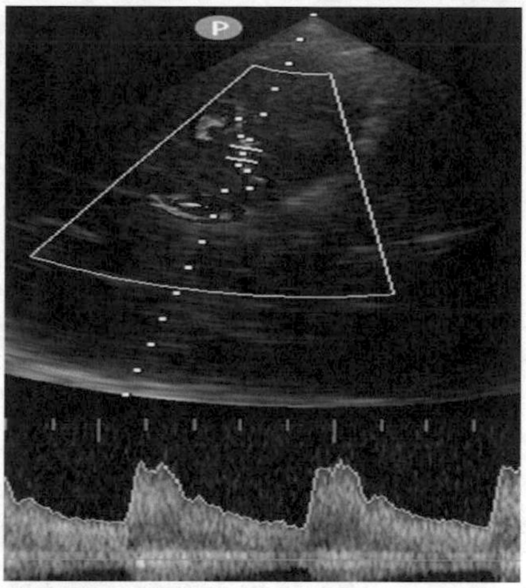	$\text{L.I.} = \dfrac{\text{FVm MCA}}{\text{FVm ICA}}$

Table 6.2 Intermediate skill

Intermediate skill		
Identification and insonation of arteries	Identification and insonation of the internal ophthalmic artery	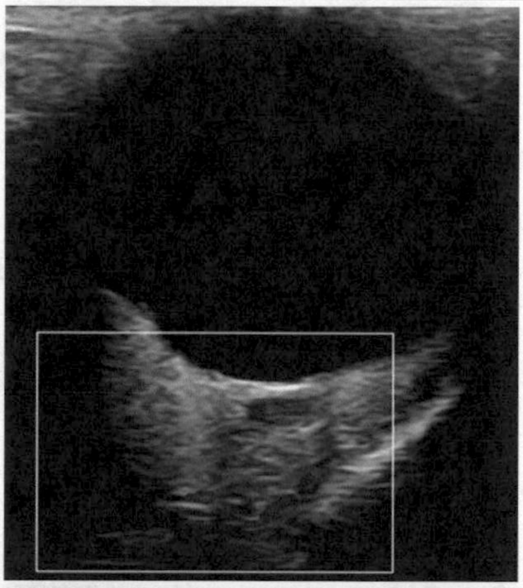
Identification of other anatomical structures	Lateral ventricles	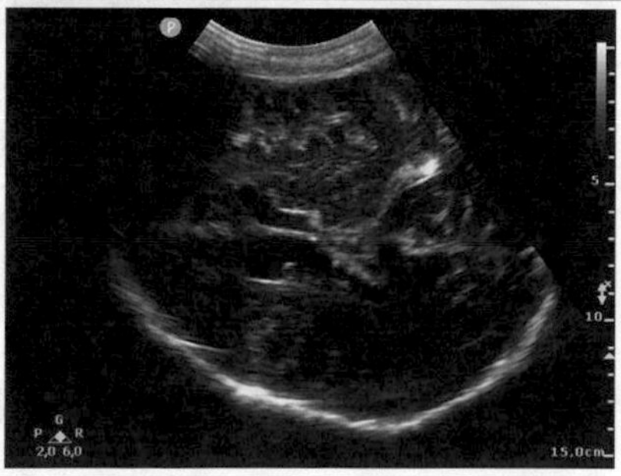

(continued)

Table 6.2 (continued)

Intermediate skill			
Diagnosis of brain pathologies	Diagnosis of cerebral hyperemia and Lindegaard Index (L.I.)	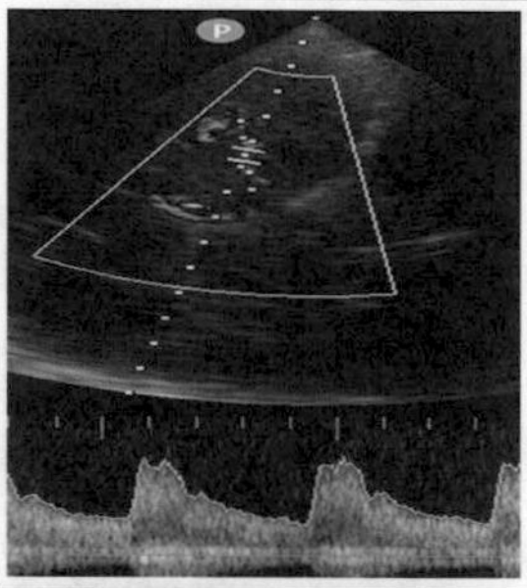	$\text{L.I.} = \frac{\text{FVm MCA}}{\text{FVm ICA}}$
	Intracerebral hemorrhages (sub, extradural hemorrhage, intracranial hemorrhage) (red line)	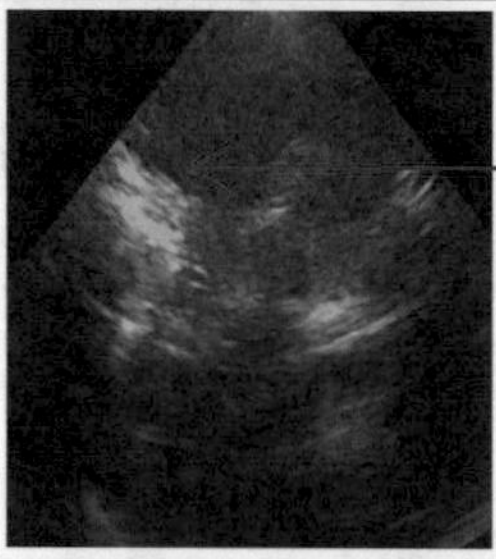	
	Diagnosis of cerebral circulatory arrest for the confirmation of brain death	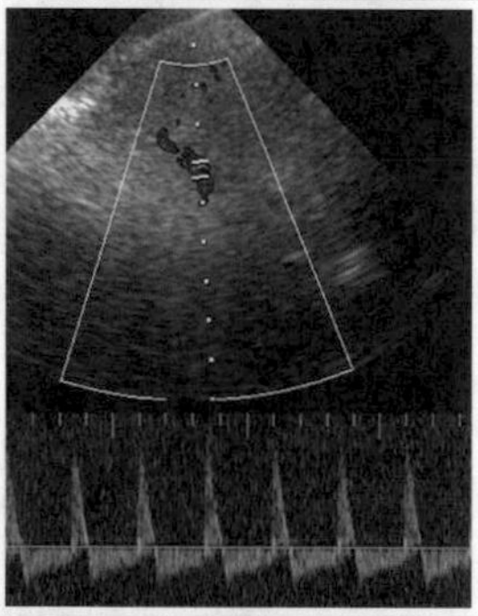	
	Assessment of cerebrovascular autoregulation: CO2 reactivity	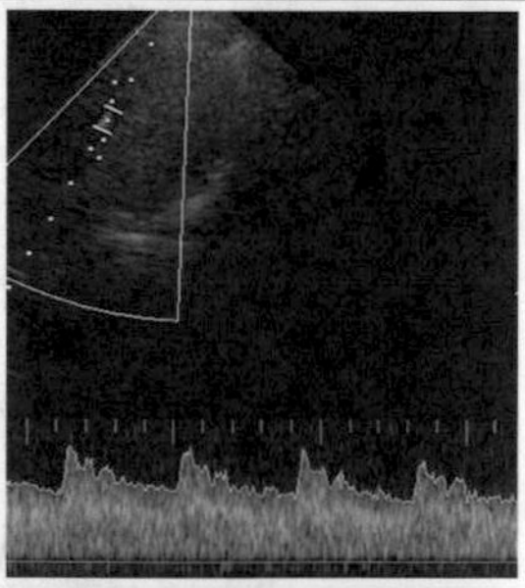	Absolute CO_2 reactivity = ΔCBFV/$\Delta PaCO_2$
	Diagnosis of hydrocephalus Third ventricle (red line)	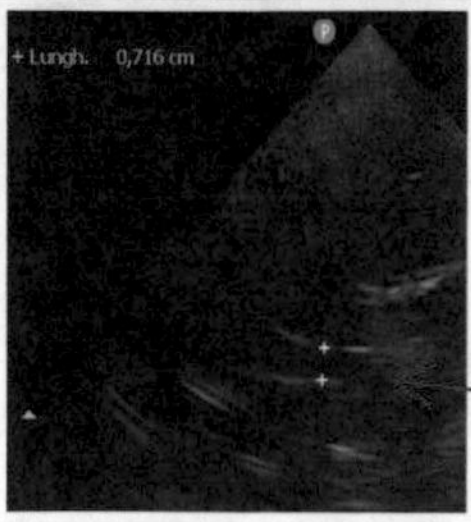	

ΔCBFV change in CBFV in cm/s per mmHg, *ΔPaCO2* change in PaCO2 tension

Table 6.3 Advanced skill

Advanced skill			
Diagnosis of brain pathologies	Assessment of critical closing pressure	$\mathrm{CrCP} = \mathrm{ABP} \cdot \left[1 - \frac{1}{\sqrt{\left(\mathrm{CVR} \cdot \mathrm{Ca} \cdot \mathrm{HR} \cdot 2\pi\right)^2 + 1}} \right]$	Critical closing pressure is the arterial blood pressure threshold, below which small arterial vessels collapse and cerebral blow flow ceases
	Assessment of cerebrovascular time constant (τ)	$\tau = C_a \bullet \mathrm{CVR}$	The cerebrovascular time constant represents the product of compliance of cerebral arterial bed and the vascular resistance distal to the place of insonation
	Diagnosis of venous pathology (straight sinus)		

τ cerebral arterial time constant (seconds), C_a cerebral arterial compliance, *CVR* cerebrovascular resistance, *CrCP* critical closing pressure, *ABP* arterial blood pressure, *HR* heart rate

$$\mathrm{CrCP} = \mathrm{ABP} \cdot \left[1 - \frac{1}{\sqrt{\left(\mathrm{CVR} \cdot \mathrm{Ca} \cdot \mathrm{HR} \cdot 2\pi\right)^2 + 1}} \right]$$

In the advanced level the expert sonographer is capable of performing the most difficult tests and monitoring techniques which use BUS, such as evaluation of cerebral compliance, cerebrovascular time constant, and venous insonation. At this point the sonographer is experienced enough to act as a tutor and teach BUS to other students (Table 6.3).

6.4 Learning Through Technological Aid

We are at present living in an era of technological simulation, not only in medicine but also in sports, military, commercial pilot training, and so on. In medicine, simulators are being used for surgical procedures, anesthesia (difficult intubation for example), CPR, and obstetrics. Ultrasound teaching may also be guided through the use of simulators [14] for example:

- Simulators
- Automatic signal retriever
- Smartphone probes and software
- Integration with other monitoring systems or imaging devices (EEG, intraoperative MRI, MMM)
- Improvements in signal quality (3D imaging)

6.5 Learning Through Guidelines and Practice Standards

Practice parameters and technical standards are not inflexible rules or requirements of practice and are not intended to be used in order to establish a legal standard of care.

It should be recognized that adherence to practice parameters will not assure an accurate diagnosis or a successful outcome. All that should be expected is that the practitioner will follow a reasonable course of action based on current knowledge, available resources, and consensus. The sole purpose of practice parameters is to assist practitioners in achieving an improvement in outcome.

Factors such as qualification, responsibilities of the physician, and written request for the examination may differ between countries, cities, and even hospitals within the same city itself. A fair example of variation in guidelines is present for the use of BUS for the diagnosis of cerebral circulatory arrest. In a recent paper [15] the authors highlight the great deal of variability which exists among centers and countries regarding brain death (BD) determination and state. Although consensus guidance is available to standardize national processes for the diagnosis of BD, the current variation and inconsistency in European practice make it imperative that an international consensus is developed.

Regarding BUS, many societies have created task forces in an attempt to unify guidelines and practice standards. The *American Academy of Neurology* (*AAN*), for example, published the 2004 Guidelines for the use of TCD and provide the indications, sensitivity, specificity, and reference standards for the most common pathologies evaluated by TCD [16]. However, this document has been retired by the Guideline Development, Dissemination, and Implementation Subcommittee on February 23, 2018, due to no updates or reaffirmation in 5 years or less after the previous publication. Hence, the recommendations and conclusions in all retired guidelines are considered no longer valid and no longer supported by the *AAN*.

More recently, the *American Society of Neurophysiologic Monitoring* (*ASNM*) and *American Society of Neuroimaging* (*ASN*) Guidelines Committees formed a joint task force and developed guidelines to assist in the use of transcranial Doppler (TCD) monitoring in the surgical and intensive care settings [17].

Specifically, these guidelines delineate the objectives of TCD monitoring, characterize the responsibilities and behaviors of the sonographer during monitoring, and describe methodological and ethical issues uniquely relevant to monitoring. They stress that in order to perform a quality examination, the acquisition and interpretation of intraoperative TCD ultrasonograms be performed by qualified individuals, and that the service providers define their diagnostic criteria and develop ongoing self-validation programs of these performance criteria in their practice.

In 2010, a multidisciplinary panel of experts reviewed the published literature on TCD from 1982 through December 2009. Given the emphasis on accreditation of vascular laboratories [18] they emphasize a need for standardization of scanning and interpretation processes and initiated the development of a series of standards and guidelines by experts in transcranial Doppler and members of the *American Society of Neuroimaging Practice Guidelines Committee* as well as international neuro-sonological organizations.

Despite the increasing use of brain ultrasound, this technique still remains underused. An example is presented for one of TCD's most common indications in the intensive care unit, aneurysmal subarachnoid hemorrhage (aSAH) for surveillance of cerebral vasospasm (CV) [19]. The authors in this study performed an analysis of nationwide trends in TCD prevalence by using Nationwide Inpatient Sample (NIS) data from 2002 to 2011. Teaching hospitals were examined separately for TCD utilization rates. The objective was to estimate the proportion of patients with aSAH receiving TCD monitoring using the NIS. In teaching hospitals, 2% of the aSAH patients (95% CI 1.0–4.0) underwent TCD examination. TCD utilization increased from <1% during the 2002–2005 period to ≥1.5% during the 2006–2011 period (odds ratio 2.3, 95% CI 1.0–5.7), an increase also seen in nonteaching hospitals. They concluded that TCD is underused nationally in the care of aSAH and that the prevalence of TCD is nearly nonexistent in nonteaching hospitals.

The *Intersocietal Commission on Accreditation of Vascular Laboratories* (ICAVL) [18] has established guidelines for the certification of laboratories making or interpreting diagnostic ultrasonic measurements of cerebral blood flow velocity (CBFV) with transcranial Doppler (TCD) ultrasonography. However, of the more than 950 ICAVL-approved facilities, less than 2% are certified for intracranial or TCD measurements.

Numerous training programs pertaining to various scientific societies are available and technological advances in both hardware and software are making it much easier to obtain the necessary competence. These include simulators, certification courses, and user-friendly ultrasound machines.

6.6 Competence

Competence for transcranial color-coded duplex sonography is rapidly acquired [2].

A broad spectrum of usage scenarios has been proposed for transcranial Doppler sonography (TCD) in the intensive care setting (ICU) as a method to assess intracerebral hemodynamics, including detection of vasospasm in subarachnoid hemorrhage, arterial steno-occlusive disease, estimation of intracranial pressure, and determination of brain death.

As a bedside, easy-to-access, and noninvasive method, TCD is an attractive tool.

In one study, untrained as compared to trained TCD operators estimated blood flow velocity with wide variation, impairing the clinical usefulness of TCD when performed by untrained operators. In contrast, no similar studies have been performed in TCCD [20].

It has been shown that TCCD applied to measure the mean flow velocity (MFA) in the MCA is an easy-to-learn tool yielding accurate and reliable measurements in volunteers even in the hands of untrained operators. Competence for transcranial color-coded duplex sonography is rapidly acquired [2]. Overall, there was a good agreement between measurements of untrained and trained operators. A short-term learning program including an introduction session followed by either five supervised and five non-supervised examinations (supervised group) or ten non-supervised examinations (non-supervised group) was assessed. The supervised program yielded a more rapid and accurate learning curve due to active supervision in addition to the effect of repetitive measurements.

Neulen et al. [21] in a recently published study examined the aspect of "image guidance," where acquired image data were combined with a TCD system allowing anatomic orientation. Experienced operators were asked to identify cerebral vessels by conventional TCD while inexperienced operators were challenged with the same task supported by "image guidance." While TCD performed by experienced operators was determined with a mislabeling rate of 37%, image guidance reduced the mislabeling rate to 10%. Anatomic orientation and visual guidance facilitate the correct identification of the vessel of interest. Especially in the setting of inexperienced operators, this advantage may facilitate the performance of reliable measurements and may very well explain the favorable learning curve of TCCD we found in the present study.

References

1. https://www.asnweb.or/i4a/pages/index.cfm?pageID=4028&acriveFuII=true
2. Klinzing S, Steiger P, Schüpbach RA, et al. Competence for transcranial color-coded duplex sonography is rapidly acquired. Minerva Anestesiol. 2015;81(3):298–304.
3. Echocardiography. Accreditation in adult critical care echocardiography. https://www.bsecho.org/media/161652/cc_accreditation_pack_2015.pdf.
4. Bartels E. Transcranial color-coded duplex ultrasound possibilities and limits of this method in comparison with conventional transcranial Doppler ultrasound. Ultraschall Med. 1993;14:272–8.
5. Schoning M, Buchholz R, Walter J. Comparative study of transcranial color duplex sonography and transcranial Doppler sonography in adults. J Neurosurg. 1993;78:776–84.
6. Rasulo F, et al. Visualizing impending cerebral circulatory arrest caused by intracranial hypertension following aneurysmal subarachnoid hemorrhage. J Neurosurg Anesthesiol. 2017;29(1):64–6.
7. Becker G, Bogdahn U, Strassburg HM, et al. Identification of ventricular enlargement and estimation of intracranial pressure by transcranial color-coded real-time sonography. J Neuroimaging. 1994;4:17–22.
8. Seidel G, Gerriets T, Kaps M, Missler U. Dislocation of the third ventricle due to space-occupying stroke evaluated by transcranial duplex sonography. J Neuroimaging. 1996;6:227–30.
9. Cardim D, Robba C, Bohdanowicz M, et al. Non-invasive monitoring of intracranial pressure using transcranial Doppler ultrasonography: is it possible? Neurocrit Care. 2016;25:473–91.
10. Robba C, Santori G, Czosnyka M, et al. Optic nerve sheath diameter measured sonographically as non-invasive estimator of intracranial pressure: a systematic review and meta-analysis. Intensive Care Med. 2018;44:1284–94.
11. Robba C, Cardim D, Tajsic T, et al. Ultrasound non-invasive measurement of intracranial pressure in neurointensive care: a prospective observational study. PLoS Med. 2017;14:e1002356. https://doi.org/10.1371/journal.pmed.1002356.
12. Rasulo FA, Bertuetti R, Robba C, et al. The accuracy of transcranial Doppler in excluding intracranial hypertension following acute brain injury: a multicenter prospective pilot study. Crit Care. 2017;21(1):44.
13. Robba C, Poole D, Citerio G, et al. Brain ultrasonography consensus on skill recommendation and competence levels within the critical care setting. Neurocrit Care. 2019;32:502.
14. Parks AR, Atkinson, Verheul G. Can medical learners achieve point-of-care ultrasound competency using a high-fidelity ultrasound simulator? A pilot study. Crit Ultrasound J. 2013;5:9.
15. Robba C, Iaquaniello C, Cierio G. Death by neurologic criteria: pathophysiology, definition, diagnostic criteria and tests. Minerva Anestesiol. 2019;85(7):774–8.
16. Sloan MA, Alexandrov AV, Teheler CH, et al. Assessment: transcranial Doppler ultrasonography: report of the Therapeutics and Technology Assessment Subcommittee of the American Academy of Neurology. Neurology. 2004;62(9):1468–81.
17. Edmonds HL, Isley MR, Sloan TB, et al. American Society of Neurophysiologic Monitoring and American Society of Neuroimaging joint guidelines for transcranial Doppler ultrasonic monitoring. J Neuroimaging. 2011;21(2):177–83.
18. http://www.icavl.org
19. Kumar G, Albright KC, Donnelly, et al. Trends in transcranial Doppler monitoring in aneurysmal subarachnoid hemorrhage: a 10-year analysis of the nationwide inpatient sample. J Stroke Cerebrovasc Dis. 2017;26(4):851–7.
20. McMahon CJ, McDermott P, Horsfall D, Selvarajah JR, King AT, Vail A. The reproducibility of transcranial Doppler middle cerebral artery velocity measurements: implications for clinical practice. Br J Neurosurg. 2007;21:21–7.
21. Neulen A, Greke C, Prokesch E, et al. Image guidance to improve reliability and data integrity of transcranial Doppler sonography. Clin Neurol Neurosurg. 2013;115(8):1382–8.

Part II

Basic and Advanced Parameters

7 Flow Velocity, Pulsatility Index, Autoregulation, and Critical Closing Pressure

Marta Fedriga and Marek Czosnyka

Contents

7.1 Introduction

Transcranial Doppler (TCD) has been named the 'stethoscope for the brain'. Apart from cerebral blood flow velocity and its waveform, secondary indices and derived formulae can be detected. These measurements might have several useful clinical applications which have been studied during the last decades demonstrating that brain ultrasonography has a strong potential as a safe, non-invasive repeatable device in acute brain-injured patients. However, the strength of this non-invasive technique might become even stronger when other more invasive assessments of brain haemodynamic are contraindicated, such as in hepatic failure or during infectious disease. Moreover, it can be a useful in the intraoperative and perioperative setting. Even though brain ultrasound over the years has been considered an essential part of the clinical assessment and management of patients we cannot deny that it has limitations such as the necessity of patent transcranial acoustic windows and operator dependency. TCD and transcranial colour-coded Doppler (TCCD) have been considered relatively simple methods; however specific

M. Fedriga
Brain Physics Laboratory, Division of Neurosurgery, Department of Clinical Neurosciences, University of Cambridge, Cambridge, UK

Department of Anesthesia, Critical care and Emergency, Spedali Civili University Hospital, Brescia, Italy

M. Czosnyka (✉)
Brain Physics Laboratory, Division of Neurosurgery, Department of Clinical Neurosciences, University of Cambridge, Cambridge, UK
e-mail: mc141@medschl.cam.ac.uk

C. Robba, G. Citerio (eds.), *Echography and Doppler of the Brain*,
https://doi.org/10.1007/978-3-030-48202-2_7

skills are required not only to recognise different landmarks and brain's anatomical features but first and foremost to interpret properly the number given by the machine. In addiction with transcranial Doppler, we should remember not to be stuck on a single measurement: what is more important indeed is to track the trend of measurements in the patient clinical pathway taking all the indexes and derived calculations together in order to draft a complete physiopathological picture of the patient we are studying and treating.

7.2 Flow Velocity

The velocity of red blood cells flowing through the large vessels of the brain can be detected via TCD and TCCD ultrasonography. The Doppler principle was first described by Christian Doppler in 1843 as the frequency shift, the measured difference in frequencies between the original signal (sent by the ultrasound machine), and the reflected signal. The Doppler frequency shift is directed proportionally to the flow velocity of red blood cells and is usually expressed in centimetres per second.

Flow velocity (FV) can be used as a surrogate descriptor of cerebral blood flow (CBF); it permits dynamic, non-invasive monitoring with good temporal and spatial resolution. However, we must be aware of the two main assumptions that govern the use of TCD: the constant diameter of the insonated vessel and an unchanged angle of insonation [1, 2].

The velocity measured by the probe is described by the following formula:

$$\text{measured velocity} = \text{real velocity} \times \text{cosine of angle of incidence}\left(\cos\theta\right).$$

Therefore, when the angle is 0°, the cosine is 1 and the measured velocity is equal to the real velocity. At 90°, cosine is 0, and it is not possible to detect the flow velocity. As a consequence, the detection of real velocity is limited by anatomical constraints that derive from the position and the course of the vessels with respect to the probe.

To counter this, the use of the newer, more advanced TCCD enables operators to visualise the insonated artery and modify the angle of insonation for more accurate estimation of blood velocity. However, as long as the angle of insonation remains constant, changes in the detected velocity reflect changes in the true velocity and therefore changes in cerebral blood flow.

Another crucial factor that affects the interpretation of TCD velocity is the cross-sectional area of the insonated vessel since the volume which passes through a vessel depends on both the velocity of red cells and the diameter of the vessel. The diameter of the vessel should, therefore, remain stable during the measurement if the operator wants to detect a true velocity.

The range of normal flow velocity values for adults was first determined by Aaslid et al. [2] in 1982, and was verified during direct intraoperative Doppler measurements [3]. These values have thus been adopted as the standard values used by other authors during the last decades; see Table 7.1.

Table 7.1 The table represents the normal range of values of the main brain arteries considering the mean flow velocity as determined by Aaslid et al. [2]

ARTERY	Mean velocity (cm/s)
MCA M1	46–86
ACA A1	41–76
PCA P1	33–64
EICA	37
TICA	60
OPHTHALMIC artery	20
CAROTID SIPHON	55
VERTEBRAL artery	27–55
BASILAR artery	30–57

MCA middle cerebral artery, *ACA* anterior communicating artery, *PCA* posterior communicating artery, *EICA* extracranial internal carotid artery, *TICA* terminal internal carotid artery

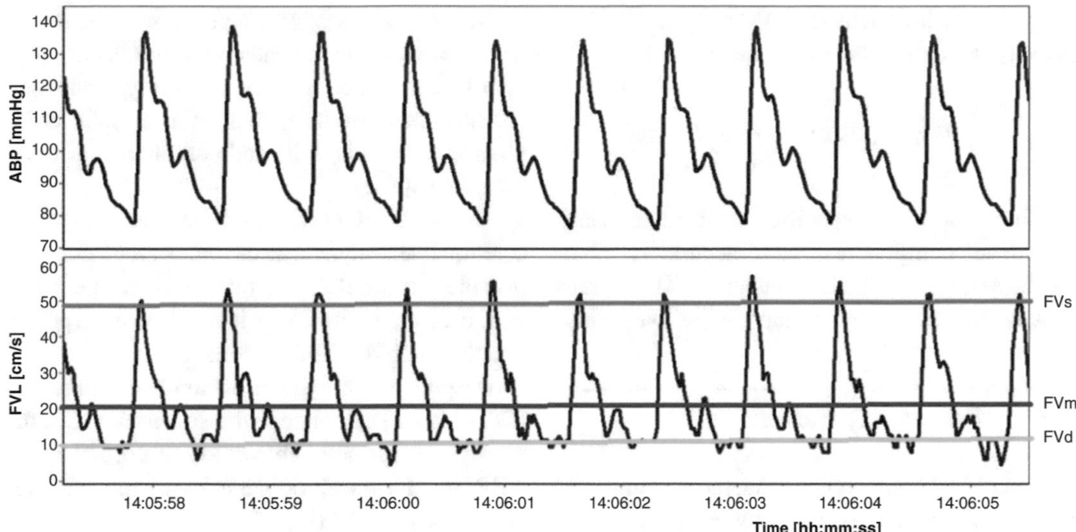

Fig. 7.1 TCD waveform is similar to the waveform of blood pressure. Landmark values are flow velocity systolic (FVs), diastolic (FVd) and mean (FVm), as indicated on a graph

Several authors have suggested that flow velocities vary between individuals, and demonstrate a "moment-to-moment" variability within the same individual in both healthy and brain-injured subjects; this consensus underscores the importance of continuous measurements rather than focusing on single values [4].

In addition, normal values are influenced not only by vessel diameter and angle of insonation, but also by the collateral flow, haematocrit, partial pressure of arterial carbon dioxide ($PaCO_2$), arterial blood pressure (ABP), intracranial pressure (ICP) and cerebrocascular resistance (CVR). Flow velocity is higher during haemodilution [5], a fact that could lead to misinterpretation of vessel stenosis and must be taken into account, particularly when evaluating subarachnoid-related vasospasm.

Flow velocity increases usually around 2.5–3% for every mm Hg increase in $PaCO_2$ [6].

Demographic factors that could affect flow velocity include age, sex, pregnancy, and arousal state. At birth, the flow velocity of the middle cerebral artery is approximately 24 cm/s, increasing to 100 cm/s by the age of 4–6 years. Thereafter, it decreases steadily to about 40 cm/s in the seventh decade of life. Women generally have a higher FV than men, although the difference is usually small (10–15%). During normal pregnancy, FV is maintained for the first two trimesters but decreases during the third. FV also drops by approximately 15% during sleep [7, 8].

Signal processing of the Doppler frequency shift with fast Fourier transform returns a TCD waveform with three components: systolic flow velocity of CBF (FVs), mean flow velocity of CBF (FVm), and diastolic flow velocity of CBF (FVd); see Fig. 7.1.

Systolic flow velocity is first and foremost dependent on systemic haemodynamics, more so on cardiac output rather than cerebral haemodynamics [9].

The clinical interpretation of diastolic flow velocity is still debated in critical care; diastolic velocity might be considered an index of cerebral hypoperfusion due to the fact that a decrease in cerebral perfusion pressure (CPP) attributed to an increase in intracranial pressure (ICP) is reflected as a decrease in diastolic flow velocity. When ICP increases to a very high value, diastolic cerebral blood flow approaches zero. With a continued rise in ICP, diastolic blood flow reappears, but it is in the opposite direction (reversed flow), which is presented as retrograde flow by TCD [10–12].

The mean flow velocity best correlates with CBF [13, 14] and is primarily used to assess cerebral arterial flow. Many TCD devices calculate FVm using systolic flow velocity (FVs) and diastolic flow velocity (FVd) with the traditional formula:

$$FVm = (FVs + 2 * FVd)/3.$$

This assumes a specific linear relationship among all components. More accurately, FVm can be assessed as the time integral of the current flow velocities divided by the integration period.

7.3 Pulsatility Index

Information about cerebral haemodynamic can be derived from the TCD waveform; the most commonly used cerebral haemodynamic parameter is that derived from Gosling's pulsatility index (gPI) which describes the pulsatility of the TCD waveform; it is calculated as (FVsystolic-FVdiastolic) divided by the FV mean. The benefit of measuring PI is that it is not affected by the angle of insonation. However, the utility of PI for the assessment of cerebrovascular resistance, non-invasive ICP, and non-invasive CPP has yielded controversial conclusions about its reliability and accuracy [15].

Normal values of PI range from 0.5 to 1 [2]; however, its value depends on a significant number of factors such as ABP pulsatility, heart rate, CPP, haematocrit, body temperature, CVR, compliance of vessels, ICP, and compliance of cerebrospinal space.

Although PI corresponds to the change in cerebral haemodynamic, the index alone does not provide meaningful information about the cause of the change; therefore it must be interpreted together with the clinical context.

Despite not being an accurate estimator of ICP, PI is still calculated when assessing ICP; for example, a PI value above 2 with normal mean ABP in a normocapnic patient may indicate elevated ICP [16–18] (Fig. 7.2).

PI can identify cerebral haemodynamic asymmetry and indicate low CPP, but it cannot be used as a reliable descriptor of cerebrovascular resistance [19].

7.4 Critical Closing Pressure

The first theoretical model demonstrating that small vessels collapse below a 'critical value' was developed by Burton in 1951 [20]. This pressure

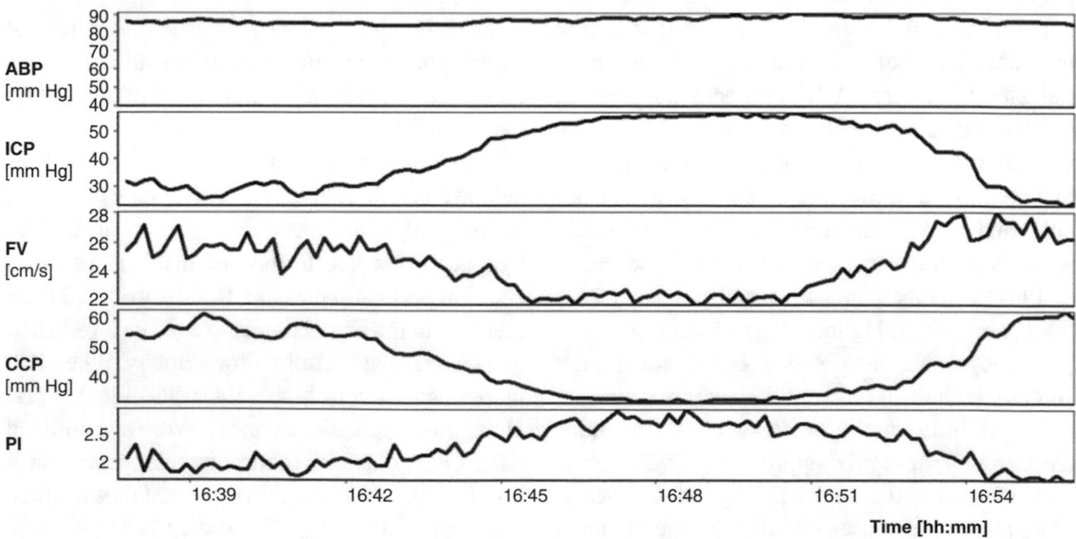

Fig. 7.2 Pulsatility index is a variable describing the shape of TCD pulse waveform. It increases when cerebral perfusion pressure (CPP) decreases. Changes in PI are observed during plateau wave of ICP, where both flow velocity (FV) and CPP decrease

value was named critical closing pressure (CrCP) and represents a lower threshold of ABP below which the CBF approaches zero. Vasomotor tone or wall tension and ICP are the major determinants of CrCP. CrCP can be described indeed as the sum of two closing forces: ICP and vascular wall tension (WT), which represents the active cerebral vasomotor tone [21]:

$$\mathrm{CrCP} = \mathrm{ICP} + \mathrm{WT}\left(\mathrm{mm\,Hg}\right).$$

The difference between the 'opening' force ABP and 'closing' force is the force that keeps vessels open and has been denoted the 'closing margin'. If this 'closing margin' is reduced to zero, vessels will collapse causing a cessation of cerebral blood flow [22].

Based on this relationship, patients at risk of developing intracranial hypertension could be identified by non-invasive estimation of CrCP (or estimation of WT from invasive ICP measurement) to derive information about vascular tone [23].

With TCD/TCCD, we can assess blood flow velocity non-invasively and compare its pulsatile waveform with the pulsatile waveform of ABP. CrCP can be then estimated as the intercept point of a regression line between arterial pressure plotted along the x-axis and the corresponding values of blood flow velocity plotted along the y-axis (see Fig. 7.3).

The intercept is the value of ABP at which the CBF (estimated through the blood flow velocity) is equal to zero [22, 24].

The most popular method for CrCP estimation uses the fundamental harmonics of the pulse waveforms of ABP and flow velocity (FV), decomposed in the frequency domain [25, 26]:

$$\mathrm{CrCP} = \mathrm{ABP} - \mathrm{AMP}_{\mathrm{ABP}} * \mathrm{FV} / \mathrm{AMP}_{\mathrm{FV}}\left(\mathrm{mm\,Hg}\right).$$

where ABP and FV are the mean values of the respective signals, while AMP denotes the amplitude of the fundamental harmonics of ABP and FV. This current method is limited by the possibility of obtaining negative values of CrCP which cannot be interpreted physiologically.

Another pressure threshold has been derived from CrCP and diastolic ABP (ABPd) which is the diastolic closing margin of the brain microvasculature (DCM = ABPd-CrCP) [27].

DCM might represent an index that provides information about the 'pressure reserve' available in order to avoid the cessation of CBF during the diastolic portion of the cardiac cycle.

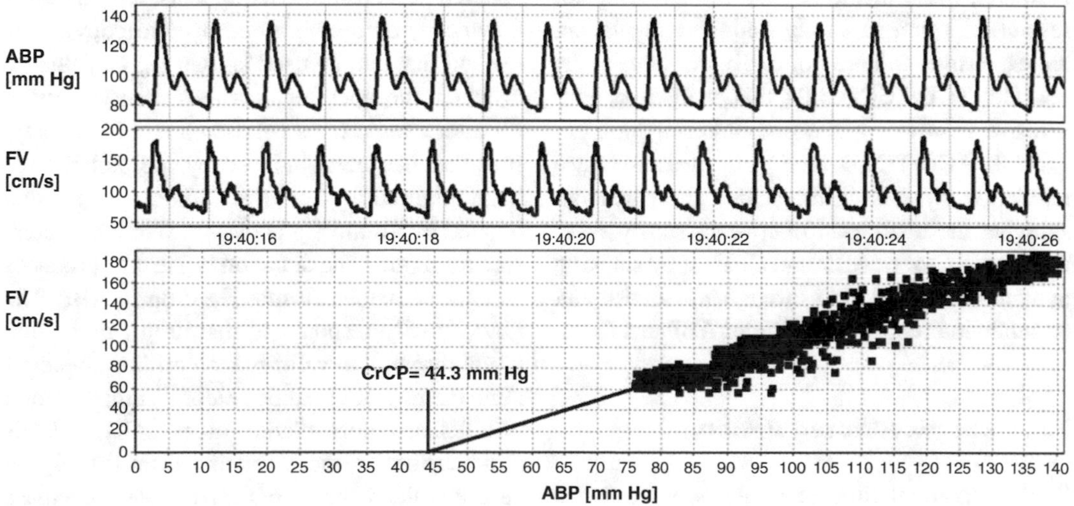

Fig. 7.3 CrCP calculated as regression between ABP and FV waveforms averaged from several heartbeats. Before regression ABP waveform is shifted backward in time (blood pressure is delayed compared to FV, as it is measured from a radial artery)

7.5 Autoregulation

Cerebral autoregulation reflects the ability of the brain to maintain a relatively constant level of cerebral blood flow (CBF) despite changes in cerebral perfusion pressure. It is an intrinsic neuroprotective mechanism which physiological bases are still not clearly understood. It was first observed by Mogens Fog in 1938 who demonstrated an inverse relationship between the rise in ABP and the diameter of pial arteries in cats [28]. The usefulness of the 'autoregulation concept' and its clinical implications have been studied for several years; during the last few years, researchers have surmised that autoregulation is not only an elegant mechanism but indeed can bring about remarkable clinical implications. Autoregulation has been demonstrated to have prognostic value [29], enables clinicians to understand the pathological state of patients, and can also influence the therapeutic strategy with the use of 'optimal cerebral perfusion pressure' [30, 31].

There are various modalities with a good spatial resolution which reliably reflect CBF, including imaging, and help to directly assess perfusion such as positron emission tomography (PET), single-photon emission computerised tomography (SPECT), xenon-enhanced CT (Xe-CT), and computerised tomography perfusion (CTP). However, these methods have limited temporal resolution, can assess only static autoregulation, are expensive, and are not easily available at the bedside. TCD/TCCD fills this void as a non-invasive, relatively low-cost monitoring tool.

With TCD/TCCD, we can measure autoregulation by measuring static autoregulation, studying the relationship between 'steady-state' changes in CPP or ABP and CBF, or by studying dynamic autoregulation through the assessment of continuous changes in CPP or ABP and CBF.

7.5.1 Static Autoregulation

Static autoregulation can be assessed by a 20 mm Hg increase in mean blood pressure (MBP) achieved through an infusion of phenylephrine 0.01% with the concurrent measurement of FV.

From MBP and FV, cerebrovascular resistance can be estimated as eCVR = MBP/FV. The static rate of autoregulation (SRoR) is the ratio of percentage change in estimated CVR to the percentage change in CPP (or the percentage change in MBP if ICP is not measured). When MBP is used rather than CPP, results may be affected by an error associated with 'false autoregulation', which occurs in the non-autoregulating brain when ICP rises consistently with MBP and leaves CPP constant.

If the percentage change in CVR was in agreement with the percentage change in MBP, then FV would remain constant. Therefore, an SROR of 0% mirrors a complete disruption of autoregulation whereas a SRoR of 100% implies perfect autoregulation.

7.5.2 Dynamic Autoregulation

Dynamic autoregulation can be assessed by rapidly varying ABP and CPP while measuring CBF. In order to measure dynamic autoregulation, the timing and magnitude of the reaction of CBF to the CPP/ABP challenge (induced or spontaneous) are observed over time, which can only be possible when using monitoring modalities with high temporal resolution (i.e. TCD, laser Doppler flowmetry, or near-infrared spectroscopy). One method that can be used is tight *leg-cuff release* in which the operator measures the recovery in FV after a rapid transient decrease in blood pressure that has been induced by the deflation of large thigh cuffs [32]. The cuffs are placed and inflated to 50 mm Hg above systolic blood pressure for 3 min. The deflation of the cuff produces an approximately 20 mm Hg drop in ABP. The flow velocity response to that drop can be analysed through a validated algorithm to determine the rate of dynamic cerebral autoregulation (dROR) or autoregulation index (ARI). ARI is a dimensionless index ranging from 0 to 9 that describes the response of CBF to a steep decrease in ABP. The threshold for good or disturbed autoregulation is an ARI value of around 5. The dRoR describes the rate of restoration of FV (percentage per second) with respect to the drop in MBP. The normal dRoR is 20%/s [32]. However, the release of the leg cuffs may also alter the CVR by the draining of vasoactive metabolites accumulated in the peripheral circulation during the cuff inflation.

Another method is the *transient hyperaemic response test*, which is performed by compressing the common carotid artery for 5–8 s before observing the change in flow velocity after the compression has ceased [33]. The transient hyperaemic response ratio (THRR: the ratio of the hyperaemic flow velocity recorded after carotid release and the precompression baseline flow velocity) is then calculated—see Fig. 7.4. Normal values in healthy volunteers range between 1.105 and 1.29. A threshold of 1.10 has been adopted as the lower limit of a normal response. However, this method could bring about some risk of releasing embolisms and extra variability of ABP.

Other methods include the squat-to-stand or sit-to-stand manoeuvres, controlled slow breathing, lower body negative pressure, Valsalva manoeuvre or analysis of spontaneous slow fluctuations of ABP.

7.5.3 Continuous Monitoring of Autoregulation

Continuous monitoring of autoregulation can be performed through the analysis over consecutive time-averaged samples of FV and CPP or ABP (thirty 10-s averages are usually taken).

Mx [34] is the correlation coefficient index calculated between FVm and CPP, and Sx is the correlation coefficient index between FVs and CPP. When either Mx or Sx is positive, there is a positive association between FV and CPP, and thus disturbed autoregulation. A negative or 0 correlation coefficient signifies intact autoregulation; see Fig. 7.5. They both describe cerebrovascular reactivity and correlate with outcome after a head injury, and therefore either can be used to guide autoregulation-oriented therapy [35].

Mxa is the correlation coefficient between ABP and FV. A Mxa close to +1 denotes that slow fluctuations of ABP produce synchronised slow changes in FV that describe deranged autoregulation. According to previous literature in TBI patients, negative values or values <0.3 of Mxa indicate intact autoregulation, whereas values >0.3 indicate the failure of cerebral autoregulation [36].

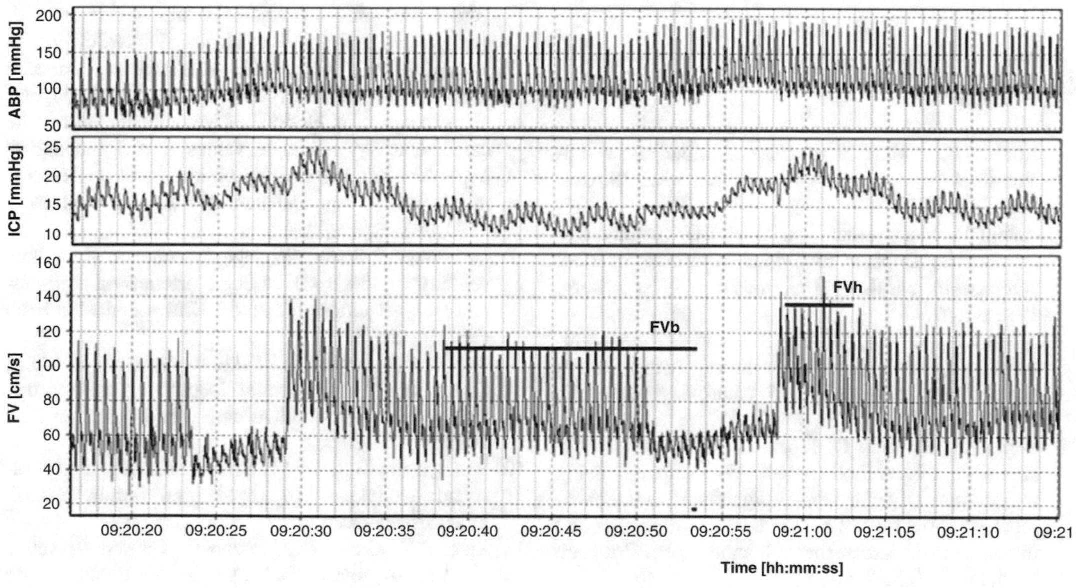

Fig. 7.4 Example of transient hyperaemic response test with autoregulation working well (FVh/FVb is above 1.15)

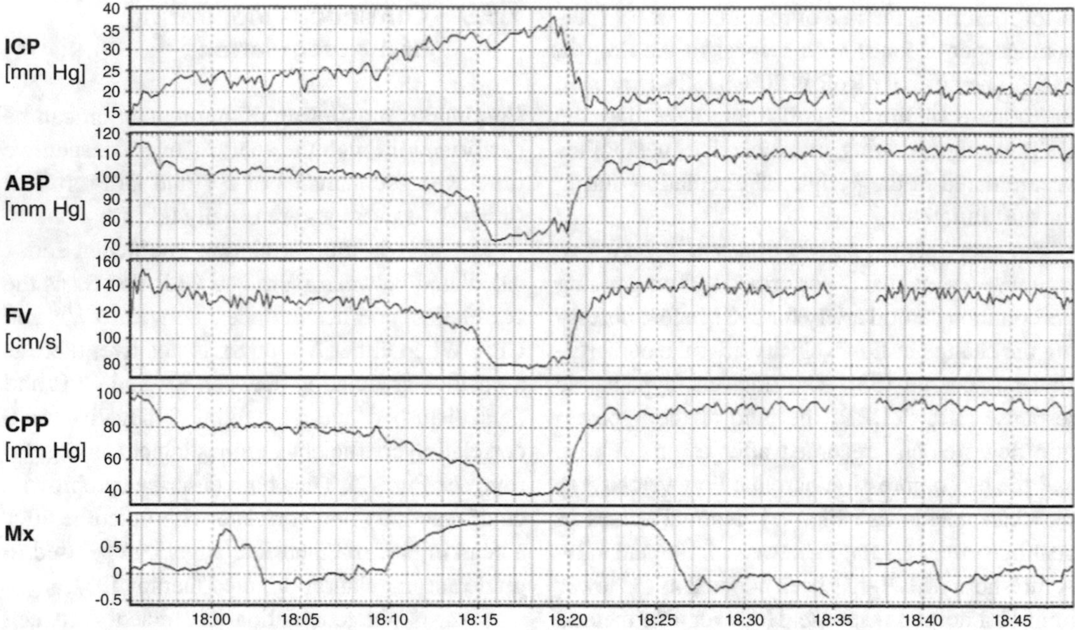

Fig. 7.5 Example of TCD, ICP, and ABP recording in TBI patient including a period of unstable ABP and ICP. During this period value of MX changed from around 0 to above 0.5—indicating the episode of short-term autoregulation failure

This index seems to be ideal for non-invasive bedside continuous monitoring of transient changes in autoregulation that could be interpreted instantaneously.

References

1. Kontos HA. Validity of cerebral blood flow calculations from velocity measurements. Stroke. 1989;20:1–3.
2. Aaslid R, Markwalder TM, Nornes H. Noninvasive transcranial Doppler ultrasound recording of flow velocity in basal cerebral arteries. J Neurosurg. 1982;57:769–74.
3. Nornes H, Grip A, Wikeby P. Intraoperative evaluation of cerebral hemodynamics using directional Doppler technique. J Neurosurg. 1979;50:570–7.
4. Venkatesh B, Shen Q, Lipman J. Continuous measurement of cerebral blood flow velocity using transcranial Doppler reveals significant moment-to-moment variability of data in healthy volunteers and in patients with subarachnoid hemorrhage*. Crit Care Med. 2002;30:563–9.
5. Brass LM, Pavlakis SG, DeVivo D, Piomelli S, Mohr JP. Transcranial Doppler measurements of the middle cerebral artery. Effect of hematocrit. Stroke. 1988;19:1466–9.
6. Markwalder T-M, Grolimund P, Seiler RW, Roth F, Aaslid R. Dependency of blood flow velocity in the middle cerebral artery on end-tidal carbon dioxide partial pressure—a transcranial ultrasound Doppler study. J Cereb Blood Flow Metab. 1984;4:368–72.
7. Brouwers PJ, Vriens EM, Musbach M, Wieneke GH, van Huffelen AC. Transcranial pulsed Doppler measurements of blood flow velocity in the middle cerebral artery: reference values at rest and during hyperventilation in healthy children and adolescents in relation to age and sex. Ultrasound Med Biol. 1990;16:1–8.
8. Grolimund P, Seiler RW. Age dependence of the flow velocity in the basal cerebral arteries—a transcranial Doppler ultrasound study. Ultrasound Med Biol. 1988;14:191–8.
9. Robba C, Cardim D, Sekhon M, Budohoski K, Czosnyka M. Transcranial Doppler: a stethoscope for the brain-neurocritical care use. J Neurosci Res. 2018;96:720–30.
10. Purkayastha S, Sorond F. Transcranial Doppler ultrasound: technique and application. Semin Neurol. 2012;32:411–20.
11. Ziegler D, Cravens G, Poche G, Gandhi R, Tellez M. Use of transcranial Doppler in patients with severe traumatic brain injuries. J Neurotrauma. 2017;34:121–7.

12. Ract C, Le Moigno S, Bruder N, Vigué B. Transcranial Doppler ultrasound goal-directed therapy for the early management of severe traumatic brain injury. Intensive Care Med. 2007;33:645–51.
13. Czosnyka M, Matta BF, Smielewski P, Kirkpatrick PJ, Pickard JD. Cerebral perfusion pressure in head-injured patients: a noninvasive assessment using transcranial Doppler ultrasonography. J Neurosurg. 1998;88:802–8.
14. Shigemori M, Kikuchi N, Tokutomi T, Ochiai S, Harada K, Kikuchi T, Kuramoto S. Monitoring of severe head-injured patients with transcranial Doppler (TCD) ultrasonography. Acta Neurochir Suppl (Wien). 1992;55:6–7.
15. Bellner J, Romner B, Reinstrup P, Kristiansson KA, Brandt L. Transcranial Doppler sonography pulsatility index (PI) reflects intracranial pressure (ICP). Surg Neurol. 2004;62:45–51.
16. Behrens A, Lenfeldt N, Ambarki K, Malm J, Eklund A, Koskinen LO Transcranial Doppler pulsatility index: not an accurate method to assess intracranial pressure. Neurosurgery. 2010;66:1050–7.
17. Figaji AA, Zwane E, Fieggen AG, Siesjo P, Peter JC. Transcranial Doppler pulsatility index is not a reliable indicator of intracranial pressure in children with severe traumatic brain injury. Surg Neurol. 2009;72:389–94.
18. Tude Melo JR, Di Rocco F, Blanot S, Cuttaree H, Sainte-Rose C, Oliveira-Filho J, Zarah M, Meyer PG. Transcranial Doppler can predict intracranial hypertension in children with severe traumatic brain injuries. Childs Nerv Syst. 2011;27:979–84.
19. De Riva N, Budohski K.P., Smielewski P, Kasprowicz M, Zweifel C, Steiner LA, Reinhard M, Fàbregas N, Pickard JD, Czosnyka M. Transcranial Doppler pulsatility index: what it is and what it isn't. Neurocrit Care. 2012;17:58–66.
20. Nichol J, Girling F, Jerrard W, Claxton EB, Burton AC. Fundamental instability of the small blood vessels and critical closing pressure in vascular beds. Am J Phys. 1951;164:330–44.
21. Dewey RC, Pieper HP, Hunt WE. Experimental cerebral hemodynamics. J Neurosurg. 1974;41:597–606.
22. Donnelly J, Czosnyka M, Harland S, Varsos GV, Cardim D, Robba C, Liu X, Ainslie PN, Smielewski P. Cerebral haemodynamics during experimental intracranial hypertension. J Cereb Blood Flow Metab. 2017;37:694–705.
23. Panerai RB. The critical closing pressure of the cerebral circulation. Med Eng Phys. 2003;25:621–32.
24. Varsos GV, Kasprowicz M, Smielewski P, Czosnyka M. Model-based indices describing cerebrovascular dynamics. Neurocrit Care. 2014;20:142–57.
25. Michel E. Gosling's Doppler pulsatility index revisited. Baseline. 1998;29:713–6.
26. Varsos GV, Richards H, Kasprowicz M, Budohoski KP, Brady KM, Reinhard M, Avolio A, Smielewski P, Pickard JD, Czosnyka M. Critical closing pressure determined with a model of cerebrovascular impedance. J Cereb Blood Flow Metab. 2013;33:235–43.
27. Varsos GV, Richards HK, Kasprowicz M, Reinhard M, Smielewski P, Brady KM, Pickard JD, Czosnyka M. Cessation of diastolic cerebral blood flow velocity: the role of critical closing pressure. Neurocrit Care. 2014;20:40–8.
28. Fog M. The relationship between the blood pressure and the tonic regulation of the pial arteries. J Neurol Psychiatry. 1938;1:187–97.
29. Czosnyka M, Smielewski P, Kirkpatrick P, Laing RJ, Menon D, Pickard JD. Continuous assessment of the cerebral vasomotor reactivity in head injury. Neurosurgery. 1997;41:11–7.
30. Donnelly J, Aries MJ, Czosnyka M. Further understanding of cerebral autoregulation at the bedside: possible implications for future therapy. Expert Rev Neurother. 2014;15:169–85.
31. Panerai RB, Kerins V, Fan L, Yeoman PM, Hope T, Evans DH. Association between dynamic cerebral autoregulation and mortality in severe head injury. Br J Neurosurg. 2004;18:471–9.
32. Tiecks FP, Lam AM, Aaslid R, Newell DW. Comparison of static and dynamic cerebral autoregulation measurements. Stroke. 1995;26:1014–9.
33. Smielewski P, Czosnyka M, Kirkpatrick P, Pickard JD. Evaluation of the transient hyperemic response test in head-injured patients. J Neurosurg. 1997;86:773–8.
34. Czosnyka M, Smielewski P, Kirkpatrick P, Menon DK, Pickard JD. Monitoring of cerebral autoregulation in head-injured patients. Stroke. 1996;27:1829–34.
35. Czosnyka M, Smielewski P, Piechnik S, Steiner LA, Pickard JD. Cerebral autoregulation following head injury. J Neurosurg. 2001;95:756–63.
36. Czosnyka M, Brady K, Reinhard M, Smielewski P, Steiner LA. Monitoring of cerebrovascular autoregulation: facts, myths, and missing links. Neurocrit Care. 2009;10:373–86.

8 Transcranial Doppler and Optic Nerve Ultrasonography for Non-invasive ICP Assessment

Danilo Cardim and Chiara Robba

Contents

D. Cardim (✉)
Department of Neurology and Neurotherapeutics, University of Texas Southwestern Medical Center, Dallas, TX, USA

Institute for Exercise and Environmental Medicine, Texas Health Presbyterian Hospital Dallas, Dallas, TX, USA

C. Robba
Anesthesia and Intensive Care, Policlinico San Martino, IRCCS for Oncology and Neuroscience, Genoa, Italy

8.1 Introduction

Brain ultrasonography has been explored as a technique for non-invasive estimation of intracranial pressure (nICP) basically through two main modalities: transcranial Doppler (TCD) ultrasonography of the middle cerebral artery (MCA) and measurement of the optic nerve sheath diameter (ONSD).

C. Robba, G. Citerio (eds.), *Echography and Doppler of the Brain*,
https://doi.org/10.1007/978-3-030-48202-2_8

TCD-derived nICP methods are based on the relationship between ICP and indices derived from cerebral blood flow velocity. Increased pressure in the intracranial compartment affects the physiologic relationship between blood flow velocity and pressure in cerebral vessels with compliant walls, producing marked changes in cerebral blood flow velocity (FV) waveform resulting in low diastolic FV, peaked waveform, and higher pulsatility index (PI) [1, 2]. Such indications of disturbed cerebral blood flow (CBF) have been applied in a variety of methods describing the cerebral haemodynamics as well as for nICP monitoring [3]. TCD-based nICP methods are originated from quantitative relationships between ICP and TCD-derived cerebrovascular parameters. Methodologically, they can be divided into three categories: (1) methods based on the TCD-derived PI; (2) methods based on the calculation of non-invasive cerebral perfusion pressure (nCPP); and (3) methods based on mathematical models associating cerebral blood flow velocity and arterial blood pressure.

The optic nerve sheath is an extension of the dura which contains cerebrospinal fluid (CSF) and optic nerve within the perineural subarachnoid space. In conditions of brain injury and cerebral oedema, volume changes in the intracranial compartment producing ICP elevation shift CSF into the optic nerve sheath, causing the ONSD to increase [4–6]. In particular, ONSD measurements can be obtained with the transcranial colour-coded duplex (TCCD) technique.

This chapter presents a compilation of the main approaches for nICP assessment based on brain ultrasonography.

8.2 TCD-Derived Pulsatility Index

Methods based on TCD-derived pulsatility index rely on the observation that ICP and PI are positively correlated. PI quantifies morphological changes in the TCD waveform resulting from varying CPP. It is represented by the difference between systolic and diastolic flow velocities divided by the mean velocity, initially described by Gosling in 1974 [7]:

$$PI = \frac{FV_s - FV_d}{FV_m} (\text{a.u.})$$

PI has been reported as inversely proportional to mean CPP, directly proportional to pulse amplitude of arterial blood pressure (ABP) and non-linearly proportional to the compliance of the cerebral arterial bed (C_a), cerebrovascular resistance (CVR) and heart rate (HR) [8]. In Gosling's original work, normal PI values were reported between 0.5 and 1.19 [7]. Proximal stenosis or occlusion may lower PI below 0.5 due to downstream arteriolar vasodilation, whereas distal occlusion or constriction may increase PI above 1.19 [9]. A PI less than 0.5 may also indicate an arteriovenous malformation as the resistance in proximal vessels is reduced due to continuous distal venous flow [10].

More recently, a larger study including more than 350 healthy individuals has reported normative values for TCD assessment of arteries in the circle of Willis [11]. Normal PI values have been reported as 0.82 ± 0.16 (mean ± standard deviation) and 0.81 ± 0.13 for distal and proximal middle cerebral arteries, respectively. As a ratio, PI is not affected by the angle of insonation and therefore may be a sensitive parameter for early detection of intracranial haemodynamic changes [11].

The usefulness of PI to predict ICP and CPP is still controversial. This controversy results from the fact that changes in PI are not strictly specific to changes in ICP. PI can be modulated by CPP and arterial blood pressure (ABP), and variations in partial pressure of CO_2 or in the pulsatility of the ABP waveform [8]. nICP methods based on TCD-derived pulsatility index are listed in Table 8.1.

Table 8.1 nICP methods based on TCD-derived pulsatility index ($nICP_{PI}$)

Method	Author	Study purpose	Sample size and disease	Invasive ICP monitoring	nICP method accuracy and correlation measures with ICP	Sensitivity (%)	Specificity (%)	AUC
$nICP_{PI}$	Steiger [54]	Investigate PI in TBI patients and compare them to healthy volunteers.	9, TBI	NA	PI analysis revealed values from 1.5 to 2.0 in control subjects, showing a gradual increase in patients with post-traumatic brain oedema. PI values ≥3 were associated with severe intracranial hypertension			
	Chan et al. [15]	Examine the relationships between FV, SJO_2 and alterations in ABP, ICP and CPP.	41, TBI	Subdural	Rises in ICP or drops in ABP were associated with a reduction in FV, particularly with FVd falling more than FVs. PI was strongly correlated with ICP ($R = 0.9^{a}$)			
	Homburg et al. [55]	Investigate the PI-ICP relation so as to evaluate TCD as an alternative to invasive ICP.	10, TBI	Epidural	Correlation between PI and ICP was $R = 0.82$			
	Martin et al. [56]	Assess PI in three distinct haemodynamic phases (hypoperfusion, hyperaemia and vasospasm).	125, TBI	Intraventricular/ intraparenchymal	Higher PI values were found in all haemodynamic phases during the first 2 weeks after injury (on day 0, compared to days 1 through 3 and days 4 through 14 post-trauma)			
	McQuire et al. [57]	Investigate the incidence of early abnormalities in the cerebral circulation after TBI by relating the results of CT scan with TCD-PI.	22, TBI	NM	Ten patients presented increased PI in conditions indicative of ICH (space-occupying haematomas or brain swelling indications on CT)			
	Moreno et al. [58]	Investigate the correlation between TCD, ICP and CPP in TBI patients.	125, TBI	NA	Correlation between PI and ICP was $R^2 = 0.69$. Elevated PI (≥1.56) was predictive of poor outcome			

(continued)

Table 8.1 (continued)

Method	Author	Study purpose	Sample size and disease	Invasive ICP monitoring	nICP method accuracy and correlation measures with ICP	Sensitivity (%)	Specificity (%)	AUC
	Rainov et al. [59]	Investigate a possible relationship between PI, RI, FV and ICP changes in adult patients with hydrocephalus.	29, Hydrocephalus	Epidural	PI in patients with elevated ICP prior to shunting was significantly increased. Pre-shunting ICP and PI were not correlated ($R = 0.37$)			
	Asil et al. [60]	TCD was compared with clinical examination and neuroradiologic findings.	18, Stroke and MCA infarction	NM	Increases in PI were correlated with midline shift as indication of elevated ICP ($R = 0.66^a$)			
	Bellner et al. [61]	Investigate the relationship between ICP and PI in neurosurgical patients.	81 (SAH, TBI and other intracranial disorders)	Intraventricular	Correlation between PI and ICP was $R = 0.94^a$ (ICP = 10.93 × PI − 1.28) In the ICP range of 5–40 mmHg, the correlation formula is: ICP = 11.5 × PI − 2.23 ($R^2 = 0.73^a$) In this interval, SD for *nICP_PI* was ±2.5 mmHg in the ICP range of 5–40 mmHg 95% CI of ±4.2 mmHg	88 (threshold of 10 mmHg) 83 (threshold of 20 mmHg)	69 (threshold of 10 mmHg) 99 (threshold of 20 mmHg)	
	Voulgaris et al. [62]	Investigate TCD as a tool for detection of cerebral haemodynamic changes	37, TBI	Intraparenchymal	Overall correlation between ICP and PI was $R = 0.64^a$ For ICP ≥20 mmHg, correlation was $R = 0.82^a$ PI allows early identification of patients with low CPP and risk of cerebral ischaemia			
	Behrens et al. [63]	Validate TCD as a method for ICP determination of INPH	10, INPH	Intraparenchymal	Correlation between PI and ICP was $R^2 = 0.22^a$ (ICP = 23 × PI + 14) 95% CI for a mean ICP of 20 mmHg was −3.8 to 43.8 mmHg PI is not a reliable predictor of ICP			

	Figaji et al. [64]	Examine the relationship between PI, ICP and CPP in children with severe TBI	34 Children, TBI	NM	Marginal correlation between PI and ICP of $R = 0.36$[a] No significant relationships between PI and ICP when differences within individuals or binary examination of PI (PI <1 and ≥1) were considered PI is not a reliable non-invasive indicator of ICP in children with severe TBI	25 (threshold of 20 mmHg)	88 (threshold of 20 mmHg)	
	Brandi et al. [65]	Assess an optimal nICP and nCPP following TBI using TCD.	45, TBI	Intraventricular	Bellner's equation resulted in nICP similar to measured ICP, with nICP of 10.6 ± 4.8 and ICP of 10.3 ± 2.8 mmHg			
	Tude Melo et al. [66]	Evaluate the accuracy of TCD in emergency settings to predict intracranial hypertension and abnormal CPP in children with TBI.	117 Children, TBI	Intraparenchymal	PI ≥1.31 was observed in 94% of cases with initially elevated ICP, and 59% of those with normal initial ICP values TCD is an excellent first-line examination to screen children who need urgent treatment and continuous invasive ICP monitoring	94 (for detecting initial ICH)	95 (for detecting initial ICH)	
	Zweifel et al. [67]	Assess PI as a diagnostic tool for nICP and nCPP estimation.	290, TBI	Intraparenchymal	Correlation between PI and ICP was $R = 0.31$[a] 95% Prediction interval >±15 mmHg The value of PI to assess nICP is very limited			0.62 (ICP ≥15 mmHg) 0.74 (ICP ≥35 mmHg)
	De Riva et al. [8]	Assess the relationship between PI and CVR in situations where CVR increases (mild hypocapnia) and decreases (plateau waves of ICP) in TBI patients.	345, TBI	Intraparenchymal	Correlation between PI and ICP in such situations was $R = 0.70$[a] 95% CI of ±21 mmHg			

(continued)

Table 8.1 (continued)

Method	Author	Study purpose	Sample size and disease	Invasive ICP monitoring	nICP method accuracy and correlation measures with ICP	Sensitivity (%)	Specificity (%)	AUC
	Wakerley et al. [68]	Assess the correlation between PI with CSF pressure.	78, Miscellaneous intracranial disorders	LP	Correlation between PI and ICP (CSF pressure) was $R = 0.65^a$ Binomial logistic regression indicated a strong significant relationship between raised ICP and PI (OR: 2.44; 95% CI: 1.57–3.78)	81.1	96.3	0.84 (threshold ≥20 cmH_20)
	Wakerley et al. [69]	Present a case where TCD serves as an effective tool for nICP monitoring.	Case report, sagittal sinus thrombosis	NM	Increasing ICP was associated with rapid elevations of PI. On recording day 4, PI was reported to be 1.93 (considering a normal range of 0.6–1.2). ICP was deemed elevated according to clinical status (level of consciousness, headache) and papilledema			
	O'Brien et al. [70]	Determine the relationship between PI, FV_d and ICP in children with severe TBI.	36 Children, TBI	Intraventricular/ intraparenchymal	*Initial 24 h post-injury* Correlation between PI and ICP was $R = 0.6^a$ *Beyond 24 h post-injury* Correlation between PI and ICP was $R = 0.38^a$	*Initial 24 h post-injury* 100 (threshold ≥20 mmHg for PI of 1.3) *Beyond 24 h post-injury* 47 (threshold ≥20 mmHg for PI of 1.3)	*Initial 24 h post-injury* 82 (threshold ≥20 mmHg for PI of 1.3)	

ABP arterial blood pressure, *AUC* area under the curve, *CI* confidence interval; *CT* computerised tomography, *CSF* cerebrospinal fluid, FV_d diastolic flow velocity, *ICH* intracranial hypertension, *INPH* idiopathic normal pressure hydrocephalus, *LP* lumbar puncture, *MCA* middle cerebral artery, *NA* not available, *NM* not measured, *NPV* negative predictive value, *OR* odds ratio, *PPV* positive predictive value, *R* correlation coefficient, R^2 coefficient of determination, *RI* resistance index, *SAH* subarachnoid haemorrhage, *SD* standard deviation, SJO_2 jugular bulb venous blood oxygen saturation, *TBI* traumatic brain injury

[a]Correlation coefficient is significant at the 0.05 level

8.3 Methods Based on the Calculation of Non-invasive CPP (nCPP)

Many authors have also investigated methods based on the primarily intended calculation of non-invasive cerebral perfusion pressure (nCPP), and secondarily calculating non-invasive ICP based on the assumption that "nICP = ABP − nCPP". nICP methods based on TCD-derived cerebral perfusion pressure are listed in Table 8.2.

8.3.1 Aaslid et al. [12] (*nICP*$_{Aaslid}$)

Aaslid et al. (1986) [12] were the pioneers in the development of a mathematical model for non-invasive estimation of CPP based on TCD waveform analysis. Supported by the knowledge that increased ICP was related to decreases of the flow waveform in the internal carotid artery [13], the authors deemed feasible that less evident changes in the flow pattern could be detected by more refined methods of waveform analysis. TCD, in such a perspective, could be used to obtain an estimate of ICP. Considering CPP as the driving force to flow through the cerebral vascular bed and the main factor determining pulsatile dynamics, the flow would be approximately proportional to CPP [12].

During increases in ICP, the proportion of the systolic to the diastolic CPP increases as ICP approaches the diastolic ABP. Consequently, the pulsatile component of CPP increases proportionally to its mean value and this would also be reflected in the FV waveform. Thus, the ratio between mean FV (FVm) and pulsatile amplitude of FV (*f*1) would be expected to be related to CPP. The simplest approach, in this case, would be using this ratio as an index for CPP. However, it does not consider changes in the ratio caused by variations in the amplitude of ABP waveform. Such limitation was solved by multiplying the ratio described above by the amplitude of the first harmonic of ABP (*a*1) [12]:

$$\mathrm{nCPP}_{\mathrm{Aaslid}} = \left(\mathrm{FV}_{\mathrm{m}} / f1\right) \times a1\,\mathrm{mmHg}$$

This method was tested in patients with supratentorial hydrocephalus undergoing ventricular infusion tests. The linear regression determined for nCPP estimation considering all cases was

$$\mathrm{CPP} = 1.1\,\mathrm{nCPP}_{\mathrm{Aaslid}} - 5\,\mathrm{mmHg}$$

In the individual case, there was a strong correlation between nCPP and CPP, $R = 0.93$–0.99. The standard deviation between nCPP and CPP was 8.2 mmHg at 40 mmHg, while the mean deviation was only 1 mmHg. Overestimation occurred in two cases, 10 mmHg and 18 mmHg, respectively. Underestimation was present in other two cases, 9 and 8 mmHg, respectively. For the six remaining cases, the estimates were within ±5 mmHg of measured CPP. The method could differentiate correctly between low (<40 mmHg) and normal (>80 mmHg) CPP in all patients. At higher levels of CPP, the estimates presented with low accuracy, showing correct differentiation between CPPs of 70 and 100 mmHg in 80% of the cases.

8.3.2 Czosnyka et al. [14] (*nICP*$_{FVd}$)

Some studies have demonstrated that certain patterns of the TCD waveform, like a decrease in $\mathrm{FV_d}$, reflect impaired cerebral perfusion caused by a CPP decrease [14, 15]. Czosnyka et al. [14] described this relationship as the following formula:

$$\mathrm{nCPP}_{\mathrm{FV_d}} = \mathrm{ABP} \times \frac{\mathrm{FV_d}}{\mathrm{FV_m}} + 14\,mmHg$$

The correlation between nCPP and invasively measured CPP in traumatic brain injury (TBI) patients was $R = 0.73$, $p < 0.001$. In 71% of the examinations, the estimation error was below 10 mmHg, and in 84% of the examinations, the error was less than 15 mmHg. The method had a high positive predictive value (94%) for detecting low CPP (<60 mmHg). Estimated CPP was highly specific for detecting changes in measured CPP over time, caused by either increases in ICP (plateau waves) or systemic hypotension. In six patients presenting plateau waves, nCPP compared with measured CPP had an average goodness-of-fit coefficient R^2 of 0.82.

Table 8.2 nICP methods based on non-invasive cerebral perfusion pressure estimation

Method	Author	Study purpose	Sample size and disease	Invasive ICP monitoring	nICP/nCPP method accuracy and correlation measures with ICP/CPP	AUC	PPV (%)	NPV (%)
$nICP_{Aaslid}$	Aaslid et al. [12]	Describe and assess a method for nCPP calculation based on FV and ABP.	10, Supratentorial hydrocephalus	Intraventricular	SD for nCPP estimation of 8.2 mmHg at 40 mmHg Able to differentiate between low (≤40 mmHg) and normal (≥80 mmHg) CPP in all cases Low accuracy (80%) at higher levels of CPP (70–100 mmHg)			
	Czosnyka et al. [14]	Assess $nICP_{Aaslid}$.	96, TBI	Intraparenchymal	95% PE for nCPP estimation was >27 mmHg Sensitive to detect changes of CPP over time			
$nICP_{FVd}$	Czosnyka et al. [14]	Describe and assess a method for nCPP calculation based on FV (using the concept of FVd) and ABP.	96, TBI	Intraparenchymal	Correlation between nCPP and CPP was $R = 0.73^{a}$ Estimation error was less than 10 and 15 mmHg in 71% and 84% of the cases, respectively Highly specific for detecting changes over time: $R^2 = 0.82$ Averaged correlation considering day-by-day variability between CPP and nCPP was $R = 0.71$		94 (CPP ≤60 mmHg)	
	Schmidt et al. [71]	Assess $nICP_{FVd}$.	25, TBI	Intraparenchymal	Error for nCPP estimation was less than 10 and 13 mmHg in 89% and 92% of the cases, respectively 95% CI of ±12 mmHg			
	Gura et al. [72]	Assess $nICP_{FVd}$.	47, TBI	Intraparenchymal	Correlation between nCPP and CPP was $R = 0.92^{a}$ Mean values of nCPP and CPP were 66.10 ± 10.55 mmHg and 65.40 ± 10.03 mmHg, respectively			
	Brandi et al. [65]	Assess an optimal nICP and nCPP following TBI using TCD.	45, TBI	Intraparenchymal	*nICP*: Bias of 5.6 mmHg and 95% CI of ±17.4 mmHg *nCPP*: Bias of −5.5 mmHg and 95% CI of ±20.6 mmHg			
	Rasulo et al. [73]	Assess $nICP_{FVd}$.	38, Acute brain injury	28 Intraparenchymal, 10 intraventricular	Bias of 6.2 mmHg and 95% CI of 11.8 mmHg	0.96 (≥20 mmHg)		

	Cardim et al. [74]	Assess $nICP_{FVd}$.	100, TBI	Intraparenchymal	No correlation between ICP and nICP ($R = -0.17$)	0.34 (≥20 mmHg)		
	Cardim et al. [42]	Assess $nICP_{FVd}$.	11, Hypoxic-ischaemic brain injury after cardiac arrest	Intraparenchymal	Correlation between ICP and nICP was $R = 0.30$[a]	0.91 (≥20 mmHg)		
$nICP_{Edouard}$	Edouard et al. [16]	Describe and assess a method for nCPP calculation based on FV and ABP under stable conditions and during CO_2 reactivity test.	20, TBI	Intraparenchymal	*During normocapnia*: nCPP and CPP were correlated (slope, 0.76; intercept, 10.9; 95% CI, −3.5 to 25.4 mmHg) *During hypercapnia*: nCPP and CPP were correlated, but with increased discrepancy, as reflected in confidence interval (slope, 0.55; intercept, 32.6; 95% CI, 16.3–48.9 mmHg)			
	Brandi et al. [65]	Assess $nICP_{Edouard}$.	45, TBI	Intraparenchymal	*nICP*: Bias of 6.8 mmHg and 95% CI ±19.7 mmHg *nCPP*: Bias of −6.8 mmHg and 95% CI ±45.2 mmHg			
$nICP_{CrCP}$	Varsos et al. [18]	Describe and assess a method for nCPP calculation based on FV (using the concept of CrCP) and ABP.	280, TBI	Intraparenchymal	Correlation between nCPP and CPP was $R = 0.85$[a] Bias ± SD of 4.02 ± 6.01 mmHg nCPP estimation error was below 10 mmHg in 83.3% of the cases *Temporal analysis*: Mean correlation in time domain was $R = 0.73$ (0.23–0.99) Bias of 3.45 mmHg (range: 4.69–9.03 mmHg) Mean SD of 5.52 mmHg (range: 1.52–10.76 mmHg) and 95% CI of the SD of 1.89–5.01 mmHg	>0.8		
Spectral nCPP	Abecasis & Cardim et al. [24]	Describe and assess a method for nCPP calculation based on FV and ABP.			Correlation between nCPP and CPP was $R = 0.67$[a] Bias of 19.61 mmHg 95% CI: ± 40.1 mmHg *Temporal analysis*: Mean correlation in time domain was $R = 0.55$ (±0.42)			

AUC area under the curve, *ABP* arterial blood pressure, *CI* confidence interval, *FV* cerebral blood flow velocity, *NPV* negative predictive value, *PPV* positive predictive value, *PE* prediction error, *R* correlation coefficient, R^2 coefficient of determination, *SD* standard deviation, *SAH* subarachnoid haemorrhage, *TBI* traumatic brain injury

[a]Correlation coefficient is significant at the 0.05 level

Furthermore, nCPP was very sensitive to detecting decreases in ABP below 70 mmHg (in ten patients) with an average R^2 of 0.92. A good correlation was found between the average measured CPP and nCPP when day-by-day variability was assessed in a group of 41 patients ($R = 0.71$).

8.3.3 Edouard et al. [16] (nICP$_{Edouard}$)

This method is based on a non-invasive assessment of CPP using a combination of phasic values of both FV in the MCA and ABP. It was primarily validated in preeclamptic and healthy pregnant women by comparing nCPP with CPP measured at the epidural space [17].

In Edouard et al.'s prospective study [16], the objective was to assess the adequacy of such method for TBI patients with invasive ICP monitoring, in both a stable state and during a rapid change in cerebrovascular tone following an induced alteration in arterial blood carbon dioxide pressure ($PaCO_2$).

The non-invasive CPP (nICP$_{Edouard}$) was calculated using the following formula:

$$nCPP_{Edouard} = \left(\frac{FV_m}{FV_m - FV_d} \right) \times \left(ABP_m - ABP_d \right) \text{mmHg}$$

ABP_m and ABP_d represent the mean and diastolic ABP, respectively.

Twenty adults with bilateral and diffuse brain injuries were included in the study and subdivided into two groups. In group A ($N = 10$), the comparison was repeatedly performed under stable conditions. In group B ($N = 10$), the comparison was conducted during a CO_2 reactivity test. nICP was not estimated in this study. In group A, nCPP and measured CPP were correlated (slope, 0.76; intercept, +10.90; 95% CI, −3.50 to +25.40). The relationship persisted during ICP increase caused by the reactivity test in group B (slope, 0.55; intercept, +32.60; 95% CI, +16.30 to +48.90). However, the discrepancy between nCPP and measured CPP increased as reflected by the increase in bias and variability.

8.3.4 Varsos et al. [18] (nICP$_{CrCP}$)

The concept of critical closing pressure (CrCP) was first introduced by Burton's model, described as the sum of ICP and vascular wall tension (WT) [19]. WT represents the active cerebral vasomotor tone that combined with ICP determines the CrCP. Clinically, CrCP represents the lower threshold of ABP below which blood pressure in the brain microvasculature is inadequate to prevent the collapse and cessation of blood flow [19]. CrCP can be assessed non-invasively using TCD, by comparing the pulsatile waveforms of FV and ABP. Given the relationship with the vasomotor tone of small blood vessels, CrCP can provide information regarding the state of cerebral haemodynamics and reflect changes in CPP [19–23].

The conception and assessment of the model for the non-invasive estimator of CPP (nCPP$_{CrCP}$) were performed using a cohort of 280 TBI patients, divided into two subgroups: the formation group with 232 patients (including 455 recordings) and the validation group with 48 patients (including 325 recordings):

$$nCPP_{CrCP} = ABP \times \left[0.734 - \frac{0.266}{\sqrt{\left(CVR \cdot C_a \cdot HR \cdot 2\pi \right)^2 + 1}} \right] - 7.026 \, \text{mmHg}$$

$$\mathrm{CVR} = \frac{\mathrm{ABP}}{\mathrm{FV}}$$

$$C_a = \frac{C_a BV1}{a1}$$

CVR (mmHg/(cm/s)) represents cerebral vascular resistance, C_a (cm/mmHg) denotes compliance of the cerebral arterial bed (arteries and arterioles) and HR represents heart rate given in beat/s. $a1$ represents the pulse amplitude of the first harmonic of the ABP waveform; $f1$ the pulse amplitude of the first harmonic of the FV waveform; and C_aBV1 the pulse amplitude of the first harmonic of the cerebral arterial blood volume waveform (C_aBV). The pulse amplitude of first harmonics is determined with fast Fourier transformation (FFT).

$nCPP_{CrCP}$ was tested against invasive CPP using data from the validation group. $nCPP_{CrCP}$ was correlated with measured CPP ($R = 0.85$, $p < 0.001$), with a bias of 4.02 ± 6.01 mmHg, and in 83.3% of the cases with an estimation error below 10 mmHg. $nCPP_{CrCP}$ prediction analysis at low CPP limits (50, 60 and 70 mmHg) resulted in AUCs greater than 0.8 for all limits. $nCPP_{CrCP}$ was found to be strongly correlated with CPP changes in the time domain (mean $R = 0.73$, range 0.23–0.99). For each patient, $nCPP_{CrCP}$ presented a mean difference from CPP of 3.45 mmHg (range 4.69–19.03 mmHg), and a mean standard deviation of this difference of 5.52 mmHg (range 1.52–10.76 mmHg). $nCPP_{CrCP}$ could predict CPP between multiple recording sessions with a 95% CI of 1.89–5.01 mmHg.

8.3.5 Abecasis and Cardim et al. (Spectral nCPP) [24]

This recently proposed method is based on accounting for changes in pulsatile cerebral arterial blood volume (C_aBV) applied to the analysis of a simplified hydrodynamic model of CBF and CSF dynamics [25–27]. The spectral feature of the method has some advantages: it creates partial independence from the inaccuracy associated with zeroing ABP transducers at heart level (a common clinical practice) and partially eliminates the issue of the time delay between peripheral ABP and FV in the MCA. The dynamical model of CSF and cerebral blood circulation proposed by Ursino and Lodi [25, 26] is the theoretical basis for the spectral nCPP method; the former has also been modified by other authors to incorporate changes in cerebral blood volume and adapted to nICP or nCPP estimations. $nICP_{Heldt}$ [28] described in Sect. 8.4 is one example. Similarly to this method, spectral nCPP produces patient-specific CPP estimates and does not require calibration datasets of reference patients.

Abecasis and Cardim et al. [24] assessed spectral nCPP on a retrospective analysis from 19 children (69 TCD recordings). Spectral nCPP presented good correlation with CPP measure invasively ($R = 0.67$ ($p < 0.0001$)), and a good mean correlation in time domain ($R = 0.55 \pm 0.42$). Spectral nCPP also demonstrated strong ability to predict values of CPP below 70 mmHg (AUC of 0.908 (95% CI = 0.83–0.98)). The agreement between spectral nCPP and invasive CPP assessed by Bland-Altman analysis revealed that nCPP overestimated invasive CPP by 19.61 mmHg with a wide 95% CI of ±40.4 mmHg.

8.4 Methods Based on Mathematical Models Associating Cerebral Blood Flow Velocity and Arterial Blood Pressure

Several authors have proposed mathematical models that simulate the cerebrovascular dynamics using simultaneous FV and ABP measurements. nICP methods based on mathematical models are listed in Table 8.3.

8.4.1 Black-Box Model for ICP Estimation ($nICP_{BB}$)

In this model, the intracranial compartment is considered a black-box (BB) system, with ICP being a system response to the incoming signal ABP [29]. This mathematical model originates

Table 8.3 nICP methods based on mathematical models

Method	Author	Study purpose	Sample size and disease	Invasive ICP monitoring	nICP method accuracy and correlation measures with ICP	Sensitivity (%)	Specificity (%)	AUC
$nICP_{BB}$	Schmidt et al. [29]	Describe and assess a method for nICP calculation based on FV and ABP using a black-box model.	11, TBI	Epidural	Bias of 4.0 mmHg and SDE of 1.8 mmHg In this cohort a maximum 95% CI of ±12.8 mmHg was found			
	Schmidt et al. [75]	This study aimed at predicting the time course of raised ICP during CSF infusion tests and its suitability for estimating the R_{CSF} using $nICP_{BB}$.	21, Different types of hydrocephalus	Epidural	*Analysis across all records*: Correlation between nR_{CSF} and R_{CSF} was $R = 0.73$[a] Bias of 4.1 mmHg and SDE for R_{CSF} prediction of 2.2 mmHg minute/ml *Analysis specific to different subtypes of hydrocephalus*: Correlation between nR_{CSF} and R_{CSF} was $R = 0.89$[a] Bias of 2.7 mmHg and SDE for R_{CSF} prediction of 1.7 mmHg min/ml			
	Schmidt et al. [76]	Assess $nICP_{BB}$ during plateau waves of ICP.	17, TBI (plateau (A) waves observed in 7 patients)	Intraparenchymal	Correlation between nICP and ICP during ICP increase was $R = 0.98$[a] *Analysis considering the baseline of plateau waves*: Bias of 8.3 mmHg and SDE of 5.4 mmHg *Analysis considering the top of plateau waves*: Bias of 7.9 mmHg and SDE of 4.3 mmHg *Increases of nICP and direct ICP during plateau waves*: $R = 0.98$ ($p < 0.001$)			
	Schmidt et al. [77]	This study aimed at investigating the ability of $nICP_{BB}$ to adapt to the SCA, using Mx and PRx as parameters	145 (135 TBI, 10 stroke)	Intraparenchymal/ intraventricular	Correlation between nMx and Mx was $R = 0.90$[a] Correlation between nPRx and PRx was $R = 0.62$[a] Median bias of 6.0 mmHg *Only TBI*: Bias of 7.1 mmHg *Only stroke*: Bias of 4.3 mmHg	For Mx: 97 For PRx: 61	For Mx: 92 For PRx: 67	

nICP$_{Heldt}$	Kashif and Heldt et al. [28]	Describe and assess a method for nICP calculation based on FV and ABP.	37 (45 TCD recordings in total, 30 bilateral), TBI	Intraparenchymal	*Across all TCD records*: Correlation between nICP and ICP was $R = 0.90$ Bias of 1.6 and SDE of ±7.6 mmHg Inferred 95% CI of ±14.9 mmHg *Across bilateral TCD records*: Correlation between nICP and ICP was $R = 0.76$ Bias 1.5 and SDE 5.9 mmHg Inferred 95% CI of ±11.6 mmHg *On a patient record basis*: Correlation between nICP and ICP was $R = 0.90$ ($N = 45$ recordings)	83 90	70 80	0.83 (≥20 mmHg) 0.88 (≥20 mmHg)
Modified nICP$_{BB}$	Xu et al. [33]	Describe and assess a method for nICP calculation based on FV and ABP, using an appropriated model for *nICP*$_{BB}$.	23 (14 TBI, 9 hydrocephalus)	Intraparenchymal/ intraventricular	Biases for non-linear models were <6.0 mmHg compared to 6.7 mmHg of the $nICP_{BB}$ (linear) Inferred 95% CIs for non-linear models were ≤±10.8 mmHg, compared to 10.6 mmHg of the linear model			
Data mining	Hu et al. [38]	Describe and assess a method for nICP calculation based on FV and ABP based on the concepts of data mining.	9, TBI	Intraventricular	Median correlation between data mining nICP and ICP was $R = 0.80$			
	Kim et al. [39]	Describe and assess a method for nICP calculation based on FV and ABP based on the concepts of data mining.	57, TBI	NM	Kernel spectral regression-based method presented a median bias of 4.37 mmHg			
Semi-supervised learning	Kim et al. [40]	Describe and assess a method for nICP calculation based on FV and ABP based on the concepts of semi-supervised machine learning.	90 (44 TBI, 36 SAH, 10 NPH)	Intraparenchymal/ intraventricular	Decision curve analysis showed that the semi-supervised method is more accurate and clinically useful than the supervised or PI-based method			0.92

Inferred 95% CI was calculated as 1.96*SDE

AUC area under the curve, *CI* confidence interval, *R* correlation coefficient, R^2 coefficient of determination, *SDE* standard deviation of the error, R_{CSF} resistance to cerebrospinal fluid (CSF) outflow, R_{CSF} nICP-derived R_{CSF}; *NPH* normal pressure hydrocephalus, *TBI* traumatic brain injury, *SAH* subarachnoid haemorrhage, *SCA* state of cerebral autoregulation

[a]Correlation coefficient is significant at the 0.05 level

from systems analysis, which provides a method to describe the transmission characteristics, with input and output signals. The intracranial compartment is indirectly described by a transfer function [30, 31] which connects the assumed input signal, ABP, with the output signal, ICP. Two linear models are first established to depict the relationship between ABP and ICP and that between ABP and FV, yielding two coefficients, ***f*** and ***w***, respectively. By applying this linear mapping function, non-invasive ICP estimation can be performed by first estimating ***f*** from the coefficients ***w*** obtained from ABP and FV (TCD characteristics). An estimate of ICP can then be derived from ABP using the calculated ***f***. The output data provides a continuous full waveform of nICP (in mmHg) and constant relationship between FV and ABP.

$nICP_{BB}$ was first validated in a cohort of 11 TBI patients [29]. For each patient, measured and predicted ICP were compared during a time interval of 100 s. As a measure of the model's accuracy, the mean of the absolute values of the differences (bias) between measured and predicted ICP values (MAD-ICP) was obtained. To verify the model's capability of predicting the mean ICP averaged over one cardiac cycle (ICP_{CC}), the mean of the absolute differences (bias) between measured and predicted ICP_{CC} (MAD-ICP_{CC}) was calculated.

The MAD-ICP was smaller than 3 mmHg in four patients and smaller than 5 mmHg in eight patients, and the maximum MAD-ICP was 7.50 mmHg. The MAD-ICP_{CC} was slightly lower than the MAD-ICP; it was smaller than 3 mmHg in four patients and smaller than 5 mmHg in nine patients, and again the maximum was 7.50 mmHg. On average, the patients' MAD-ICP was 4.0 ± 1.80 mmHg, and the MAD-ICP_{CC} was 3.80 ± 1.90 mmHg. The 95% CI for ICP prediction was smaller than 5 mmHg in three patients and smaller than 10 mmHg in eight patients, and the maximum was 12.80 mmHg. The 95% CI for ICP_{CC} was smaller than 5 mmHg in four patients and smaller than 10 mmHg in 11 patients, and the maximum was 11.70 mmHg.

8.4.2 Cerebrovascular Dynamics Model for Estimation of ICP [28, 32] (nICP$_{Heldt}$)

This model-based nICP method focuses on the major intracranial compartments and their associated variables: brain tissue, cerebral vasculature and CSF. It continuously estimates and tracks ICP using measurements of peripheral ABP and FV in the MCA. This physiological model of cerebrovascular dynamics is represented by a circuit analogue and provides mathematical limits that relate the measured waveforms to ICP. Patient-specific ICP estimations are produced by an algorithm, with no calibration or training in specific populations needed. Ursino and Lodi [26] initially described the dynamical model of CSF and cerebral blood flow, and then modified by many independently working neuroscientists.

The $nICP_{Heldt}$ method was validated in a cohort of 37 TBI patients with severe closed head injury, in a total of 45 recordings. Thirty of these recordings presented bilateral FV monitoring. The correlation coefficient between $nICP_{Heldt}$ and measured ICP was $R = 0.90$ for the total data obtained on the 2665 non-overlapping estimation windows. The bias of $nICP_{Heldt}$ versus measured ICP in this case across all patients was 1.6 mmHg and standard deviation of the error (SDE) was 7.60 mmHg. The overall correlation coefficient with measured ICP (ranging up to 100 mmHg) was strong ($R = 0.90$). However, considering only the bilateral recordings, the correlation dropped to 0.76, despite the smaller SDE of 5.90 mmHg due to the narrower range of ICP variation (few points above 40 mmHg). On a patient record basis of the 45 estimates, the correlation coefficient was 0.92, reflecting the fact that the average ICP covers a range of about 75 mmHg across these records, whereas the SDE was under 6 mmHg.

The ability of the method to correctly identify elevated ICP was tested for the 2665 data pairs, considering a nICP threshold of 20 mmHg. The estimates presented a sensitivity of 83% and a specificity of 70%. A full receiver operating characteristic was obtained by varying the nICP threshold from 0 to 100 mmHg. This resulted in an AUC of 0.83. This procedure was repeated on a patient record basis using the threshold of 20 mmHg, and the sensitivity and specificity were 90% and 80%, respectively. In this case, the ROC analysis, also obtained by varying the nICP threshold, had an AUC of 0.88.

8.4.3 Models Based on Non-linear Models Between Arterial Blood Pressure and Cerebral Blood Flow Velocity

8.4.3.1 Modified $nICP_{BB}$

The previously described black-box model for ICP estimation [29] adopts a linear relationship among ABP, ICP and FV. Xu et al. [33], assuming that the relationships among these three signals are more complex than linear models and consequently not adequate to depict the relationship between $\boldsymbol{f}$ and $\boldsymbol{w}$ coefficients, investigated the adoption of several non-linear regression approaches. Considering that non-linear regressions, such as support vector machines (SVM) [34] and kernel spectral regression (KSR) [35], have been proved to be more powerful for the prediction problem than the linear ones [36, 37], the authors proposed using these approaches to model the relationship between coefficients $\boldsymbol{f}$ and $\boldsymbol{w}$.

Modified $nICP_{BB}$ showed that the mean ICP error by the non-linear approaches could be reduced to below 6 mmHg compared to 6.70 mmHg of the original approach. Moreover, the ICP estimation error by the proposed non-linear kernel approaches was statistically smaller ($p < 0.05$) than that obtained with the original linear model.

8.4.3.2 Data Mining

Hu et al. [38] initially proposed an innovative data mining framework for nICP assessment. The proposed framework explores the rules of deriving ICP from ABP and FV that are captured by a signal database without using a mathematical model. The main strategy of this framework is to provide a mapping function to quantify the uncertainty of an ICP estimate associated with each database entry, and to use this information to determine the best entry to build an ICP simulation model for an optimal ICP estimation. It achieved significant improvements regarding ICP simulation accuracy. In comparison to $nICP_{BB}$, for example, the proposed method presented a median normalised prediction error for ICP of 39% compared to 51% of $nICP_{BB}$, and its median correlation coefficient between estimated and measured normalised ICP was 0.80 compared to 0.35 of $nICP_{BB}$.

In another work, Kim et al. [39] aimed at adopting a new (linear and non-linear combination) mapping functions into the previous data mining framework to demonstrate that the performance of nICP assessment could be improved by utilising proper mapping functions. The new framework used a database of simultaneously recorded signals (ABP, FV and ICP) and dynamic models of the signals (inputs: ABP and FV, output: ICP). Two types of relevant data are drawn from this database: haemodynamic features and dissimilarity measures. Haemodynamic features are extracted from ABP and FV to capture the characteristic aspects of the cerebral haemodynamic state. Dissimilarity measures are calculated as the distance between actual ICP and its estimates, obtained by simulating the dynamic models in the database. This approach quantifies how closely each dynamic model can estimate actual ICP only using the corresponding ABP/FV signals.

The main strategy of the data mining framework is to formulate a mapping function between haemodynamic features and dissimilarity measures. The results demonstrated that a non-linear mapping function significantly improves the performance of the proposed data mining framework in comparison to other linear mapping functions, showing a median ICP estimation error of 4.37 mmHg.

8.4.4 Semi-supervised Machine Learning

Kim et al. [40] introduced a non-invasive ICH detection method based on the TCD measurement of FV alone to demonstrate its performance both in the supervised and semi-supervised learning settings.

ICH detection is a classification problem to differentiate patients with elevated ICP from those with normal (or low) ICP. The traditional approach uses only labelled samples to train a given classifier, referred to as supervised learning. The major drawback of this method is that it cannot utilise unlabelled samples even when useful information learned from them may result in the improvement of classification accuracy.

To address the ambiguity in labelling samples, the authors adopted a new classification approach, a semi-supervised learning. With this concept, labelling is not necessary since classifiers can be trained using both labelled and unlabelled samples.

Simulation results demonstrated that the predictive accuracy (AUC) of the semi-supervised method could be as high as 92%, while that of the supervised method was only around 82%. AUC of the PI-based method was as low as 59%. A decision curve analysis showed that the semi-supervised ICH detection method was not only more accurate but also clinically more useful than the supervised ICH detection method or the PI-based ICH detection method.

8.5 Optic Nerve Sheath Diameter Measurement

Increased ONSD has repeatedly been associated with elevated ICP in patients with TBI and hypoxic ischaemic injuries and suggested as a useful marker for identifying intracranial hypertension [4, 41–43]. According to a recent systematic review meta-analysis to evaluate the diagnostic accuracy of sonographic ONSD in adults [41], thresholds in the range of 4.80–6.30 mm demonstrated reliable prediction ability (AUC of 0.94) for the assessment of intracranial hypertension (considering a threshold of >20 mmHg or >25 cmH_2O). The pooled diagnostics odds ratio and positive and negative likelihood ratios also demonstrated robustness of the method, 67.5 (95% CI 29–135), 5.35 (95% CI 3.76–7.53) and 0.088 (95% CI 0.046–0.152), respectively.

Nevertheless, an ONSD cut-off value for the detection of intracranial hypertension is still under debate. Some studies even suggest that cut-off values differ in gender [44] and ethnic groups [45]. This could be explained by distinct patterns in anatomy and connective tissue elasticity on an individual basis [46]. However, most studies report this optimal cut-off in the 5.0–6.0 mm range [6, 47–49].

To complement such findings in the context of utilisation of ultrasound-based non-invasive ICP, more recently a study on the utilisation of ONSD and TCD assessments for nICP estimation applied in a clinical protocol for intracranial hypertension has demonstrated the successful management of a patient with suspected meningitis presenting with potentially raised ICP for whom invasive monitoring was contraindicated due to the risk of coagulopathy [50]. In addition, ONSD assessed at patient admission has been associated with impaired cerebral blood flow autoregulation and demonstrated reasonable prediction of sustained intracranial hypertension events during the clinical management of TBI patients [51].

Other potential applications include the evaluation of intracranial hypertension in hypoxic ischemic brain injury after cardiac arrest. In a study of Cardim et al. [42], ONSD showed a linear relationship between ICP (R = 0.53, $p < 0.0001$), with a strong ability to predict intracranial hypertension (ICP ≥20 mmHg) in this population (AUC = 0.96 (95% CI: 0.90–1.00)).

Moreover, future studies should consider the joint assessment of different parameters describing cerebral haemodynamics. For instance, it has been demonstrated that the combination of ONSD with other ultrasound modalities, like venous transcranial Doppler assessment of the straight sinus, could improve the prognostic accuracy for intracranial hypertension prediction than ONSD alone. Robba et al. [52] evaluated the combination of ONSD and straight sinus systolic flow velocity in a prediction model, showing a statistically significant improvement of AUC values compared with only ONSD (0.93 and 0.91, respectively (p = 0.01)).

8.6 Take-Home Message for Clinicians

Considering that the clinically relevant range of ICP is about 10 or 20 mmHg, the state of the art of TCD-based methods is not able to predict mean ICP values reliably since the overall intrinsic confidence interval lays around ±12 mmHg according to a recent literature review [3].

Despite the intrinsic limitations and inaccuracy to predict ICP mean absolute values, qualitative-wise, TCD-based nICP methods generally present a positive degree of agreement and acceptable correlations with measured ICP/CPP to detect changes over time. In view of this, an important concept that should be stressed is ICP is not solely an absolute value, given that dynamical features of this parameter (for instance, pulse waveform and relative changes in time) are important for a complete clinical assessment [53].

As indicated in other chapters of this book, the assessment of TCCD-derived indices and imaging findings of the intracranial anatomy may provide important bedside information regarding the onset and evolution of cerebrovascular conditions. Particularly, the sonographic measurement of ONSD can be potentially useful for identifying intracranial hypertension (present/absent) when invasive monitoring methods are not unavailable or contraindicated.

8.7 Final Remarks

Brain ultrasonography through TCD and ONSD assessments is a versatile technique for nICP estimation. However, the variability in accuracy presented by different methods precludes their use for diagnostic purposes. Despite these intrinsic limitations, ultrasound-based nICP methods may have a potential utility as an ancillary clinical tool since this technique allows the non-invasive assessment of cerebral circulation dynamics as ICP changes over time, with the possibility to track nICP/nCPP changes in real time in a variety of clinical settings (emergency rooms, ambulatories, operating theatres, etc.).

References

1. Klingelhöfer J, Conrad B, Benecke R, et al. Evaluation of intracranial pressure from transcranial Doppler studies in cerebral disease. J Neurol. 1988;235:159–62.
2. Czosnyka M, Richards HK, Whitehouse HE, Pickard JD. Relationship between transcranial Doppler-determined pulsatility index and cerebrovascular resistance: an experimental study. J Neurosurg. 1996;84:79–84. https://doi.org/10.3171/jns.1996.84.1.0079.
3. Cardim D, Robba C, Bohdanowicz M, et al. Non-invasive monitoring of intracranial pressure using transcranial Doppler ultrasonography: is it possible? Neurocrit Care. 2016; https://doi.org/10.1007/s12028-016-0258-6.
4. Geeraerts T, Launey Y, Martin L, et al. Ultrasonography of the optic nerve sheath may be useful for detecting raised intracranial pressure after severe brain injury. Intensive Care Med. 2007;33:1704–11. https://doi.org/10.1007/s00134-007-0797-6.
5. Geeraerts T, Merceron S, Benhamou D, et al. Non-invasive assessment of intracranial pressure using ocular sonography in neurocritical care patients. Intensive Care Med. 2008;34:2062–7. https://doi.org/10.1007/s00134-008-1149-x.
6. Dubourg J, Javouhey E, Geeraerts T, et al. Ultrasonography of optic nerve sheath diameter for detection of raised intracranial pressure: a systematic review and meta-analysis. Intensive Care Med. 2011;37:1059–68. https://doi.org/10.1007/s00134-011-2224-2.
7. Gosling RG, King DH. Arterial assessment by Doppler-shift ultrasound. Proc R Soc Med. 1974;67:447–9.
8. De Riva N, Budohoski KP, Smielewski P, et al. Transcranial doppler pulsatility index: what it is and what it isn't. Neurocrit Care. 2012;17:58–66. https://doi.org/10.1007/s12028-012-9672-6.
9. Nicoletto HA, Burkman MH. Transcranial Doppler series part III: interpretation. Am J Electroneurodiagnostic Technol. 2009;49:244–59.
10. Nicoletto HA, Burkman MH. Transcranial Doppler series part IV: case studies. Am J Electroneurodiagnostic Technol. 2009;49:342–60.
11. Tegeler CH, Crutchfield K, Katsnelson M, et al. Transcranial doppler velocities in a large, healthy population. J Neuroimaging. 2013;23:466–72. https://doi.org/10.1111/j.1552-6569.2012.00711.x.
12. Aaslid R, Lindegaard KF, Lundar T, et al. Estimation of cerebral perfusion pressure from arterial blood pressure and transcranial Doppler recordings. In: Miller JD, Teasdale GM R, JO et al. (eds) Intracranial Pressure VI. Berlin: SpringerVerlag; 1986. p. 226–9.
13. Greenfield JC, Tindall GT. Effect of acute increase in intracranial pressure on blood flow in the internal carotid artery of man. J Clin Invest. 1965;44:1343–51. https://doi.org/10.1172/JCI105239.

14. Czosnyka M, Matta BF, Smielewski P, et al. Cerebral perfusion pressure in head-injured patients: a noninvasive assessment using transcranial Doppler ultrasonography. J Neurosurg. 1998;88:802–8. https://doi.org/10.3171/jns.1998.88.5.0802.
15. Chan KH, Miller JD, Dearden NM, et al. The effect of changes in cerebral perfusion pressure upon middle cerebral artery blood flow velocity and jugular bulb venous oxygen saturation after severe brain injury. J Neurosurg. 1992;77:55–61. https://doi.org/10.3171/jns.1992.77.1.0055.
16. Edouard AR, Vanhille E, Le Moigno S, et al. Noninvasive assessment of cerebral perfusion pressure in brain injured patients with moderate intracranial hypertension. Br J Anaesth. 2005;94:216–21. https://doi.org/10.1093/bja/aei034.
17. Belfort MA, Tooke-Miller C, Varner M, et al. Evaluation of a noninvasive transcranial Doppler and blood pressure-based method for the assessment of cerebral perfusion pressure in pregnant women. Hypertens Pregnancy. 2000;19:331–40.
18. Varsos GV, Kolias AG, Smielewski P, et al. A noninvasive estimation of cerebral perfusion pressure using critical closing pressure. J Neurosurg. 2015;11 https://doi.org/10.3171/2014.10.JNS14613.Disclosure.
19. Nichol J, Girling F, Jerrard W, et al. Fundamental instability of the small blood vessels and critical closing pressures in vascular beds. Am J Phys. 1951;164:330–44.
20. Czosnyka M, Richards H, Pickard JD, et al. Frequency-dependent properties of cerebral blood transport—an experimental study in anaesthetized rabbits. Ultrasound Med Biol. 1994;20:391–9. https://doi.org/10.1016/0301-5629(94)90008-6.
21. Michel E, Hillebrand S, vonTwickel J, et al. Frequency dependence of cerebrovascular impedance in preterm neonates: a different view on critical closing pressure. J Cereb Blood Flow Metab. 1997;17:1127–31. https://doi.org/10.1097/00004647-199710000-00015.
22. Puppo C, Camacho J, Yelicich B, et al. Bedside study of cerebral critical closing pressure in patients with severe traumatic brain injury: a transcranial Doppler study. Acta Neurochir Suppl. 2012;114:283–8. https://doi.org/10.1007/978-3-7091-0956-4_55.
23. Varsos GV, Richards H, Kasprowicz M, et al. Critical closing pressure determined with a model of cerebrovascular impedance. J Cereb Blood Flow Metab. 2013;33:235–43. https://doi.org/10.1038/jcbfm.2012.161.
24. Abecasis F, Cardim D, Czosnyka M, et al. Transcranial Doppler as a non-invasive method to estimate cerebral perfusion pressure in children with severe traumatic brain injury. Childs Nerv Syst. 2019; https://doi.org/10.1007/s00381-019-04273-2.
25. Ursino M, Di Giammarco P. A mathematical model of the relationship between cerebral blood volume and intracranial pressure changes: the generation of plateau waves. Ann Biomed Eng. 1991;19:15–42. https://doi.org/10.1007/BF02368459.
26. Ursino M, Lodi CA. A simple mathematical model of the interaction between intracranial pressure and cerebral hemodynamics. J Appl Physiol. 1997;82:1256–69.
27. Czosnyka M, Piechnik S, Richards HK, et al. Contribution of mathematical modelling to the interpretation of bedside tests of cerebrovascular autoregulation. J Neurol Neurosurg Psychiatry. 1997;63:721–31. https://doi.org/10.1136/JNNP.63.6.721.
28. Kashif FM, Verghese GC, Novak V, et al. Model-based noninvasive estimation of intracranial pressure from cerebral blood flow velocity and arterial pressure. Sci Transl Med. 2012;4:129ra44. https://doi.org/10.1126/scitranslmed.3003249.
29. Schmidt B, Klingelhöfer J, Schwarze JJ, et al. Noninvasive prediction of intracranial pressure curves using transcranial Doppler ultrasonography and blood pressure curves. Stroke. 1997;28:2465–72. https://doi.org/10.1161/01.STR.28.12.2465.
30. Kasuga Y, Nagai H, Hasegawa Y, Nitta M. Transmission characteristics of pulse waves in the intracranial cavity of dogs. J Neurosurg. 1987;66:907–14. https://doi.org/10.3171/jns.1987.66.6.0907.
31. Marmarelis PMV. Analysis of physiological systems. New York: Plenum Press; 1978.
32. Kashif FM, Heldt T, Verghese GC. Model-based estimation of intracranial pressure and cerebrovascular autoregulation. Comput Cardiol. 2008;35:369–72. https://doi.org/10.1109/CIC.2008.4749055.
33. Xu P, Kasprowicz M, Bergsneider M, Hu X. Improved noninvasive intracranial pressure assessment with nonlinear kernel regression. IEEE Trans Inf Technol Biomed. 2010;14:971–8. https://doi.org/10.1109/TITB.2009.2027317.
34. Lin C-J. Formulations of support vector machines: a note from an optimization point of view. Neural Comput. 2001;13:307–17. https://doi.org/10.1162/089976601300014547.
35. Cai D, He X, Han J. Spectral regression for efficient regularized subspace learning. Proc IEEE Int Conf Comput Vis. 2007; https://doi.org/10.1109/ICCV.2007.4408855.
36. Melgani F, Bazi Y. Classification of electrocardiogram signals with support vector machines and particle swarm optimization. IEEE Trans Inf Technol Biomed. 2008;12:667–77. https://doi.org/10.1109/TITB.2008.923147.
37. Bates DM, Watts DG. Nonlinear regression analysis and its applications: Wiley; 2007. http://eu.wiley.com/WileyCDA/WileyTitle/productCd-0470139005.html. Accessed 9 Sep 2015
38. Hu X, Nenov V, Bergsneider M, Martin N. A data mining framework of noninvasive intracranial pressure assessment. Biomed Signal Process Control. 2006;1:64–77. https://doi.org/10.1016/j.bspc.2006.05.003.
39. Kim S, Scalzo F, Bergsneider M, et al. Noninvasive intracranial pressure assessment based on a data-mining approach using a nonlinear mapping function.

IEEE Trans Biomed Eng. 2012;59:619–26. https://doi.org/10.1109/TBME.2010.2093897.

40. Kim S, Hamilton R, Pineles S, et al. Noninvasive intracranial hypertension detection utilizing semisupervised learning. IEEE Trans Biomed Eng. 2013;60:1126–33. https://doi.org/10.1109/TBME.2012.2227477.
41. Robba C, Santori G, Czosnyka M, et al. Optic nerve sheath diameter measured sonographically as non-invasive estimator of intracranial pressure: a systematic review and meta-analysis. Intensive Care Med. 2018;44:1284–94. https://doi.org/10.1007/s00134-018-5305-7.
42. Cardim D, Griesdale DE, Ainslie PN, et al. A comparison of non-invasive versus invasive measures of intracranial pressure in hypoxic ischaemic brain injury after cardiac arrest. Resuscitation. 2019; https://doi.org/10.1016/j.resuscitation.2019.01.002.
43. Robba C, Goffi A, Geeraerts T, et al. Brain ultrasonography: methodology, basic and advanced principles and clinical applications. A narrative review. Intensive Care Med. 2019;45:913–27. https://doi.org/10.1007/s00134-019-05610-4.
44. Goeres P, Zeiler FA, Unger B, et al. Ultrasound assessment of optic nerve sheath diameter in healthy volunteers. J Crit Care. 2016;31:168–71. https://doi.org/10.1016/j.jcrc.2015.10.009.
45. Maude RR, Hossain MA, Hassan MU, et al. Transorbital sonographic evaluation of normal optic nerve sheath diameter in healthy volunteers in Bangladesh. PLoS One. 2013; https://doi.org/10.1371/journal.pone.0081013.
46. Hansen HC, Helmke K. The subarachnoid space surrounding the optic nerves. An ultrasound study of the optic nerve sheath. Surg Radiol Anat. 1996;18:323–8. https://doi.org/10.1007/BF01627611.
47. Ebraheim AM, Mourad HS, Kishk NA, et al. Sonographic assessment of optic nerve and ophthalmic vessels in patients with idiopathic intracranial hypertension. Neurol Res. 2018; https://doi.org/10.1080/01616412.2018.1473097.
48. Kimberly HH, Shah S, Marill K, Noble V. Correlation of optic nerve sheath diameter with direct measurement of intracranial pressure. Acad Emerg Med. 2008;15:201–4. https://doi.org/10.1111/j.1553-2712.2007.00031.x.
49. Soldatos T, Karakitsos D, Chatzimichail K, et al. Optic nerve sonography in the diagnostic evaluation of adult brain injury. Crit Care. 2008;12:R67. cc6897 [pii]\r10.1186/cc6897
50. Sheehan JR, Liu X, Donnelly J, et al. Clinical application of non-invasive intracranial pressure measurements. Br J Anaesth. 2018; https://doi.org/10.1016/j.bja.2018.04.017.
51. Robba C, Donnelly J, Cardim D, et al. Optic nerve sheath diameter ultrasonography at admission as a predictor of intracranial hypertension in traumatic brain injured patients: a prospective observational study. J Neurosurg. 2019:1–7. https://doi.org/10.3171/2018.11.JNS182077.
52. Robba C, Cardim D, Tajsic T, et al. Ultrasound non-invasive measurement of intracranial pressure in neurointensive care: a prospective observational study. PLoS Med. 2017;14:e1002356. https://doi.org/10.1371/journal.pmed.1002356.
53. Czosnyka M, Smielewski P, Timofeev I, et al. Intracranial pressure: more than a number. Neurosurg Focus. 2007;22:E10. https://doi.org/10.3171/foc.2007.22.5.11.
54. Steiger HJ. Carotid Doppler hemodynamics in posttraumatic intracranial hypertension. Surg Neurol. 1981;16:459–61.
55. Homburg AM, Jakobsen M, Enevoldsen E. Transcranial Doppler recordings in raised intracranial pressure. Acta Neurol Scand. 1993;87:488–93. https://doi.org/10.1111/j.1600-0404.1993.tb04142.x.
56. Martin NA, Patwardhan RV, Alexander MJ, et al. Characterization of cerebral hemodynamic phases following severe head trauma: hypoperfusion, hyperemia, and vasospasm. J Neurosurg. 1997;87:9–19. https://doi.org/10.3171/jns.1997.87.1.0009.
57. McQuire JC, Sutcliffe JC, Coats TJ. Early changes in middle cerebral artery blood flow velocity after head injury. J Neurosurg. 1998;89:526–32. https://doi.org/10.3171/jns.1998.89.4.0526.
58. Moreno JA, Mesalles E, Gener J, et al. Evaluating the outcome of severe head injury with transcranial Doppler ultrasonography. Neurosurg Focus. 2000;8:e8.
59. Rainov NG, Weise JB, Burkert W. Transcranial Doppler sonography in adult hydrocephalic patients. Neurosurg Rev. 2000; https://doi.org/10.1007/s101430050029.
60. Asil T, Uzunca I, Utku U, Berberoglu U. Monitoring of increased intracranial pressure resulting from cerebral edema with transcranial Doppler sonography in patients with middle cerebral artery infarction. J Ultrasound Med. 2003;22:1049–53.
61. Bellner J, Romner B, Reinstrup P, et al. Transcranial Doppler sonography pulsatility index (PI) reflects intracranial pressure (ICP). Surg Neurol. 2004;62:45–51. https://doi.org/10.1016/j.surneu.2003.12.007.
62. Voulgaris SG, Partheni M, Kaliora H, et al. Early cerebral monitoring using the transcranial Doppler pulsatility index in patients with severe brain trauma. Med Sci Monit. 2005;11:CR49-R52.
63. Behrens A, Lenfeldt N, Ambarki K, et al. Transcranial Doppler pulsatility index: not an accurate method to assess intracranial pressure. Neurosurgery. 2010;66:1050–7. https://doi.org/10.1227/01.NEU.0000369519.35932.F2.
64. Figaji AA, Zwane E, Fieggen AG, et al. Transcranial Doppler pulsatility index is not a reliable indicator of intracranial pressure in children with severe traumatic brain injury. Surg Neurol. 2009;72:389–94. https://doi.org/10.1016/j.surneu.2009.02.012.
65. Brandi G, Béchir M, Sailer S, et al. Transcranial color-coded duplex sonography allows to assess cerebral perfusion pressure noninvasively following severe

traumatic brain injury. Acta Neurochir. 2010;152:965–72. https://doi.org/10.1007/s00701-010-0643-4.
66. Melo JRT, Di Rocco F, Blanot S, et al. Transcranial Doppler can predict intracranial hypertension in children with severe traumatic brain injuries. Childs Nerv Syst. 2011;27:979–84. https://doi.org/10.1007/s00381-010-1367-8.
67. Zweifel C, Czosnyka M, Carrera E, et al. Reliability of the blood flow velocity pulsatility index for assessment of intracranial and cerebral perfusion pressures in head-injured patients. Neurosurgery. 2012;71:853–61. https://doi.org/10.1227/NEU.0b013e3182675b42.
68. Wakerley BR, Kusuma Y, Yeo LLL, et al. Usefulness of transcranial Doppler-derived cerebral hemodynamic parameters in the noninvasive assessment of intracranial pressure. J Neuroimaging. 2014:1–6. https://doi.org/10.1111/jon.12100.
69. Wakerley B, Yohana K, Luen Teoh H, et al. Non-invasive intracranial pressure monitoring with transcranial Doppler in a patient with progressive cerebral venous sinus thrombosis. J Neuroimaging. 2014;24:302–4. https://doi.org/10.1111/j.1552-6569.2012.00745.x.
70. O'Brien NF, Maa T, Reuter-Rice K. Noninvasive screening for intracranial hypertension in children with acute, severe traumatic brain injury. J Neurosurg Pediatr. 2015:1–6. https://doi.org/10.3171/2015.3.PEDS14521.
71. Schmidt EA, Czosnyka M, Gooskens I, et al. Preliminary experience of the estimation of cerebral perfusion pressure using transcranial Doppler ultrasonography. J Neurol Neurosurg Psychiatry. 2001;70:198–204. https://doi.org/10.1136/jnnp.70.2.198.
72. Gura M, Silav G, Isik N, Elmaci I. Noninvasive estimation of cerebral perfusion pressure with transcranial doppler ultrasonography in traumatic brain injury. Turk Neurosurg. 2012;22:411–5. https://doi.org/10.5137/1019-5149.JTN.4201-11.1.
73. Rasulo FA, Bertuetti R, Robba C, et al. The accuracy of transcranial Doppler in excluding intracranial hypertension following acute brain injury: a multicenter prospective pilot study. Crit Care. 2017;21:44. https://doi.org/10.1186/s13054-017-1632-2.
74. Cardim D, Robba C, Czosnyka M, et al. Noninvasive intracranial pressure estimation with transcranial Doppler: a prospective observational study. J Neurosurg Anesthesiol. 2019;1 https://doi.org/10.1097/ANA.0000000000000622.
75. Schmidt B, Czosnyka M, Schwarze JJ, et al. Evaluation of a method for noninvasive intracranial pressure assessment during infusion studies in patients with hydrocephalus. J Neurosurg. 2000;92:793–800. https://doi.org/10.3171/jns.2000.92.5.0793.
76. Schmidt B, Czosnyka M, Klingelhöfer J. Clinical applications of a non-invasive ICP monitoring method. Eur J Ultrasound. 2002;16:37–45. https://doi.org/10.1016/S0929-8266(02)00044-7.
77. Schmidt B, Czosnyka M, Raabe A, et al. Adaptive noninvasive assessment of intracranial pressure and cerebral autoregulation. Stroke. 2003;34:84–9. https://doi.org/10.1161/01.STR.0000047849.01376.AE.

9 Cerebral Perfusion: Practical Contributions of Transcranial Doppler at Bedside

Carla B. Rynkowski and Marcel J. Aries

Contents

9.1 Introduction

The use of Doppler ultrasound to estimate cerebral blood flow velocity (CBFV) was described in 1960 but it was only in the 1980s that it was appreciated that sufficient ultrasound would pass through the skull to allow the detection of cerebral blood flow (CBF) within the intracranial circulation. Transcranial Doppler (TCD) is an ultrasonographic noninvasive method of bedside neurological evaluation applied in a wide spectrum of elective and urgent intensive care unit (ICU) circumstances. It has the limitation of not measuring directly the CBF as the diameter of the insonated vessels is unknown. It detects the velocity of the red blood cell (CBFV) movement in the large vessels of circle of Willis [1, 2]. It offers—in a semicontinuous way—detection of

C. B. Rynkowski
Intensive Care Unit, Cristo Redentor Hospital, Porto Alegre, Brazil

M. J. Aries (✉)
Department of Intensive Care, University of Maastricht, Maastricht University Medical Centre, Maastricht, The Netherlands
e-mail: marcel.aries@mumc.nl

C. Robba, G. Citerio (eds.), *Echography and Doppler of the Brain*,
https://doi.org/10.1007/978-3-030-48202-2_9

dynamic perfusion changes and calculation of perfusion-related vasoreactivity, autoregulation, and/or brain compliance indices without requiring transport of potentially unstable patient [3]. The Doppler spectral pattern acquired by classical ("blind" method) TCD or B-mode transcranial color-coded duplex sonography (TCCD) provides vital information regarding different arterial segments' flow characteristics.

Blood flow in the basal cerebral arteries has a prominent diastolic component and reflects the downstream vascular resistance. The systolic component depends on upstream determinants like the cardiac output, carotid blood flow, and arterial blood pressure (ABP). For applications in emergency settings, point-of-care testing may be limited to middle cerebral artery (MCA) measurements due to the ease of access through the temporal window, quality of the signal, and very limited (insonation) angle correction needed. The MCA carries approximately 50–60% of the ipsilateral carotid artery blood flow and thus can be taken to represent CBF to the hemisphere. The mean CBFV is the weighted velocity that takes into account the different velocities of the formed elements in the blood vessel insonated and decreases with low CBF [4].

CO2 reactivity provides an indirect estimate of cerebral vasoregulation using TCD CBFV, but more frequently TCD has been used to estimate cerebral autoregulation directly. Classical methods of determining cerebral autoregulation usually require complex measurements of CBF, and manipulation of ABP with pharmacological agents. A direct estimate can also be obtained by comparing the rate of change of CBFV with that of ABP, after a sudden (induced by inflation and deflation of tight cuffs) step reduction in ABP. All these manipulations—CO2, induced changes by medications, and tight cuffs—are not well tolerated in ICU patients [5]. Therefore, different frequency or time correlation-based methods have been studied for the influence of "spontaneous" oscillations in ABP on CBFV measurements. This relies on the assumption that the CBFV returns to baseline much more rapidly than ABP as the brain wants to keep volume and flow constant. These methods provide a unique tool to explore the importance of impaired dynamic autoregulation in different diseases. We provide some examples of the correlation-based autoregulation methods below.

9.2 TCD: Velocity or Flow?

It should always be remembered that Doppler ultrasound measures velocity rather than flow, and therefore provides an estimation of CBF only if vessel diameter of the insonated vessels remains unchanged. In the majority of TCD papers, the parochial acknowledgment of this major TCD limitation (diameter constancy) tends to read like this:

Under the assumption of a Poiseuille flow, an estimate of CBF can be obtained from the TCD measurement of the centerline velocity ("v") through

$$\mathrm{CBF}_{\mathrm{TCD}} = \frac{\pi R^2}{M}\frac{v}{2\cos\theta},$$

where R is a characteristic value of the vessel radius, M the mass of the territory under consideration (here, the territory of different circle of Willis vessels), and θ the insonation angle (i.e., the angle between the ultrasound probe and the vessel). The values of M and θ can, in principle, be estimated and corrected for using TCCD features for each patient. In particular, the θ correction is very limited for the horizontal MCA (M1 part) with flow ±180° opposite to the transducer signal (cosinus 180° = −1). The formula, in particular, illustrates the importance of the radius of the conducting artery when attempting to use CBFV as a surrogate for CBF. The quadratic dependency of the flow on the radius and the possibility of varying radii during measurement are at the origin of the most strident dismissals of CBFV as a possible surrogate for CBF. The literature has not provided a definite answer to this question [6]. Yet, over the last 8 years, more than 2000 studies have relied on measurements of CBFV for diagnostic evaluation of CBF, vasoreactivity to CO2, and autoregulatory blood pressure challenges.

The underlying assumption is that vasoreactivity of small vessels and perfusion in the corresponding vascular territory can be inferred from CBFV measurements in the larger conducting arteries of circle of Willis.

9.3 Detection of Conditions That Affect Cerebral Perfusion

Some findings of CBFV measurements—related to the spectral curve shape and related indexes—are common in different pathologies [7]. These findings detect a pathological condition that cannot allow to differentiate its etiology.

9.3.1 Noninvasive Estimation of Intracranial Pressure (ICP)

At the bedside, the cerebral perfusion pressure (CPP) is seen as the driving pressure for the global CBF and calculated as the ABP minus the ICP. Although ICP can guide patient management in the intensive care unit, it is not commonly monitored in many clinical conditions due to the invasiveness nature of the continuous monitors and their associated patients' risks (mainly infection and hemorrhage). TCD-based ICP/CPP measurements are based on approximate semiquantitative relationships between cerebrovascular hemodynamics and ICP. With increasing ICP, initially there is an increase in systolic velocity (peak systolic flow) as the ICP externally compresses cerebral vessels, causing the intraluminal diameter to narrow. Successively, diastolic flow becomes blunted, as intracranial hypertension becomes the predominant external pressure opposing forward arterial flow during diastole (Fig. 9.1). The pulsatility index (PI) is higher in this case [1, 2]. These observations can serve as an "alert" that might prelude important changes in CBF [7]. In extreme cases, ICP can exceed normal forward flow during diastole, leading to diastolic flow reversal and catastrophic ischemia. It is important to notice that PI levels are not directly related to absolute ICP numbers—because the index also depends on ABP and CO2 levels—being therefore probably much more representative of changes in CPP [3, 7]. The CBFV can also be used to estimate a noninvasive ICP (nICP) with different published formulas of varying accuracies [8].

9.3.2 Cerebral Vasospasm

Different pathological conditions—like subarachnoid hemorrhage (SAH)—are complicated by severe (transient) narrowing of the large cerebral arteries. The exact cause of this vasospasm is not known, but its presence is associated with development of delayed cerebral ischemia (DCI) due to compromised CBF. TCD can be used to detect the vessel narrowing by showing an increase in focal CBFV according to the Bernoulli principle [9]. In order to detect focal intracranial narrowing—instead of general conditions like hyperemia—the Lindegaard and Sloan ratios are used by comparing intracranial and extradural carotid and basilar artery CBFV values (Fig. 9.2). Cerebral vasospasm can be present not only in aneurysmal SAH but also in traumatic SAH as well as in traumatic brain injury (TBI) without subarachnoid blood visible on brain CT [10]. The presence of vasospasm should always be taken into consideration when reporting (changes in) cerebral perfusion in individual patients in the intensive care unit.

9.3.3 Hyperperfusion

Hyperemia is a condition of increased CBF(V) detected by TCD that does not meet the criteria of focal vasospasm [1, 2, 9]. An increase in CBFV alone is not a sufficient basis for confidently diagnosing hyperperfusion. In global hyperperfusion, the Lindegaard ratio is less than 3. Physiological conditions such as hyperemia (in combination with impaired autoregulation) due to nonconvulsive status epilepticus or hypercapnia might be suspected. Also induced systemic conditions such as severe hypertension and/or hypervolemia may lead to an increase in CBFV in SAH patients [7]. Generally, the increased CBFV is found in more than one

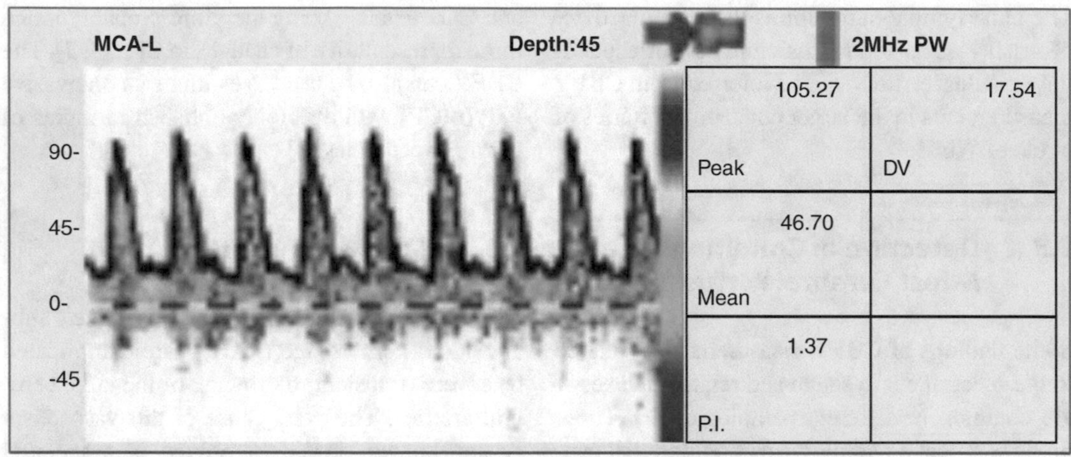

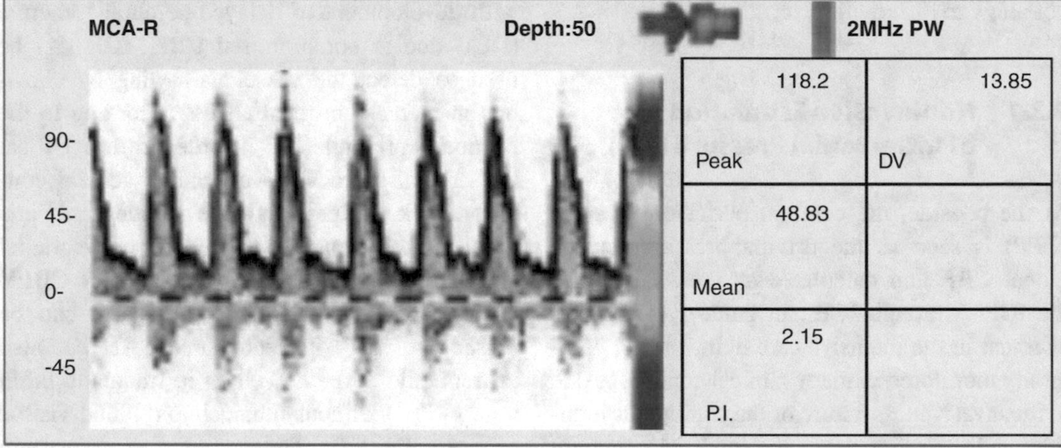

Fig. 9.1 Bilateral transcranial Doppler (TCD) recordings in middle cerebral arteries (MCA) showing high systolic, low diastolic, and high pulsatility index (PI) values. This bilateral pattern can be seen with intracranial hypertension and low cerebral perfusion state

vessel territory (Fig. 9.3A). TCD can be used for diagnosis and treatment of the postcarotid endarterectomy "hyperperfusion syndrome" which usually warrants aggressive ABP lowering [11].

9.3.4 Hypoperfusion

A reduced CBFV can be found in different conditions like severe TBI, severe intracranial hemorrhage, severe heart failure, and acute or chronic large vessel stroke (Fig. 9.3b). TCD might identify patients with initially asymptomatic vessel stenosis who cannot tolerate hypotensive periods and may develop watershed infarctions [7]. In out-of-hospital cardiac arrest (OHCA) TCD recordings may reveal individual cerebral hemodynamic patterns that are associated with worse outcome. The critical closing pressure (CrCP, mmHg) is high together with high PI and low CBFV values in the first 24 h after ictus. The CrCP of the cerebral circulation indicates the ("hypothetical") value of ABP at which CBF approaches zero and can be estimated with different TCD-based models [12]. Even short periods of hypoperfusion have been associated with worse clinical outcome and this relationship is much stronger for hypoperfusion in comparison to hyperperfusion. This suggests that individual ABP levels should be maintained at a sufficiently high level to avoid secondary ischemic brain injury.

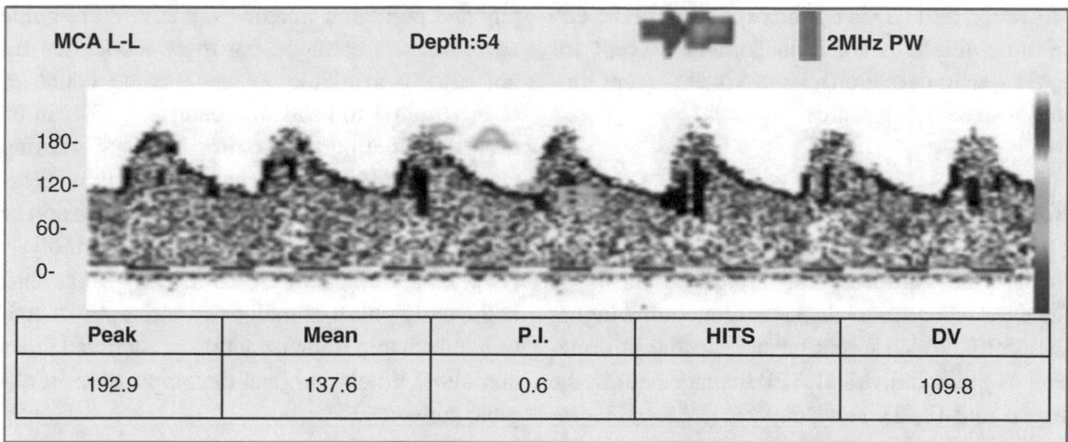

Peak	Mean	P.I.	HITS	DV
192.9	137.6	0.6		109.8

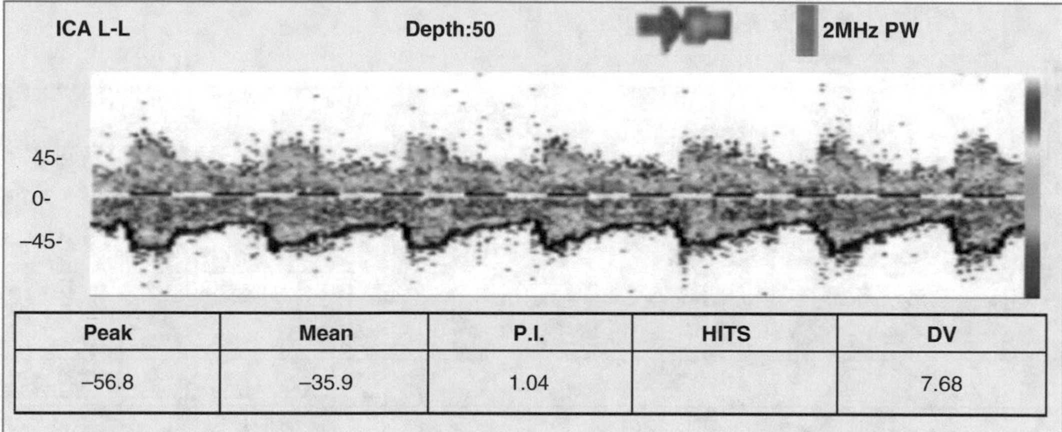

Peak	Mean	P.I.	HITS	DV
–56.8	–35.9	1.04		7.68

Fig. 9.2 Transcranial Doppler measurements in bilateral middle cerebral arteries (MCA) and distal internal carotid arteries (ICA). High mean CBFV values are found in the left MCA with normal values in the other arteries. This is suspicious for (mild) vasospasm of the left MCA

9.3.5 Brain Death

When investigating brain death, TCD/TCCD can show flow patterns that occur with cerebral circulatory arrest (Fig. 9.4). The most important pattern is the disappearance (or even negative appearance) of diastolic flow in both MCA and vertebral arteries (VA). However, these findings are only valid in patients with a neurological exam that points towards brain death [2]. TCD has a similar diagnostic power to CT angiography and EEG for brain death confirmation. In catastrophic brain injuries—before herniation—flow patterns tend to mirror the cerebral circulatory arrest pattern. Generally, it resembles situations of extreme intracranial hypertension, with an extremely high systolic CBFV and a very low diastolic CBFV.

9.4 Applications of TCD Evaluating Cerebral Perfusion in Common ICU Pathologies

In this section we provide examples on how TCD can be used in acute stroke, severe TBI, OHCA, and hepatic encephalopathy to evaluate cerebral perfusion or cerebral autoregulation.

However, as TCD is not incorporated in the different guidelines for management (except for SAH spasm detection), its use is at present limited to research practice.

9.4.1 Acute Stroke

With TCD intracerebral arterial stenosis is detected when vessel diameter reduction is higher than 50%, which might be an essential information to guide individual ABP management in the stroke unit [1, 2]. Nowadays, CT/MR angiography and perfusion imaging are advised to guide acute stroke treatment, but these modalities are not always available in low-income countries or are limited to academic centers. TCD can be used in a continuous monitoring mode—during or after IV/IA thrombolysis—to confirm successful vessel recanalization, to detect reocclusion or low-flow states, and to enhance clot fibrinolysis [13]. TCCD can be used to identify brain shift in the early phase of malignant MCA stroke and/or hemorrhagic transformation of infarcted areas and allow timely surgical decompression in eligible patients [13].

a1

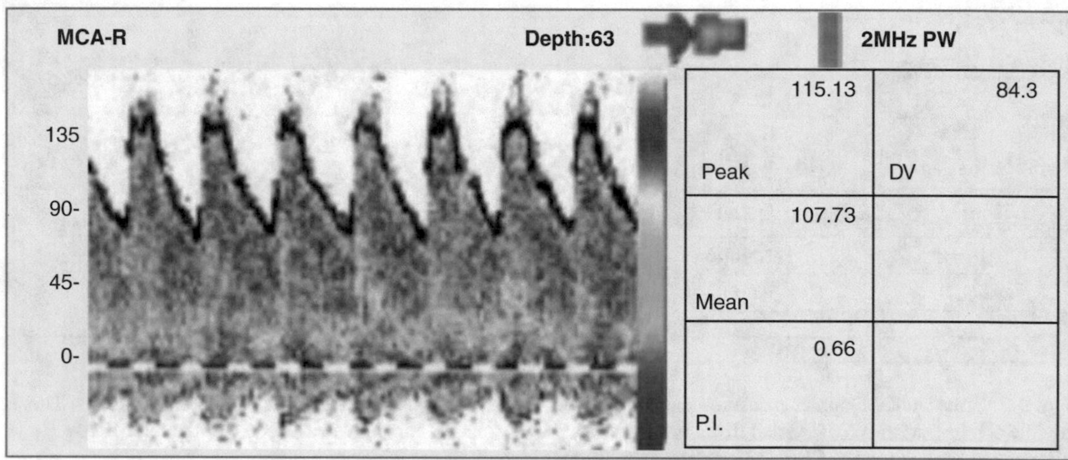

a2

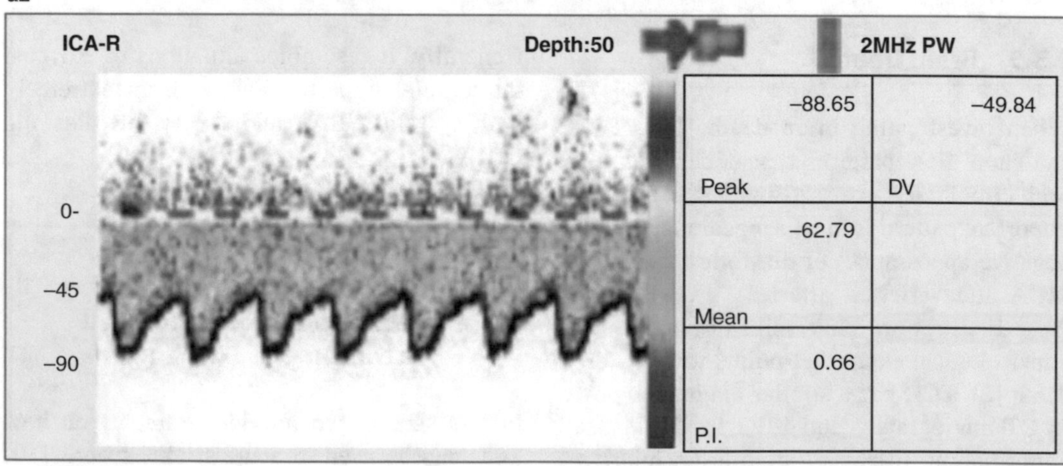

Fig. 9.3 Transcranial Doppler (TCD) measurements in patient with subarachnoid hemorrhage (SAH) (**a**) and intracerebral hemorrhage (**b**). High cerebral blood flow velocity (CBFV) values are found in the middle cerebral artery (MCA) (**a**.1) and distal internal carotid artery (dICA) (**a**.2) in SAH patient indicating hyperemia in the anterior cerebral circulation. Low CBFV values are found in both vessels (**b**.1 and **b**.2) in the intracerebral hemorrhage patient indicating low perfusion status which needs (urgent) further evaluation of its cause

b1

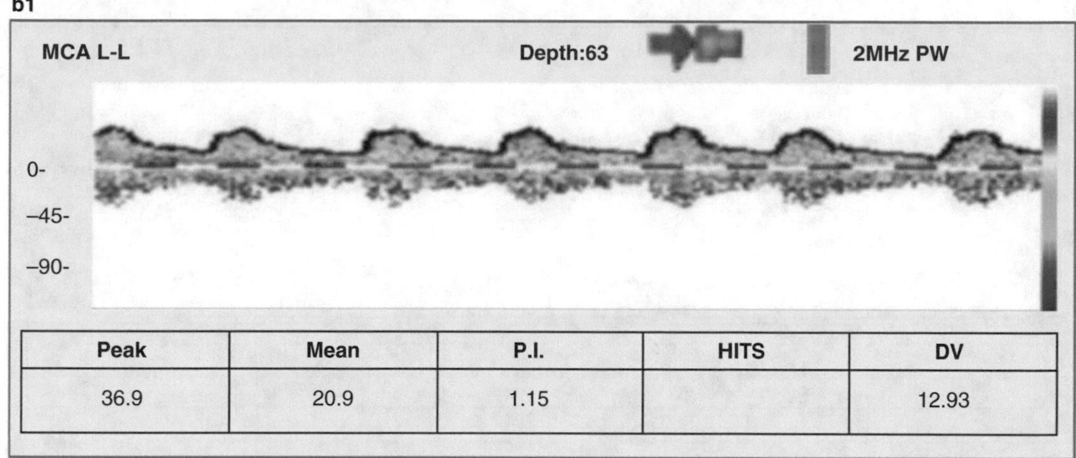

Peak	Mean	P.I.	HITS	DV
36.9	20.9	1.15		12.93

b2

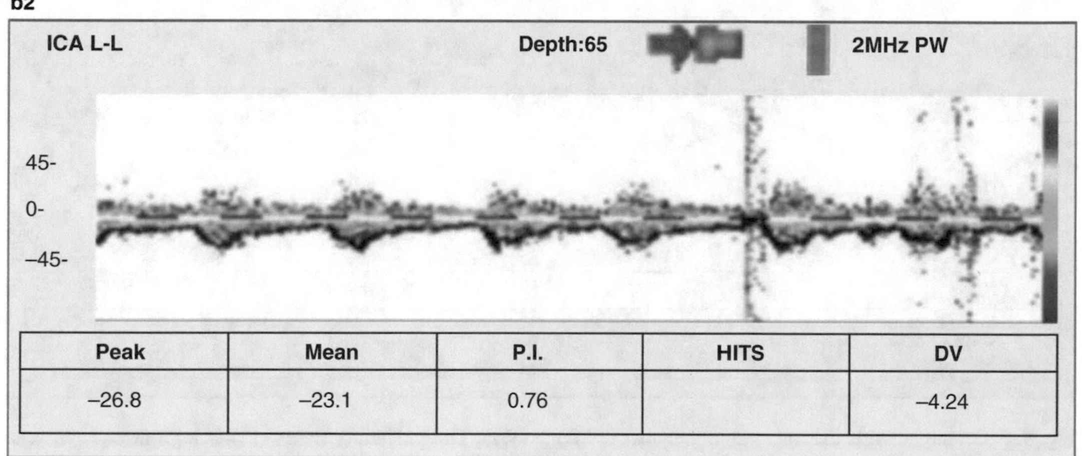

Peak	Mean	P.I.	HITS	DV
–26.8	–23.1	0.76		–4.24

Fig. 9.3 (continued)

In combination with continuous (noninvasive or invasive) ABP recordings, TCD can inform clinicians about cerebral autoregulation. Most studies relied on linear (cross-spectral or time correlation-based) methods to assess the integrity of autoregulation. Time correlation methods use a moving linear correlation between slow waves (10 s averages) of ABP and CBFV (Mxa index). A positive correlation is indicative of passive cerebral vasculature and impaired autoregulation. Zero or negative correlation is indicative of reactive vasculature and intact autoregulation [14]. Dynamic autoregulation might be impaired during the acute, subacute, and chronic stroke phase with altered CA over the infarcted side, the contralateral, or both. Impaired autoregulation is associated with clinical deterioration and poor clinical outcome [15]. Especially in comatose patients with large infarcts, neurological worsening might go unnoticed and intermittent neuromonitoring might fine-tune therapies for optimizing CBF with augmentation of ABP or regulation of CO_2 levels [16]. An “optimal” ABP range likely exists, but probably depends on an individual autoregulation variability, temporal and spatial heterogeneity of stroke pathophysiology, and stroke subtype [14].

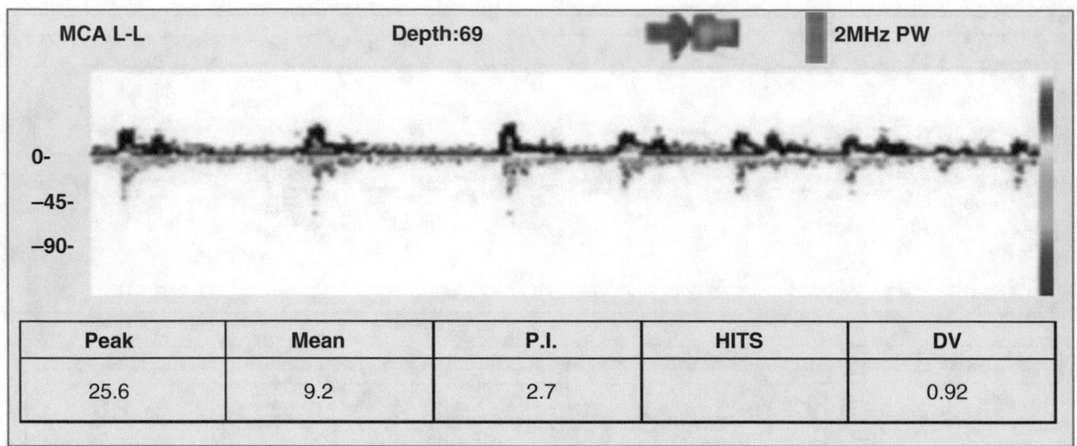

Peak	Mean	P.I.	HITS	DV
25.6	9.2	2.7		0.92

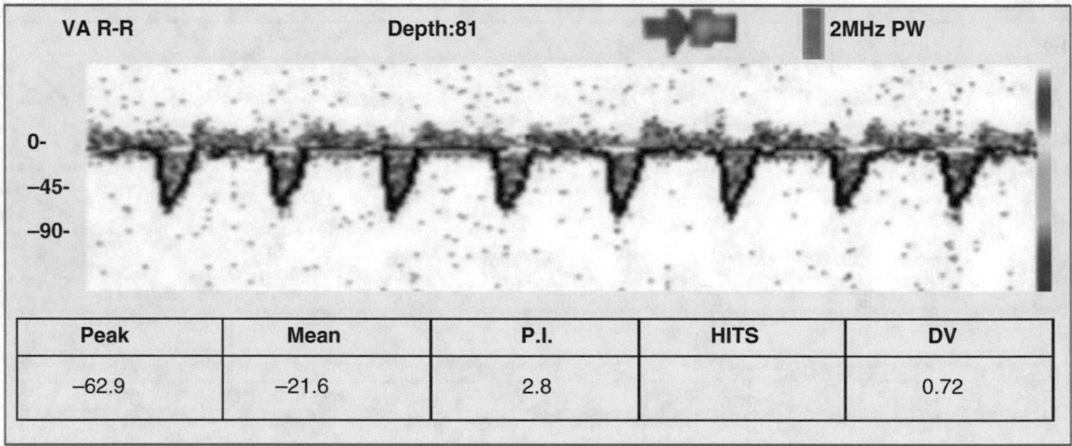

Peak	Mean	P.I.	HITS	DV
–62.9	–21.6	2.8		0.72

Fig. 9.4 On the left side the transcranial Doppler (TCD) spectrum shows a short systolic peak in the left middle cerebral artery (MCA) without diastolic flow. On the right side the same pattern is observed in the vertebral artery (VA). The pulsatility index (PI) is high in both vessels. The absence of diastolic flow is characteristic of irreversible cerebral circulatory arrest

9.4.2 Severe Traumatic Brain Injury

Although validated pharmacological interventions to treat TBI patients are still lacking, CBF manipulations and optimization remain the mainstay of therapy. However, measuring of real-time CBF changes during interventions cannot be achieved by imaging techniques. Nowadays neuromonitoring is often limited to continuous invasive ICP/CPP recordings as estimates of CBF [7]. Different TCD flow patterns have been observed during different phases after the trauma ictus. Authors have reported cerebral hypoperfusion (28%, mean CBFV < 35 cm/s), normal perfusion (45%), or vasospastic periods (27%) [17]. The abnormal patterns as well as low diastolic CBFV (defined as <20 cm/s) and high PI (defined as >1.4) are all associated with more aggressive treatments and unfavorable clinical outcome [10, 18]. Early TCD goal-directed therapy may restore normal cerebral perfusion, can detect inadvertent hypocapnia due to hyperventilation, and can limit secondary injury. The autoregulation Mx index—the moving correlation index between mean CBFV and CPP—is lower than 0.05 in patients with impaired autoregulation, whereas values greater than 0.3 reflex high dependency of CBFV on ABP [19]. Impaired cerebral autoregulation has consistently been associated with unfavorable outcome [17]. Therefore, different research groups have proposed to manipulate CPP cautiously to improve CBFV and limit secondary injury in the initial hypoperfusion phase [5]. At the moment a feasibility and effectiveness study is undertaken to guide CPP—as the driving force for CBF—by invasive autoregulation monitoring (e.g., pressure reactivity index, PRx) results in TBI patients with invasive ICP monitoring [20]. The PRx index is calculated as the moving correlation index between 10 s values of ABP and ICP. A positive phase II study might definitively extend the options for intermittent TCD monitoring and goal-directed therapy at the bedside in the near future [21]. Figure 9.5 displays an example of a multimodal monitoring recording of 4 h in a severe TBI patient with robotic TCD probe application (Fig. 9.5). An individual "optimal" CPP (CPPopt) could be estimated using both invasive ICP-derived autoregulation indices (i.e., PRx) and noninvasive TCD-derived autoregulation indices (e.g., Mx). The different autoregulation indices are plotted against 2.5 mmHg bins of CPP and with an automated curve fitting method: a CPP value with best preserved autoregulation (most negative value using these indices) can be determined and displayed at the bedside as the CPPopt value [21, 22].

9.4.3 Post-out-of-hospital Cardiac Arrest Syndrome

Despite recent improvements in the management of OHCA, the survival at hospital discharge is still below 10%. Neurological injury is not only the result of the anoxic period of cardiac arrest, but can also be exacerbated during the post-resuscitation phase due to changes in CBF [12]. Recently, it has been demonstrated with TCD and noninvasive optic nerve sheath diameter (ONSD) measurements that some patients might experience periods of intracranial hypertension that probably contributes to the low CBF state and poor outcome [23]. In that way TCD should be able to identify in advance patients under risk of generalized cerebral edema that might benefit from longer or more aggressive sedation or targeted temperature management.

Recent studies have divided the first 72 h of return after spontaneous circulation (ROSC) in three phases. Immediately after ROSC, CBFV is characterized by hyperemia for 30 min, followed by a hypoperfused phase lasting 6–12 h. The third period, from 12 to 72 h after ROSC, shows restoration of normal CBFV, increased CBFV, or persistent decreased CBF [12]. Rafi et al. reported that patients with poor neurological outcome had a lower diastolic CBFV and higher PI (CBFV 17 cm/s, PI 1.49) compared to patients with good outcome (CBFV 26 cm/s, PI 1.12), despite the absence of differences in systemic ABP. Patients who died prematurely from multiorgan failure were excluded from the outcome analysis [24]. Cerebral autoregulation status might be seen as an important explanation for the observed phases with general impairment in the initial phase and recovery in some patients in a 24–72-h period after ROSC. However, autoregulation measurements are hampered by the fact that ABP is kept very stable and therefore not able to challenge the autoregulation process.

9.4.4 Acute Liver Failure

Around half of comatose patients with acute liver failure (ALF) and hepatic encephalopathy develop intracranial hypertension with high (around 25%) mortality rates. In 80% of the patients with ALF, the brain ultrasonography will demonstrate initially hyperemia that probably precedes and/or contributes to the dangerous cerebral edema. With progressing encephalopathy low perfusion states and higher PI values dominate. Multiple mechanisms contribute to the pathogenesis, including circulating neurotoxins, systemic inflammation, and loss of cerebral autoregulation [25]. Global impaired cerebral autoregulation was found with intermittent TCD measurements in ALF patients, which recovered after hepatic function improvement or transplantation. In patients with ALF invasive ICP/CPP monitoring is not advised mainly due to lack of evidence, the associated coagulopathy, and the bad clinical condition not allowing most available ICP-lowering therapies. Recently, noninvasive ICP assessment has gained interest with intermittent estimation of ICP/CPP using

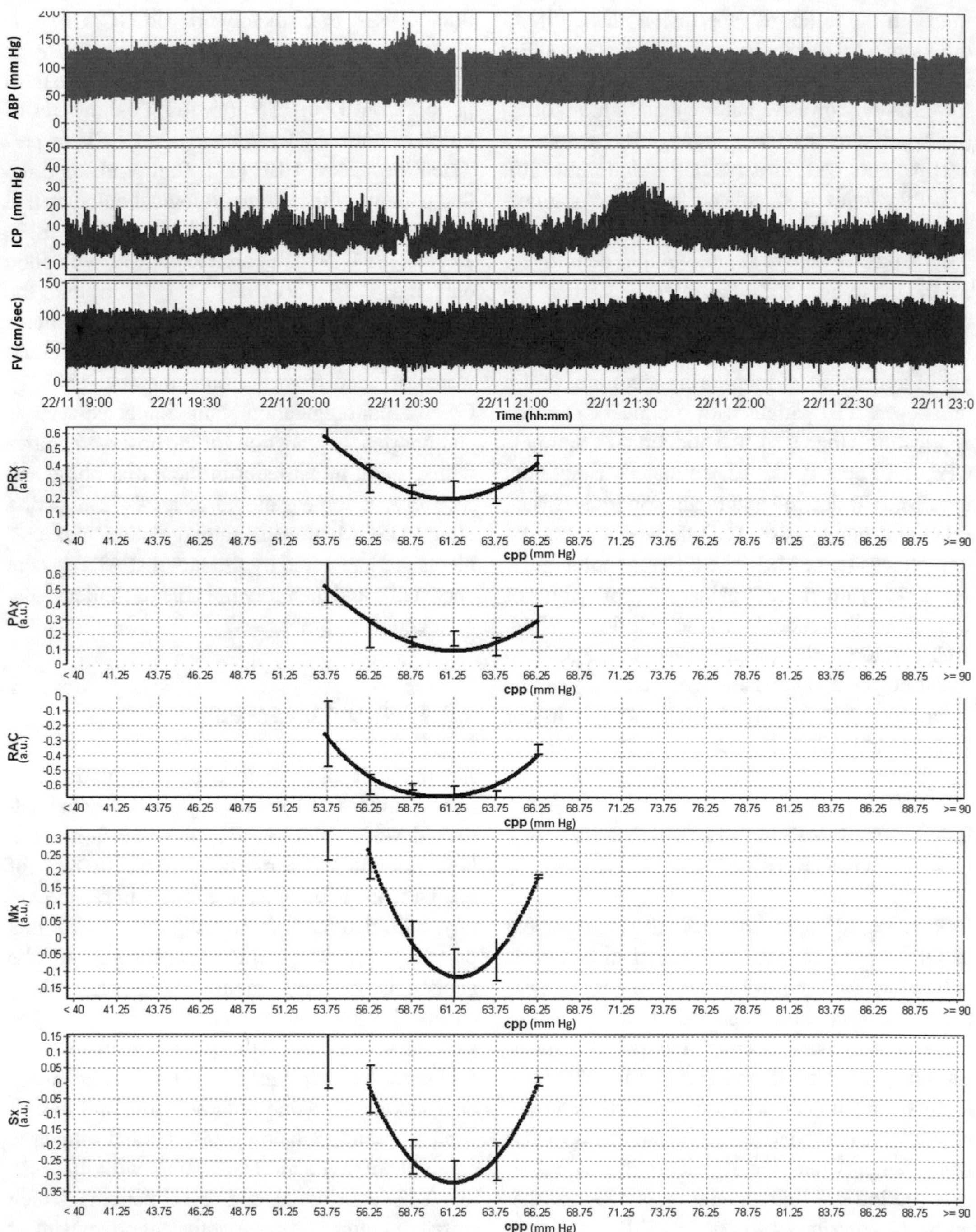

Fig. 9.5 Patient example of "optimal" CPP (CPPopt) estimation using intracranial pressure (ICP)- and transcranial Doppler (TCD)-based indices. Top 3 panels display raw (high frequency) signals for arterial blood pressure (ABP), ICP, and cerebral blood flow velocity (CBFV) over 4-h monitoring period, demonstrating stable continuous TCD recordings. The bottom five panels display CPPopt plots for (1) invasive ICP-derived autoregulation indices PRx, PAx, and RAC and (2) noninvasive TCD-derived autoregulation indices Mx and Sx. All the different autoregulation indices seem to indicate that the CPPopt is probably around 61 mmHg. Mx is calculated as the moving correlation between mean CBFV and CPP; Sx as the correlation between systolic CBFV and CPP; PAx as the moving correlation between amplitude of ICP and ABP; PRx as the moving correlation between ICP and ABP; RAC as the correlation between amplitude of ICP and CPP. TCD assessment of middle cerebral artery (MCA) CBFV was conducted via a robotic TCD system [21]

TCD parameters. The authors were able to show good negative predictive value with the applied methodology to exclude intracranial hypertension. The noninvasive measurements could be an important future bedside tool to identify intracranial hypertensive ALF patients and test out brain-protective therapies [25].

9.5 Conclusion

Both TDC and TCCD are useful to assess non-invasively individual cerebral hemodynamics in critical care patients at the bedside. Innovations like robotic probe vessel tracking might guarantee reliable measurements for longer periods and will extend the bedside applications to alarm the clinical team for hypo- and hyperperfusion periods and complications like vasospasm or autoregulation impairment. Neurological complications in critically ill patients are very common and focused assessment with TCD/TCCD is an attractive option to improve clinical management and improve clinical outcome.

References

1. Alexandrov AV, Sloan MA, Wong LK, et al. Practice standards for transcranial Doppler ultrasound: part I—test performance. J Neuroimaging. 2007;17(1):11–8.
2. Alexandrov AV, Sloan MA, Tegeler CH, et al. Practice standards for transcranial Doppler (TCD) ultrasound. Part II. Clinical indications and expected outcomes. J Neuroimaging. 2012;22(3):215–24.
3. Robba C, Cardim D, Sekhon M, Budohoski K, Czosnyka M. Transcranial Doppler: a stethoscope for the brain-neurocritical care use. J Neurosci Res. 2018;96(4):720–30.
4. Bouzat P, Oddo M, Payen JF. Transcranial Doppler after traumatic brain injury: is there a role? Curr Opin Crit Care. 2014;20(2):153–60.
5. Donnelly J, Aries MJ, Czosnyka M. Further understanding of cerebral autoregulation at the bedside: possible implications for future therapy. Expert Rev Neurother. 2015;15(2):169–85.
6. Ainslie PN, Hoiland RL. Transcranial Doppler ultrasound: valid, invalid, or both? J Appl Physiol (1985). 2014;117(10):1081–3.
7. Robba C, Goffi A, Geeraerts T, et al. Brain ultrasonography: methodology, basic and advanced principles and clinical applications. A narrative review. Intensive Care Med. 2019;45(7):913–27.
8. Rasulo FA, Bertuetti R, Robba C, et al. The accuracy of transcranial Doppler in excluding intracranial hypertension following acute brain injury: a multicenter prospective pilot study. Crit Care. 2017;21(1):44.
9. Aaslid R. Transcranial Doppler assessment of cerebral vasospasm. Eur J Ultrasound. 2002;16(1–2):3–10.
10. Ziegler D, Cravens G, Poche G, Gandhi R, Tellez M. Use of transcranial Doppler in patients with severe traumatic brain injuries. J Neurotrauma. 2017;34(1):121–7.
11. Pennekamp CW, Moll FL, de Borst GJ. The potential benefits and the role of cerebral monitoring in carotid endarterectomy. Curr Opin Anaesthesiol. 2011;24(6):693–7.
12. van den Brule JMD, van der Hoeven JG, Hoedemaekers CWE. Cerebral perfusion and cerebral autoregulation after cardiac arrest. Biomed Res Int. 2018;2018:4143636.
13. Tsivgoulis G, Alexandrov AV, Sloan MA. Advances in transcranial Doppler ultrasonography. Curr Neurol Neurosci Rep. 2009;9(1):46–54.
14. Xiong L, Liu X, Shang T, et al. Impaired cerebral autoregulation: measurement and application to stroke. J Neurol Neurosurg Psychiatry. 2017;88(6):520–31.
15. Aries MJ, Elting JW, De KJ, Kremer BP, Vroomen PC. Cerebral autoregulation in stroke: a review of transcranial Doppler studies. Stroke. 2010;41(11):2697–704.
16. Petersen NH, Silverman A, Wang A, et al. Association of personalized blood pressure targets with hemorrhagic transformation and functional outcome after endovascular stroke therapy. JAMA Neurol. 2019;76:1256.
17. Le RP, Menon DK, Citerio G, et al. Consensus summary statement of the international multidisciplinary consensus conference on multimodality monitoring in Neurocritical care: a statement for healthcare professionals from the Neurocritical Care Society and the European Society of Intensive Care Medicine. Intensive Care Med. 2014;40(9):1189–209.
18. Santbrink van H, Schouten JW, Steyerberg EW, Avezaat CJ, Maas AI. Serial transcranial Doppler measurements in traumatic brain injury with special focus on the early posttraumatic period. Acta Neurochir. 2002;144(11):1141–9.
19. Sorrentino E, Diedler J, Kasprowicz M, et al. Critical thresholds for cerebrovascular reactivity after traumatic brain injury. Neurocrit Care. 2012;16(2):258–66.
20. Beqiri E, Smielewski P, Robba C, et al. Feasibility of individualised severe traumatic brain injury management using an automated assessment of optimal cerebral perfusion pressure: the COGiTATE phase II study protocol. BMJ Open. 2019;9(9):e030727.
21. Zeiler FA, Smielewski P. Application of robotic transcranial Doppler for extended duration recording in moderate/severe traumatic brain injury: first experiences. Crit Ultrasound J. 2018;10(1):16.
22. Aries MJ, Czosnyka M, Budohoski KP, et al. Continuous determination of optimal cerebral perfu-

sion pressure in traumatic brain injury. Crit Care Med. 2012;40(8):2456–63.

23. Cardim D, Griesdale DE, Ainslie PN, et al. A comparison of non-invasive versus invasive measures of intracranial pressure in hypoxic ischaemic brain injury after cardiac arrest. Resuscitation. 2019;137:221–8.
24. Rafi S, Tadie JM, Gacouin A, et al. Doppler sonography of cerebral blood flow for early prognostication after out-of-hospital cardiac arrest: DOTAC study. Resuscitation. 2019;141:188–94.
25. Raghavan M, Marik PE. Therapy of intracranial hypertension in patients with fulminant hepatic failure. Neurocrit Care. 2006;4(2):179–89.

Part III

Pathology and Clinical Applications: Emergency Department

10 Emergency Department and Prehospital Brain US as Part of POCUS and US Multiorgan Evaluation

Gabriele Via, Tomislav Petrovic, and Frank A. Rasulo

Contents

10.1 Introduction

Despite relatively scarce publications in this specific area, transposing established or novel applications of brain ultrasound (BUS) to the very early management of the critically ill outside the specific setting of the neuro-ICU is the object of growing scientific interest and practice [1–5]. This applies to BUS both as stand-alone diagnostic test within the early clinical-diagnostic workup of acute neuro-critical patients and as part of a wider multi-organ, clinically integrated, point-of-care ultrasound (PoCUS) approach. Recent evidence shows in fact how the combination of ultrasound patterns derived from the investigation of multiple organs/apparatuses yields accurate information for diagnosis and patient management [6–10].

The bedside availability and dynamic nature of ultrasound techniques make them appealing in the emergency department and/or prehospital scenarios as potential sources of real-time information on cerebral physiology especially in:

G. Via (✉)
Cardiac Anesthesia and Intensive Care Dept., Fondazione Cardiocentro Ticino, Lugano, Switzerland
e-mail: gabriele.via@cardiocentro.org

T. Petrovic
Prehospital Emergency Medical Unit Avicenne Hospital, Bobigny, France

F. A. Rasulo
Department of Anesthesia, Critical Care and Emergency, Spedali Civili University Hospital, Piazzale Ospedali Civili, Brescia, Italy

Department of Medical and Surgical Specialties, Radiological Sciences and Public Health, University of Brescia, Brescia, Italy

C. Robba, G. Citerio (eds.), *Echography and Doppler of the Brain*,
https://doi.org/10.1007/978-3-030-48202-2_10

1. Stroke
2. Cardiac arrest, and the immediate post-cardiac arrest syndrome
3. Traumatic brain injury, with or without multiple trauma

Although yet to be proven, BUS has the potential to provide early information on brain perfusion, intracranial hypertension, and intracranial lesions in the time-sensitive prehospital and emergency department scenarios. BUS findings may thus trigger earlier treatment (e.g., second-tier ICP-directed interventions, such as hyperosmolar therapy or hyperventilation in traumatic brain injury when intracranial hypertension is detected) and faster triage (e.g., earlier activation of neurosurgery), or even guide ongoing resuscitation maneuvers (e.g., cerebral perfusion assessment during external chest compressions in cardiac arrest). The current, limited, evidence in these settings is here presented, and provides a conceptual framework for further development and validation of these applications.

10.2 BUS in Stroke

It is important to perform a concise and expeditious etiologic investigation during the initial evaluation of an acute stroke patient in order to enable early introduction of secondary prevention and treatment strategies which may potentially influence the prognosis.

It is well known that acute stroke therapy, of any type, should start as soon as possible, since it is estimated that up to two million neurons are lost per minute during ischemic stroke, strengthening the need for early diagnosis and treatment [11].

Brain ultrasound (BUS) has greatly expanded to assume an important role in the study of cerebrovascular disorders and has been suggested as a valuable tool to assist clinical investigation in the emergency department (ED) in patients with acute stroke. It is a noninvasive, portable, and fast imaging technique that, performed by experienced neurosonologists, offers reliable and reproducible information on the morphological and hemodynamic status of cervical and intracranial vessels. In this context, it can be used either for diagnostic purposes or as a guidance to treatments.

- Major BUS applications for acute ischemic stroke are represented by (Fig. 10.1):
  - Early diagnosis of stenosis
  - Evaluation of the collateral circulation
  - Monitoring of arterial recanalization during and after thrombolytic therapy
  - US-based decision-making for intra-arterial therapies and blood pressure augmentation
  - Noninvasive estimation of ICP following acute stroke
  - Sonothrombolysis guidance

Early diagnosis of stenosis. The use of BUS for the diagnosis of arterial stenosis is being more frequently applied during the very early phase following stroke symptom onset. From the ER, effort has been towards shifting initial application to the prehospital period, on the field or during transportation with air service or ambulance [12].

This is now possible due to the rapidly increasing technological development, whether it be portable laptops or digital tablets, providing new opportunities for early diagnosis before hospitalization and guaranteeing monitoring of vessel patency and possibly reducing the "door-to-needle" time of thrombolytic therapy (Figs. 10.2 and 10.3).

Monitoring arterial recanalization during and after thrombolytic therapy. Early reperfusion therapies are becoming more widely used in clinical practice. Intravenous thrombolysis with recombinant tissue plasminogen activator (rtPA), for example, is generally regarded as "first-line" therapy, and when started within 3 h of symptom onset, patients with ischemic stroke are 30% more likely to have minimal or no disability [13].

Despite its increasing use, rtPA is not normally given in the prehospital setting due mostly to the lack of imaging capabilities. Besides its use in distinguishing ischemic from hemorrhagic stroke, during this acute phase imaging would be helpful for identification of vessel and definition of the entity of occlusion.

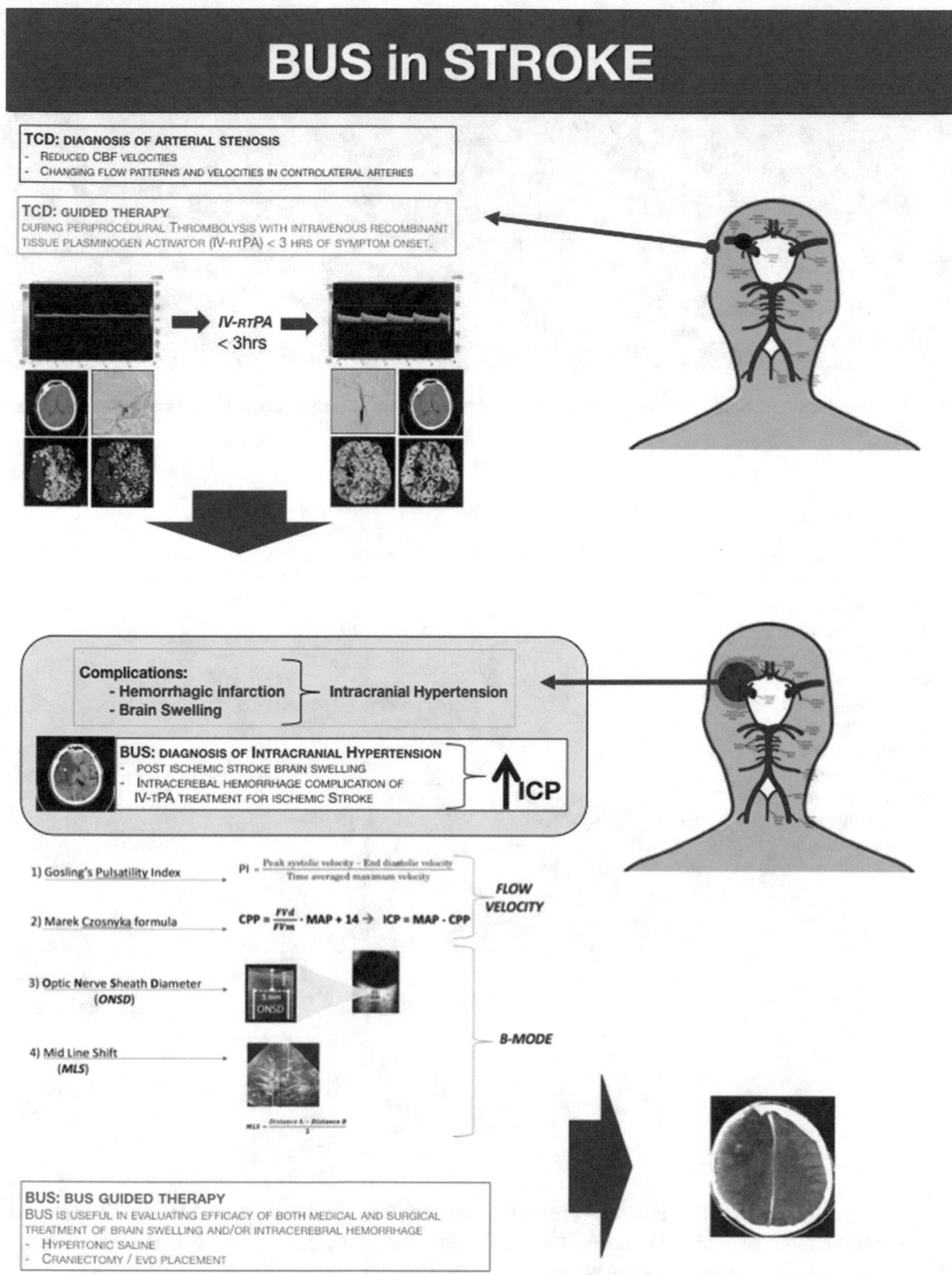

Fig. 10.1 Diagram depicting major brain ultrasound (BUS) applications in stroke management in the prehospital and emergency department settings. Modified from Robba et al. Intensive Care Medicine 2019

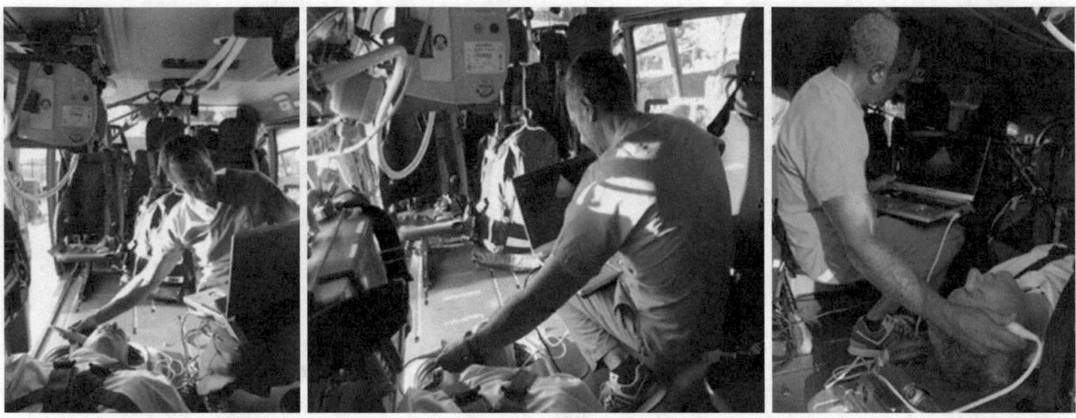

Fig. 10.2 Application scenario of early, prehospital, brain ultrasound for ischemic stroke. Pictures taken just before air transportation

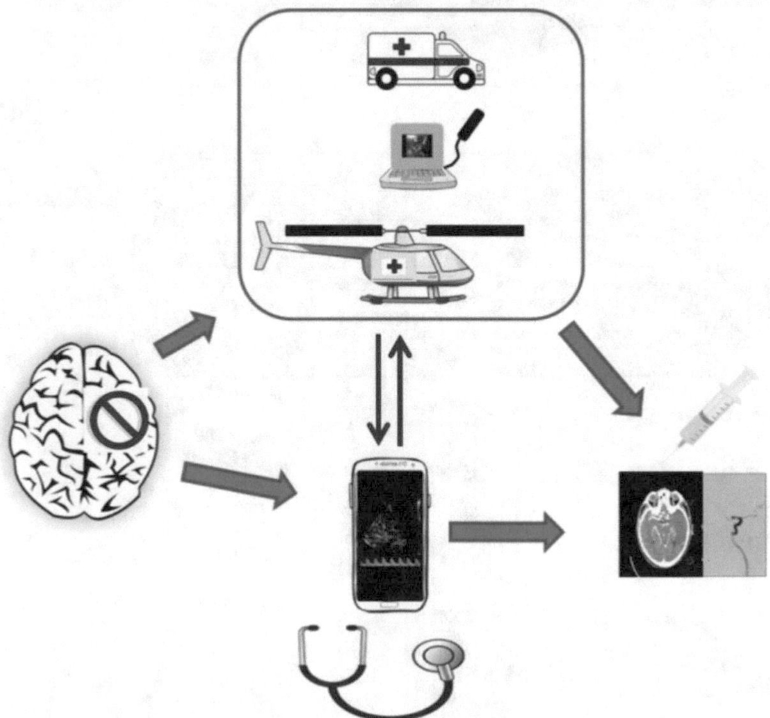

Fig. 10.3 Diagram illustrating the potential role of prehospital brain ultrasound (BUS) in the management of ischemic stroke, consistently with a "door-to-needle" time-dependent approach: BUS could hasten thrombolytic treatment, guide patient triage, and monitor noninvasively both cerebral perfusion and intracranial pressure

Within this setting, BUS may also represent a useful tool capable of verifying the efficacy of rTPA thrombolytic therapy, very early after the stroke onset. A confrontation between BUS exams of the thrombosed vessel performed before and after treatment provides important information regarding the efficacy of the procedure (Fig. 10.4). Furthermore, due to its noninvasiveness and applicability, it enables continuous bedside monitoring of patency through repeated evaluations.

Scores also exist which may help grade flow velocity and categorize the occlusion or recanalization. Two examples are the COGIF score (Consensus on Graduation of Intracranial flow) and the TIBI (Thrombolysis in Brain Ischemia)

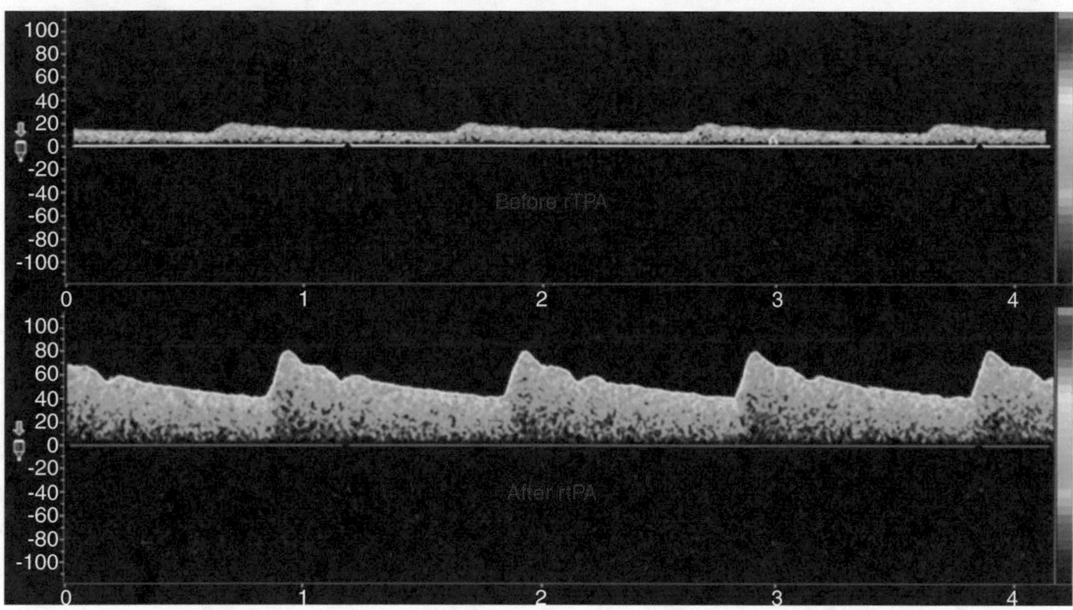

Fig. 10.4 Flow velocity of the right thrombosed MCA before (top) and after (bottom) rtPA therapy

Category	Appearance	Description
TIBI 0 COGIF 1		**ABSENT FLOW** No flow signal
TIBI 1 COGIF 2		**MINIMAL FLOW** Systolic spikes with variable velocity and duration; zero EDV; reverberating flow
TIBI 2 COGIF 3		**BLUNTED FLOW** Systolic upstroke delayed (duration >0,20 sec); EDV>0; PI<1,2
TIBI 3 COGIF 3		**DAMPENDED FLOW** Vmean decrease greater than 30% of contralateral value; upstroke normal; EDV>0
TIBI 4 COGIF 4c		**HYPEREMIC FLOW** Segmentally increased flow velocities (Vmean >80 cm/s and/or >30% compared to the control side, no turbulence; low PI; no harmonics; low degree spectral broadening.
TIBI 4 COGIF 4b		**PSEUDOSTENOTIC FLOW** Focally increased flow velocities (Vmean >30% compared to the control side; EDV>0; Significant turbulence or flow disturbance.
TIBI 5 COGIF 4a		**NORMAL FLOW** Flow velocities normal or in the range of ±%30 of the control side. [*Bar: 50 cm/sec]

COGIF grade	Hemodynamic pattern	Example
1	No flow	
2	Low flow velocities without diastolic flow	
3	Low flow velocities with diastolic flow	
4	**Established perfusion**	
	a. Flow velocities equal to contralateral side	
	b. High focal flow velocities (i.e. stenosis)	
	c. High segmental flow velocities (hyperperfusion)	

Hemodynamic Alteration	Effect on COGIF Score
1. Reflow	Improvement by ≥ 1 grade
A. Partial recanalization	
B. Complete recanalization	
2. No change	Baseline COGIF grade persists
3. Worsening	Deterioration by ≥ 1 grade

Fig. 10.5 Comparison between COGIF (Consensus on Graduation of Intracranial flow) and TIBI (Thrombolysis in Brain Ischemia) scores, which grade cerebral artery flow velocity and allow categorization of occlusion and recanalization (with permission from [15])

grade, which both provide comparable information [14] (Fig. 10.5).

Evaluation of collateral circulation. There is wide variability regarding the severity of clinical manifestations caused by the occlusion of vessels pertaining to the Willis circle, ranging from asymptomatic to fatal ischemic stroke. The collateral circulation has been recognized as an important aspect of cerebral circulation affecting the risk of stroke as well as other features of stroke presentation, such as stroke patterns in patients with cerebral arterial thrombotic disease. Through cerebrovascular autoregulation, the cerebral circulation attempts to maintain constant cerebral perfusion despite changes in systemic conditions. In case that one of the major cerebral arteries is compromised by occlusive disease, the cerebral collateral circulation plays an important role in preserving cerebral perfusion through enhanced recruitment of blood flow. With the advent of techniques, such as BUS, which allow rapid assessment of cerebral perfusion, the collateral circulation of the brain and its effectiveness may also be investigated, allowing for prompt evaluation of patients with acute stroke due to acute arterial occlusion.

TCD can determine flow patterns suggestive of collateral circulation (Fig. 10.6). In mean cerebral artery (MCA) occlusion, flow is commonly diverted from the distal internal carotid artery (ICA) to the anterior cerebral artery (ACA). This flow diversion can be detected using TCD, where typically a higher velocity flow in the ipsilateral ACA can be measured as compared with that of the contralateral ACA.

TCD is also used for the evaluation of vasomotor reactivity (VMR) to CO2, a surrogate marker of cerebrovascular reserve and autoregulation. A reduced vasoreactive response suggests impaired cerebral perfusion and poor collateral circulation [15].

BUS-based therapeutic decision-making. The first hours after an acute ischemic stroke are the most critical, when most of the treatments with greater clinical impact are applied, like the use of intravenous thrombolytics or endovascular treatments. Patients eligible for IV alteplase should receive IV alteplase even if EVTs are being considered [16]. BUS may be useful in helping other imaging techniques as demonstrated by a recent study which showed that even if patients have been already studied with advanced neuroimaging vascular techniques like brain and cervical CTA, TCD at this time provides additional information in one out of two patients, and changes in management were indicated in one out of six cases [17].

Intracranial Vessels		**Connected Arteries**	**Connecting Arteries**
Willis Circle		ICA, BA, PCA	PCoA
		ACA	ACoA
Vertebrobasilar and Willis Circle		ICA, VA, BA	Trigeminal, Hypoglossal Arteries
Tectal Plexus		PCA, SCA	Tectal rami, supra and infratentorial arteries
Cerebral Artery Branches		MCA, ACA, PCA Branches	Anastomosis of terminal branches within and between arterial territories
Leptomeningeal	Pial Plexus	Neighboring branches of the major cerebral arteries	Arterioles from branches of adjacent arteries
	Meningeal	Cerebral and Meningeal Arteries	
Extracranial Vessels		**Connected Arteries**	**Connecting Arteries**
Orbital Plexus		Ophthalmic and Middle Meningeal Maxcillary, Ethmoidal Arteries	Terminal Branches
Rete Mirabile Caroticum		ICA, ECA	

Fig. 10.6 Synopsis of the collateral cerebral circulation that can blunt the effect of main cerebral artery occlusion: arterial system (left column), corresponding to connected arteries (central column), arteries that made the connection between the former possible (right column). *ICA* internal carotid artery, *BA* basal artery, *PCA* posterior cerebral artery, *ACA* anterior cerebral artery, *VA* vertebral artery, *SCA* superior cerebellar artery, *ECA* external carotid artery, *PCoA* posterior connecting artery, *ACoA* anterior connecting artery

Although other imaging techniques are well suited to guide initial patient selection by identifying likely "responders" for reperfusion therapy by giving information on the characteristics of vessel occlusion, the collateral flow, and the extent of both hypoperfusion and established infarction, they are less effective in identifying "nonresponders" to intravenous thrombolysis [18]. However BUS has a role in guiding acute stroke therapy, where correlation is possible between ultrasonic characteristics and important clinical surrogates such as reperfusion and infarct core growth, which may help identify who most likely will or will not benefit from treatment [15]. Transcranial Doppler is well suited to the task of identifying both collateralization and time course and completeness of recanalization of the arteries of the circle of Willis. Numerous studies have examined characteristics and patterns of recanalization and its association with early neurological improvement.

Noninvasive estimation of ICP following acute stroke. Current recommendations of stroke treatment favor a moderately elevated blood pressure in the acute phase, based on the concept of an improved cerebral perfusion. BUS can help verify the efficacy of BP augmentation of CBF through the assessment of adequate cerebral perfusion. Cerebrovascular autoregulation is frequently compromised in the early phase of acute stroke [18], and this has led to the current treatment guidelines of permissive hypertension in the hyperacute phase [15]. However, stroke patients with compromised cerebrovascular autoregulation are more prone in developing either hypoperfusion or hyperperfusion, both of which can lead to brain edema and increased intracranial pressure. Furthermore, cerebral infarcts may also be complicated due to hemorrhagic infarction of the ischemic area. The latter may also lead to intracranial hypertension [19–21].

There are controversies surrounding ICP monitoring in patients with stroke [19–21]. Early studies showed that ICP monitoring was useful for predicting clinical outcomes after acute hemispheric stroke. ICP often correlated with clinical deterioration, final outcome, and computed tomography findings. However, a subsequent study of patients with malignant middle cerebral artery (MCA) infarctions showed that pupillary abnormalities and signs of severe brainstem compression were sometimes present despite normal ICP. Randomized clinical trials of ICP monitoring have not been performed in patients with stroke. An RCT of ICP monitoring in patients with traumatic brain injury failed to show superior efficacy of ICP monitoring over serial neurological examinations and repeated neuroimaging studies [19–21].

Therefore, routine ICP monitoring without careful interpretation, neurological examination, and a neuroimaging study cannot be recommended in patients with cerebral and cerebellar infarct with swelling. However, with the development of novel techniques for noninvasive measurement of ICP this type of monitoring becomes more applicable in the context of ischemic stroke, even in awake patients. BUS-derived measurements and parameters can effectively be used to assess ICP and the effect of ICP changes on cerebrovascular dynamics (Figs. 10.7 and 10.8).

Role of BUS for sonothrombolysis. Sonothrombolysis consists of the continuous ultrasound insonation of an intra-arterial occlusive thrombus during systemic or local intra-arterial thrombolysis to enhance recanalization and tissue reperfusion. Sonolysis is defined by the use of this technology as the sole thrombolytic therapy [22].

In the past literature there have been some studies showing that rtPA infusion combined with transcranial low-frequency ultrasound waves targeted on the occluded arterial segment (sonothrombolysis) alone and/or in combination with ultrasound contrast agent microbubbles may have the potential to improve transcranial thrombolysis as well [23–28].

However, a recent RCT sonothrombolysis as adjuvant therapy for IV thrombolysis has shown no clinical benefit and therefore the recent 2018 Guidelines for the Early Management of Patients with Acute Ischemic Stroke do not recommend its use [29].

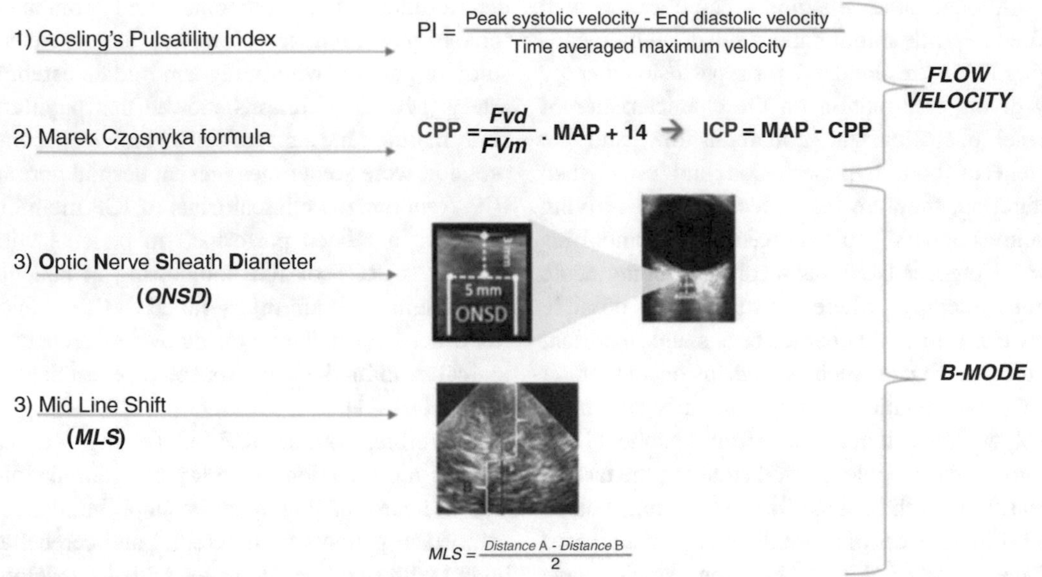

Fig. 10.7 Brain ultrasound-derived measurements and parameters used in clinical practice to measure/estimate intracranial pressure. *ICP* intracranial pressure, *MAP* mean arterial pressure; *CPP* cerebral perfusion pressure, *FVd* flow velocity, diastole, *FVm* flow velocity, mean, *MLS* midline shift

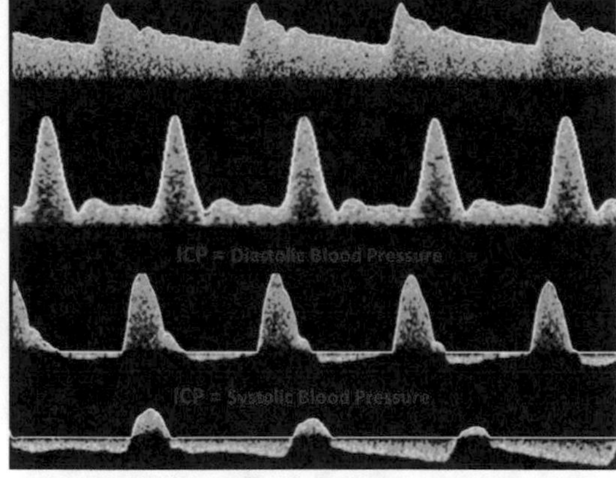

Fig. 10.8 Right MCA TCD flow pattern of an 85-year-old patient who gradually had increasing intracranial pressure following left hemispheric stroke due to occlusion of the left MCA. When ICP reaches the equivalent diastolic blood pressure, cerebral blood flow is only partially present during systole. When ICP reaches the equivalent systolic blood pressure, reverberating flow indicates cerebral circulatory arrest

It is important however to realize that BUS does not replace clinical judgment and has to be used as a complementary tool to what is currently accepted as a standard of care. Nevertheless, ultrasound presents several features of an ideal complement to our monitoring devices.

10.3 BUS Within Whole-Body Ultrasound in Cardiac Arrest and the Post-resuscitation Syndrome

Current ACLS recommendations focus on early and effective external cardiac compressions aimed at maximizing cerebral perfusion, while arrhythmias and other cardiac arrest (CA) causes are diagnosed and treated [30]. Indeed, in the setting of non-shockable CA presentation rhythms the search for, and treatment of, potentially treatable causes becomes pivotal, as the only way to ensure recovery of spontaneous circulation (ROSC), and increase survival chances [30]. Recent evidence shows that external chest compressions performed according to recommended superficial chest landmarks may be inadequate in providing effective heart chamber compression and ventricular passive ejection [31, 32]. Monitoring the hemodynamic and perfusing effect of CPR has thus become of interest, in order to assess and improve its efficacy. Besides the established clinical and monitoring tools currently available to assess CPR quality (EtCO2 [33, 34] and invasive diastolic blood pressure measurement [33, 35]), novel ultrasound applications have been proposed. Focused cardiac ultrasound has clearly a place in this context, both with a transthoracic approach [36] and with a transesophageal one [37, 38]. Very preliminary data suggest that according to the ultrasound information obtained, a greater efficacy of CPR could be obtained, as shown by higher EtCO2 values upon an ultrasound-guided choice of the chest area compressed [39]. Likewise, TCD sampling of the mean cerebral artery (MCA) flows during CPR could provide an even more targeted information on the cerebral flow generated by chest compressions [5, 40]. Although MCA velocities may correlate with better cerebral perfusion during CPR [41, 42], current literature remains limited to case reports and small case series [5, 40, 43].

The role of ultrasound during CA resuscitation has the potential to be expanded beyond the initial concept of cardiac ultrasound for the diagnosis of mechanical PEA causes (profound hypovolemia, dramatic LV systolic dysfunction, acute cor pulmonale, tamponade) as conceived by the FEEL (Focused Echocardiographic Evaluation in Life support) approach [36, 44]. The addition of lung ultrasound for the diagnosis of pneumothorax [45], of vascular ultrasound for the procedural approach to arterial and central venous cannulation [46], or of ECMO cannulas positioning in E-CPR [47, 48] could be complemented by TCD and transesophageal cardiac ultrasound for the detection of inadequate CPR quality, in a multi-organ ultrasound fashion [Fig. 10.9], with potential relevant management implications. The concept of a cerebral flow-focused assessment with carotideal Doppler sampling within the FEEL approach to resuscitation has also been proposed [49].

Another area of application of BUS within the wider multi-organ PoCUS approach in the emergency department is the use of TCD and ONSD within the primary survey of the resuscitated CA patient, as part of the demanding post-cardiac arrest syndrome (PCAS) management [50]. In the approach to PCAS, multi-organ PoCUS is invaluable in providing explanation of the causes of persistent cardiovascular instability (myocardial stunning, hypovolemia, tamponade) [51] and of hypoxemia (pulmonary edema, aspiration pneumonia, dysventilation) [52], and in screening for potential side effects of prolonged CPR (rib fractures, sternal fractures [53], lung contusions, pneumothorax, hemothorax [52], accidental liver/spleen rupture with hemoperitoneum [54, 55]). Furthermore, ultrasound can effectively guide procedural aspects of post-resuscitation care (arterial and venous line insertion [46], pleural effusion or pneumothorax drainage, lung recruitment [52]).

In this context, a potential role for BUS in neuro-prognostication has been suggested. High ONSD has been associated to poor neurological outcome, although only with moderate accuracy [3, 56–58], unless particularly high ONSD values are detected: Chelly et al. found with a small study that day 1 post-arrest ONSD was larger in nonsurvivors (7.2 mm [interquartile: 6.8–7.4] versus 6.5 mm [interquartile: 6.0–6.8]; $p = 0.008$), and associated to higher in-hospital mortality (OR 6.3; 95% CI [1.05–40] per mm of ONSD 1 above 5.5 mm; $p = 0.03$) [3]. The utility of ONSD measurement for post-CA neuro-prognostication was recently confirmed by Ertl et al.: measurements performed at admission found that nonsurvivors showed significantly higher ONSD values ($p < 0.001$), and a highly specific (100%) threshold of 5.75 mm was calculated for predicting mortality. ONSD appeared not to be influenced by hypothermia ($p = 0.70$) [56].

Additionally, the features of MCA flow assessed with TCD in the post-ROSC have been used to provide insights into cerebral hemodynamics of the reperfusion phase, and investigate potential correlations with patient outcome. Two conflicting phenomena have been described for cerebral perfusion immediately after vital circulation is restored with ROSC: a macroscopic hyperemic reperfusion in the very early phase (due to transient loss of autoregulation) [59], and a subsequent reduced microcirculatory flow (due to potentially persisting vasospasm and microthrombosis) [60]. The net effect on cerebral tissue perfusion is likely determined by the interplay between systemic hemodynamics (cardiac output and mean arterial pressure [61]), global and

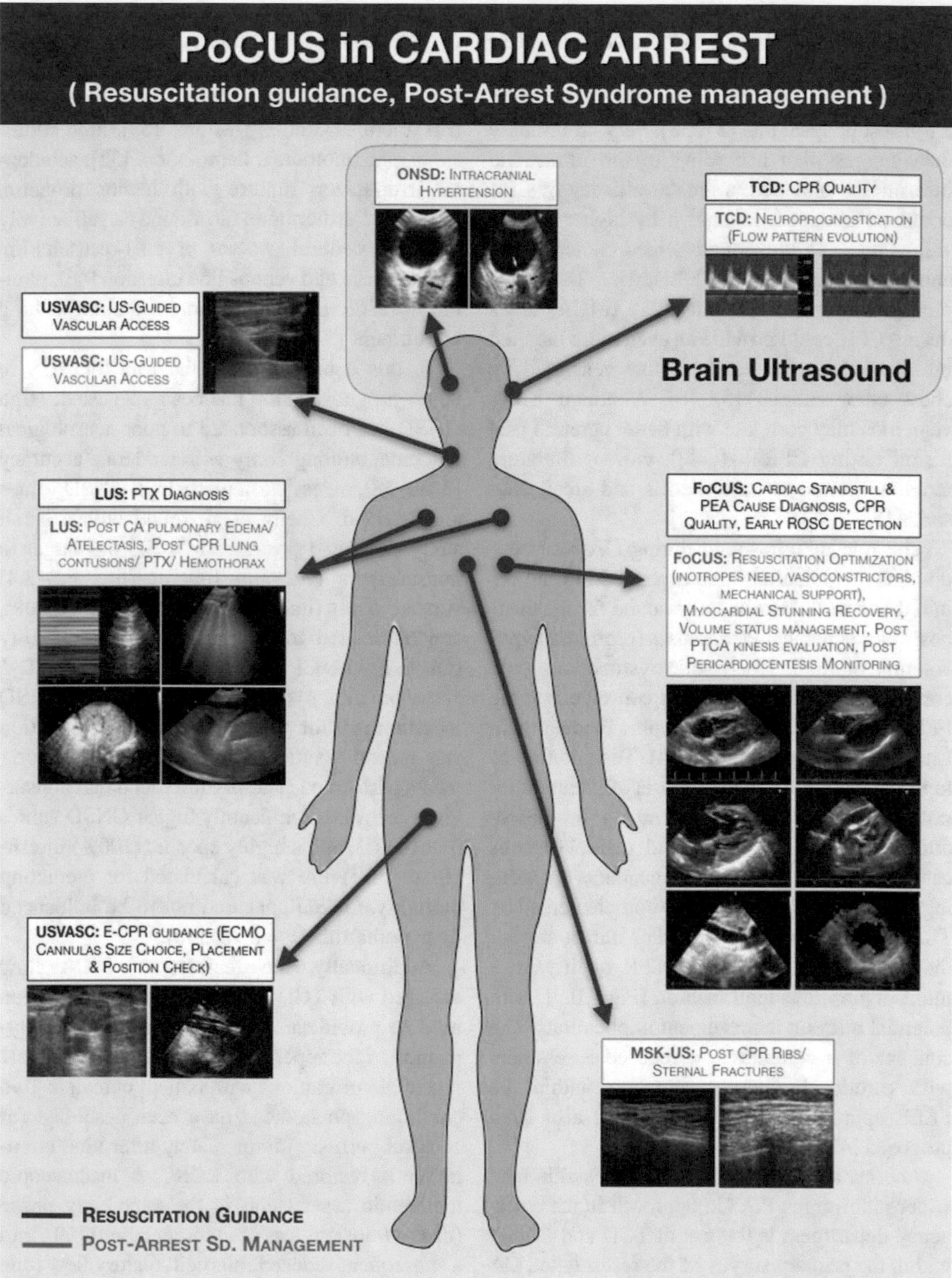

Fig. 10.9 Diagram describing the integration of brain ultrasound (BUS) applications within the multi-organ approach to cardiac arrest, both during resuscitation and in the post-ROSC phase

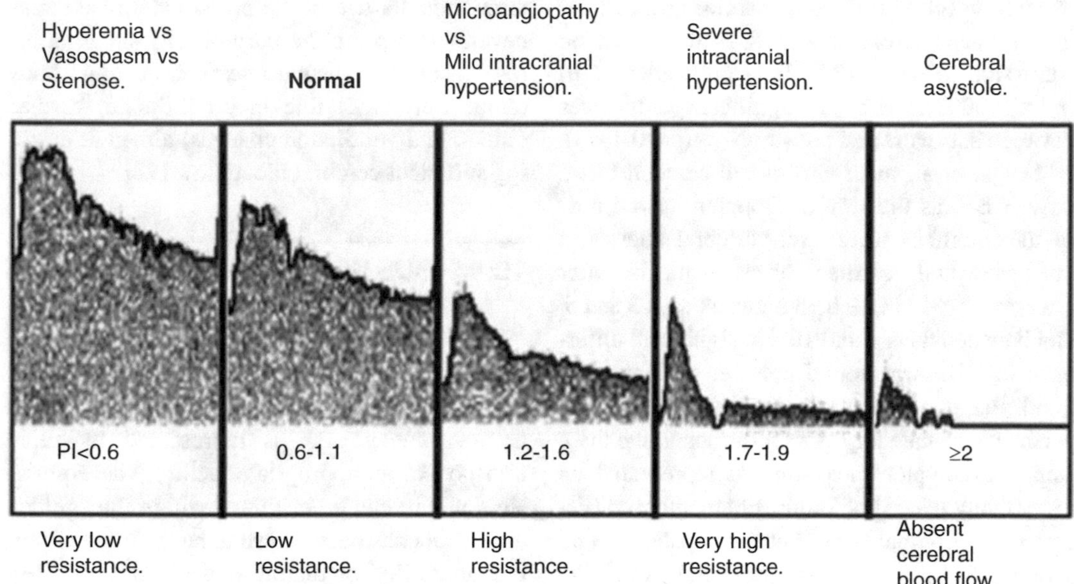

Fig. 10.10 Mean cerebral artery (MCA) TCD flow patterns (with their respective different peak and diastolic velocities and PI indexes) that can be detected in the post-resuscitation phase. PoCUS can serve both as diagnostic and monitoring tool and as procedural guidance (with permission from [42])

regional cerebral vascular resistances, and degree of cerebral edema.

Several MCA TCD flow patterns, with different peak and diastolic velocities and PI indexes, can be detected in the post-resuscitation phase, and are associated to different conditions of cerebral perfusion [41] [Fig. 10.10].

Global cerebral flow may remain reduced up to 6 h after ROSC, in association to heterogeneous multifocal hypoperfusion [62], but is expected to subsequently increase, within 72 h after ROSC [63, 64]. Return to a normal flow pattern in this time frame has been described to represent a favorable post-arrest evolution, while persistence of a low velocity-high PI pattern (reduced perfusion), or a presence of a hyperemic pattern (loss of autoregulation), to portend a negative outcome.

Studies on post-resuscitation neuroprognostication by means of TCD yielded known conflicting results. Wessels et al. found that MCA, ACA, and PCA average velocities 4 h after CPR were significantly higher in survivors (MCA flows 82 peak/31 diast cm/s in patients who survived to hospital discharge without persistent vegetative state, vs. 67 peak/24 diast cm/s in patients who subsequently died; $p < 0.05$); they thus identified within the first 24 h patients with severely disabling or fatal outcome. At 72 h after CPR average MCA systolic velocity was also significantly higher in survivors (101 vs. 80 cm s^{-1}; $p = 0.03$) [65]. With sequential MCA TCD measurements in post-ROSC patients, Lemiale et al. described a significant increase of MCA flows from the low ones at admission (27.3 [21.5–33.6] cm/s) to normal values after 72 h (50.5 [36.7–58.1] cm/s) in their whole population. Initial PI values were high (1.6 [1.3–1.9]) but reached normal values too after 72 h (1.04 [0.82–1.2]). While cerebral oxygen extraction decreased significantly only in nonsurvivors, MCA flows at 72 h showed no difference between survivors and nonsurvivors, but MCA end diastolic velocity was higher in survivors at 72 h (39.6 vs. 29.3 cm s^{-1}; $p = 0.013$) [66]. Also Hoedmaeker et al. described an increase in MCA mean flow velocities in post-cardiac arrest comatose patients (from 26.0 [18.6–40.4] cm/s on admission to 63.9 [48.3–73.1] cm/s after 72 h) ($p < 0.0001$), with no significant differences between survivors and nonsurvivors ($p = 0.4853$).

Doepp et al. measured global cerebral blood flow (CBF) as the sum of Doppler-derived flow of the internal carotid and vertebral arteries in out-of-hospital cardiac arrest patients after rewarming, within 48 h, at between days 3 and 5, and between days 7 and 10. No significant difference in CBF was found between patients with good and poor outcome, expressed as cerebral performance category (CPC) (although the three steps of Doppler measurement represented an excessively wide time frame, not to affect consistency of comparisons between patients and groups) [67]. Also Heimburger et al. (MCA TCD measured at admission, and at 24 h, during hypothermia) found no difference in MCA peak, mean, and diastolic flow velocities between patients with CPC 1–2 and CPC 3–5 [68], nor did Bisschops et al. describe any difference between survivors and nonsurvivors in sequential MCA TCD flows and PI determinations (at 12, 24, 36, 48, 60, 72, 84, 96, and 108 h after admission) in small populations of CA patients submitted to prolonged (72 h) mild hypothermia [69]. Van der Brule et al. found that MCA mean flow velocity was similar in survivors and nonsurvivors upon admission to the ICU, and increased in all patients (from 28.0 [25.0–39.0] upon ICU admission to 78.0 [65.0–123.0] cm/s after 72 h, $p < 0.001$), but the increase was greater in nonsurvivors compared to survivors ($p < 0.001$) [64]. The same group interestingly also described that MCA Doppler mean flow velocities showed significantly smaller spontaneous fluctuations in the observation period (72 h) in nonsurvivors [70]. It has also been anecdotally reported that the asymmetry in MCA flows may indicate post-arrest cerebral ischemic stroke [41, 71].

In conclusion, although TCD use for post-cardiac arrest neuro-prognostication has solid pathophysiological background, current evidence altogether speaks to an unclear role of this promising tool. Its use in the post-ROSC phase may nevertheless serve the purpose of evaluating the response to therapeutic interventions (e.g., body temperature, systemic blood pressure, cardiac output, and ventilation changes) aimed at ensuring sufficient cerebral blood flow [72].

10.4 BUS Within Whole-Body Ultrasound in Multiple Trauma

The core of prehospital and emergency room trauma management is represented by rapid transport to an appropriate facility where provision of care can be instituted within the "golden hour": this has been shown to be the most important mortality predictor in acute trauma [73]. Since the introduction of the Focused Assessment with Sonography in Trauma (FAST) protocol [74] and the further development of its paradigm into a multi-organ approach [75, 76], point-of-care ultrasound (PoCUS) has become a widespread used and taught technique in the rapid evaluation of acute trauma patients by means of multi-site investigation, encompassing cardiothoracic and abdominal [77], vascular, and skeletal scans (Fig. 10.11). This approach aims at detection of life-threatening lesions (e.g., occult hemorrhages in the pericardial, pleural, peritoneal cavities, and tension pneumothorax) and assessment of the pathophysiology of hemodynamic compromise during the primary Advanced Trauma Life Support (ATLS) survey [75]. During the secondary survey, ultrasound can be used to help detect abdominal organ injuries (liver or spleen hematomas in patients in whom hemoperitoneum is not identified, pneumoperitoneum, kidney rupture), lung contusions, soft-tissue hematomas, ocular lesions, and fractures easily obscured on radiography, such as rib and sternal fractures [75]. Indeed, PoCUS in trauma can assist/guide emergency procedures and treatment at the bedside (airway management, chest drainage, venous and arterial line placement, fluid therapy and overall hemodynamic management,

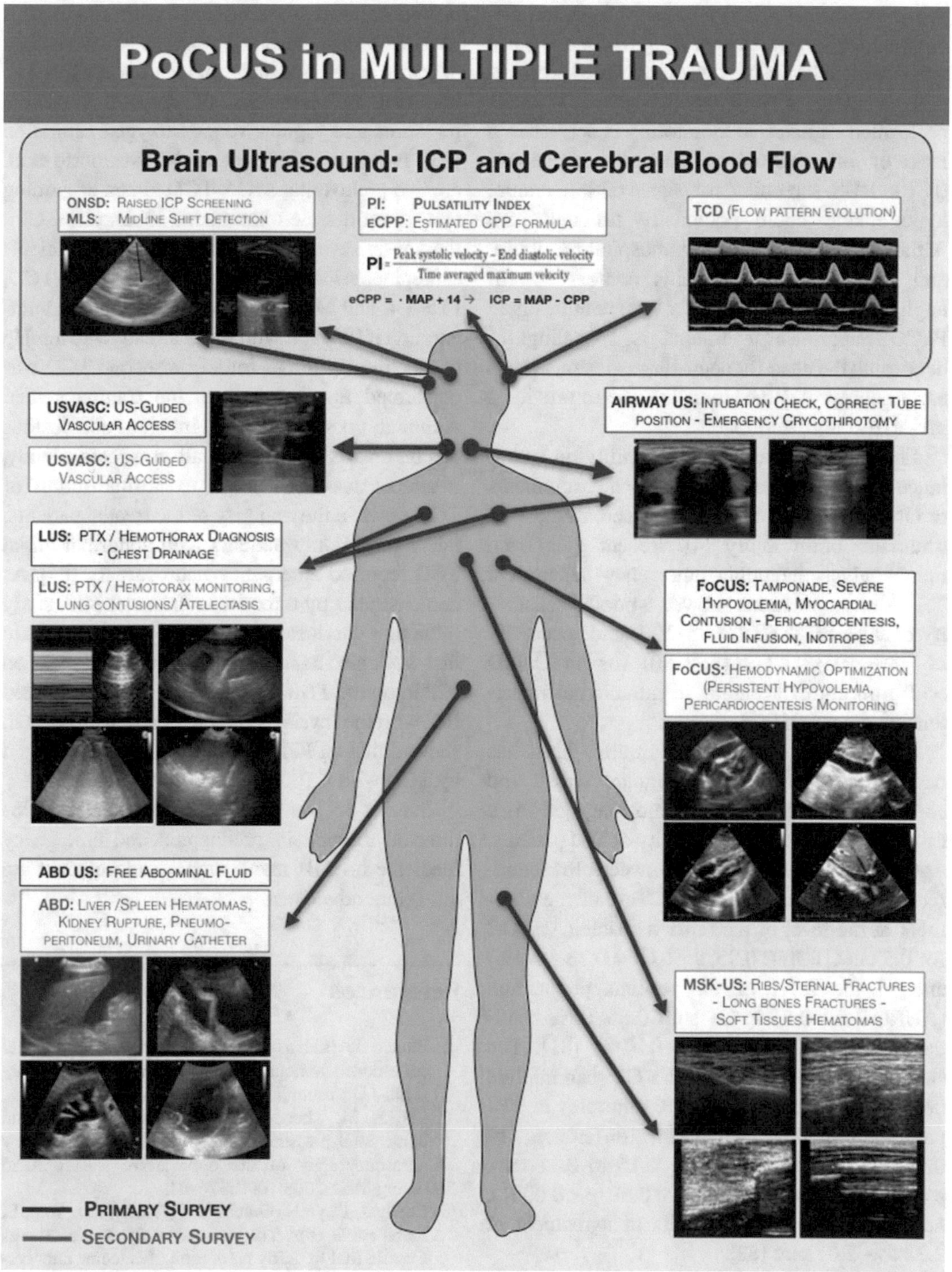

PoCUS in MULTIPLE TRAUMA

Brain Ultrasound: ICP and Cerebral Blood Flow

ONSD: Raised ICP Screening
MLS: Midline Shift Detection

PI: Pulsatility Index
eCPP: Estimated CPP formula

$$PI = \frac{\text{Peak systolic velocity} - \text{End diastolic velocity}}{\text{Time averaged maximum velocity}}$$

eCPP = · MAP + 14 → ICP = MAP - CPP

TCD (Flow pattern evolution)

USVASC: US-Guided Vascular Access

USVASC: US-Guided Vascular Access

Airway US: Intubation Check, Correct Tube position - Emergency Crycothirotomy

LUS: PTX / Hemothorax Diagnosis - Chest Drainage

LUS: PTX / Hemotorax monitoring, Lung contusions/ Atelectasis

FoCUS: Tamponade, Severe Hypovolemia, Myocardial Contusion - Pericardiocentesis, Fluid Infusion, Inotropes

FoCUS: Hemodynamic Optimization (Persistent Hypovolemia, Pericardiocentesis Monitoring

ABD US: Free Abdominal Fluid

ABD: Liver /Spleen Hematomas, Kidney Rupture, Pneumo-peritoneum, Urinary Catheter

MSK-US: Ribs/Sternal Fractures - Long bones Fractures - Soft Tissues Hematomas

Primary Survey

Secondary Survey

Fig. 10.11 Diagram describing the integration of brain ultrasound (BUS) applications within the multi-organ approach to multiple trauma, both during the primary and the secondary survey and during management

urinary catheterization) as part of both the primary and the secondary survey [78]. Due to obvious technical limitations, the prehospital scenario and the emergency department (until a CT scan is performed or invasive monitoring is set) share a lack of information on intracranial pressure (ICP): BUS screening for signs of intracranial hypertension could potentially fill that gap. Although the evidence on prehospital feasibility and benefit of BUS in this context is still negligible, its role as part of this multi-organ PoCUS approach to trauma is appealing: to determine the need for neurosurgical care, to start early neuroprotective strategies, and to provide a pre-arrival notification.

Preliminary data show a feasibility on ambulance or helicopter of high-quality measurements of ONSD, to estimate the risk of increased ICP in traumatic brain injury [4]. Recent data from meta-analysis including emergency department TBI adult populations showed a pooled sensitivity of 99% (95% CI 1/4 96–100) and specificity of 73% (95% CI 1/4 65–80) for an ONSD >5.0 mm cutoff accuracy in intracranial hypertension detection [79].

Ultrasound assessment of midline shift has been studied mostly in malignant stroke and supratentorial intracerebral hemorrhage [80]. In a mixed population with a majority of TBI patients, a good correlation was found between ultrasound-measured midline shift and CT scan measurement at the level of the third ventricle (AUROC for 0.5 cm CT shift 0.85, 95% CI = 0.73–0.94%) and at the level of the septum pellucidum (AUROC for 0.5 cm CT shift 0.86, 95% confidence interval (CI) = 0.74–0.94%) [81]. The same technique compared with CT scan midline detection (center of the third ventricle) in TBI patients yielded a mean difference of 0.12 ± 1.08 mm (95% CI – 0.15 to 0.41 mm, $p = 0.36$), a linear correlation of 0.88 ($p < 0.0001$), no significant bias, and limits of agreement of 2.33 to −2.07 mm [82].

TCD allows early detection of low cerebral blood flow by detecting low MCA diastolic flow velocities and high PI: TCD was used in the emergency room to initiate treatment (mannitol, vasopressors, and an emergency neurosurgical procedure) for adult patients with severe TBI with FVd less than 20 cm/s, FVm less than 30 cm/s, and pulsatility index greater than 1.4, obtaining normalization of cerebral perfusion pressures and jugular venous oxygen saturation [83]. In a feasibility pilot study, Tazarourte et al. applied prehospital MCA TCD aimed at guiding early goal-directed treatment to increase CPP therapy in severe traumatic brain injury patients (norepinephrine infusion if pathological TCD, PI > 1.4, and MAP <80 mmHg; mannitol administration if PI > 1.4, with MAP already >80 mmHg or reactive mydriasis found): a second TCD was performed upon arrival at the trauma center. Although no statistically significant conclusions can be drawn from this small prospective study, treatment was associated to normalization of TCD flows in the majority of the treated patients; interestingly only patients with abnormal initial TCD required emergency neurosurgery [84]. As demonstrated by a recent multicenter pilot study (although conducted in the ICU), TCD could in fact work also as an early rule-out tool for raised ICP in severe TBI: by comparing TCD-estimated ICP with the invasive gold standard, Rasulo et al. showed that an ICP > 20 mmHg can be detected by TCD with a 100% sensitivity [85].

Studies to prove the impact of early BUS-directed therapy in prehospital and emergency medicine on TBI management and outcome are altogether advocated.

References

1. Blanco P, Blaivas M. Applications of transcranial color-coded sonography in the emergency department. J Ultrasound Med. 2017;36(6):1251–66.
2. Blaivas M, Theodoro D, Sierzenski PR. Elevated intracranial pressure detected by bedside emergency ultrasonography of the optic nerve sheath. Acad Emerg Med. 2003;10(4):376–81.
3. Chelly J, Deye N, Guichard JP, Vodovar D, Vong L, Jochmans S, et al. The optic nerve sheath diameter as a useful tool for early prediction of outcome after cardiac arrest: a prospective pilot study. Resuscitation. 2016;103:7–13.
4. Houze-Cerfon CH, Bounes V, Guemon J, Le Gourrierec T, Geeraerts T. Quality and feasibility of sonographic measurement of the optic nerve sheath diameter to estimate the risk of raised intracranial

pressure after traumatic brain injury in prehospital setting. Prehosp Emerg Care. 2019;23(2):277–83.

5. Lewis LM, Gomez CR, Ruoff BE, Gomez SM, Hall IS, Gasirowski B. Transcranial Doppler determination of cerebral perfusion in patients undergoing CPR: methodology and preliminary findings. Ann Emerg Med. 1990;19(10):1148–51.
6. Laursen CB, Sloth E, Lassen AT, Christensen R, Lambrechtsen J, Madsen PH, et al. Point-of-care ultrasonography in patients admitted with respiratory symptoms: a single-blind, randomised controlled trial. Lancet Respir Med. 2014;2(8):638–46.
7. Nazerian P, Vanni S, Volpicelli G, Gigli C, Zanobetti M, Bartolucci M, et al. Accuracy of point-of-care multiorgan ultrasonography for the diagnosis of pulmonary embolism. Chest. 2014;145(5):950–7.
8. Volpicelli G, Lamorte A, Tullio M, Cardinale L, Giraudo M, Stefanone V, et al. Point-of-care multiorgan ultrasonography for the evaluation of undifferentiated hypotension in the emergency department. Intensive Care Med. 2013;39(7):1290–8.
9. Mayo P, Volpicelli G, Lerolle N, Schreiber A, Doelken P, Vieillard-Baron A. Ultrasonography evaluation during the weaning process: the heart, the diaphragm, the pleura and the lung. Intensive Care Med. 2016;42(7):1107–17.
10. Pivetta E, Goffi A, Lupia E, Tizzani M, Porrino G, Ferreri E, et al. Lung ultrasound-implemented diagnosis of acute decompensated heart failure in the ED: a SIMEU multicenter study. Chest. 2015;148(1):202–10.
11. Saver JL. Time is brain—quantified. Stroke. 2006;37(1):263–6.
12. Holscher T, Schlachetzki F, Zimmermann M, Jakob W, Ittner KP, Haslberger J, et al. Transcranial ultrasound from diagnosis to early stroke treatment. 1. Feasibility of prehospital cerebrovascular assessment. Cerebrovasc Dis. 2008;26(6):659–63.
13. National Institute of Neurological D, Stroke rt PASSG. Tissue plasminogen activator for acute ischemic stroke. N Engl J Med. 1995;333(24):1581–7.
14. Sobrino-Garcia P, Garcia-Pastor A, Garcia-Arratibel A, Dominguez-Rubio R, Rodriguez-Cruz PM, Iglesias-Mohedano AM, et al. Diagnostic, prognostic and therapeutic implications of transcranial color-coded duplex sonography in acute ischemic stroke: TIBI and COGIF scores validation. Rev Neurol. 2016;63(8):351–7.
15. Castro P, Azevedo E, Sorond F. Cerebral autoregulation in stroke. Curr Atheroscler Rep. 2018;20(8):37.
16. Powers WJ, Rabinstein AA, Ackerson T, Adeoye OM, Bambakidis NC, Becker K, et al. 2018 guidelines for the early management of patients with acute ischemic stroke: a guideline for healthcare professionals from the American Heart Association/American Stroke Association. Stroke. 2018;49(3):e46–e110.
17. Brunser AM, Mansilla E, Hoppe A, Olavarria V, Sujima E, Lavados PM. The role of TCD in the evaluation of acute stroke. J Neuroimaging. 2016;26(4):420–5.
18. Ragoschke-Schumm A, Walter S. DAWN and DEFUSE-3 trials: is time still important? Radiologe. 2018;58(Suppl 1):20–3.
19. Schwab S, Aschoff A, Spranger M, Albert F, Hacke W. The value of intracranial pressure monitoring in acute hemispheric stroke. Neurology. 1996;47(2):393–8.
20. Poca MA, Benejam B, Sahuquillo J, Riveiro M, Frascheri L, Merino MA, et al. Monitoring intracranial pressure in patients with malignant middle cerebral artery infarction: is it useful? J Neurosurg. 2010;112(3):648–57.
21. Chesnut RM, Temkin N, Carney N, Dikmen S, Rondina C, Videtta W, et al. A trial of intracranial-pressure monitoring in traumatic brain injury. N Engl J Med. 2012;367(26):2471–81.
22. Alexandrov AV, Barlinn K. Taboos and opportunities in sonothrombolysis for stroke. Int J Hyperth. 2012;28(4):397–404.
23. Molina CA, Ribo M, Rubiera M, Montaner J, Santamarina E, Delgado-Mederos R, et al. Microbubble administration accelerates clot lysis during continuous 2-MHz ultrasound monitoring in stroke patients treated with intravenous tissue plasminogen activator. Stroke. 2006;37(2):425–9.
24. Culp WC, Porter TR, Lowery J, Xie F, Roberson PK, Marky L. Intracranial clot lysis with intravenous microbubbles and transcranial ultrasound in swine. Stroke. 2004;35(10):2407–11.
25. Alexandrov AV, Molina CA, Grotta JC, Garami Z, Ford SR, Alvarez-Sabin J, et al. Ultrasound-enhanced systemic thrombolysis for acute ischemic stroke. N Engl J Med. 2004;351(21):2170–8.
26. Barlinn K, Alexandrov AV. Sonothrombolysis in ischemic stroke. Curr Treat Options Neurol. 2013;15(2):91–103.
27. Tsivgoulis G, Eggers J, Ribo M, Perren F, Saqqur M, Rubiera M, et al. Safety and efficacy of ultrasound-enhanced thrombolysis: a comprehensive review and meta-analysis of randomized and nonrandomized studies. Stroke. 2010;41(2):280–7.
28. Ricci S, Dinia L, Del Sette M, Anzola P, Mazzoli T, Cenciarelli S, et al. Sonothrombolysis for acute ischaemic stroke. Cochrane Database Syst Rev. 2012;10:CD008348.
29. Nacu A, Kvistad CE, Naess H, Oygarden H, Logallo N, Assmus J, et al. NOR-SASS (Norwegian Sonothrombolysis in Acute Stroke Study): randomized controlled contrast-enhanced sonothrombolysis in an unselected acute ischemic stroke population. Stroke. 2017;48(2):335–41.
30. Monsieurs KG, Nolan JP, Bossaert LL, Greif R, Maconochie IK, Nikolaou NI, et al. European Resuscitation Council Guidelines for Resuscitation 2015: Section 1. Executive summary. Resuscitation. 2015;95:1–80.
31. Hwang SO, Zhao PG, Choi HJ, Park KH, Cha KC, Park SM, et al. Compression of the left ventricular outflow tract during cardiopulmonary resuscitation. Acad Emerg Med. 2009;16(10):928–33.

32. Shin J, Rhee JE, Kim K. Is the inter-nipple line the correct hand position for effective chest compression in adult cardiopulmonary resuscitation? Resuscitation. 2007;75(2):305–10.
33. Soar J, Nolan JP, Bottiger BW, Perkins GD, Lott C, Carli P, et al. European Resuscitation Council Guidelines for Resuscitation 2015: Section 3. Adult advanced life support. Resuscitation. 2015;95:100–47.
34. Paiva EF, Paxton JH, O'Neil BJ. The use of end-tidal carbon dioxide (ETCO2) measurement to guide management of cardiac arrest: a systematic review. Resuscitation. 2018;123:1–7.
35. Morgan RW, French B, Kilbaugh TJ, Naim MY, Wolfe H, Bratinov G, et al. A quantitative comparison of physiologic indicators of cardiopulmonary resuscitation quality: diastolic blood pressure versus end-tidal carbon dioxide. Resuscitation. 2016;104:6–11.
36. Breitkreutz R, Walcher F, Seeger FH. Focused echocardiographic evaluation in resuscitation management: concept of an advanced life support-conformed algorithm. Crit Care Med. 2007;35(5 Suppl):S150–61.
37. Parker BK, Salerno A, Euerle BD. The use of transesophageal echocardiography during cardiac arrest resuscitation: a literature review. J Ultrasound Med. 2019;38(5):1141–51.
38. Blaivas M. Transesophageal echocardiography during cardiopulmonary arrest in the emergency department. Resuscitation. 2008;78(2):135–40.
39. Anderson KL, Castaneda MG, Boudreau SM, Sharon DJ, Bebarta VS. Left ventricular compressions improve hemodynamics in a swine model of out-of-hospital cardiac arrest. Prehosp Emerg Care. 2017;21(2):272–80.
40. Blumenstein J, Kempfert J, Walther T, Van Linden A, Fassl J, Borger M, et al. Cerebral flow pattern monitoring by transcranial Doppler during cardiopulmonary resuscitation. Anaesth Intensive Care. 2010;38(2):376–80.
41. Alvarez-Fernandez JA, Martin-Velasco MM, Igeno-Cano JC, Perez-Quintero R. Transcranial Doppler ultrasonography usefulness in cardiac arrest resuscitation. Med Intensiva. 2010;34(8):550–8.
42. Lewis LM, Stothert JC Jr, Gomez CR, Ruoff BE, Hall IS, Chandel B, et al. A noninvasive method for monitoring cerebral perfusion during cardiopulmonary resuscitation. J Crit Care. 1994;9(3):169–74.
43. Belohlavek J, Skalicka H, Boucek T, Kovarnik T, Fichtl J, Smid O, et al. Feasibility of cerebral blood flow and oxygenation monitoring by continuous transcranial Doppler combined with cerebral oximetry in a patient with refractory cardiac arrest treated by extracorporeal life support. Perfusion. 2014;29(6):534–8.
44. Breitkreutz R, Price S, Steiger HV, Seeger FH, Ilper H, Ackermann H, et al. Focused echocardiographic evaluation in life support and peri-resuscitation of emergency patients: a prospective trial. Resuscitation. 2010;81(11):1527–33.
45. Volpicelli G. Sonographic diagnosis of pneumothorax. Intensive Care Med. 2011;37(2):224–32.
46. Troianos CA, Hartman GS, Glas KE, Skubas NJ, Eberhardt RT, Walker JD, et al. Special articles: guidelines for performing ultrasound guided vascular cannulation: recommendations of the American Society of Echocardiography and the Society of Cardiovascular Anesthesiologists. Anesth Analg. 2012;114(1):46–72.
47. Ahn HJ, Lee JW, Joo KH, You YH, Ryu S, Lee JW, et al. Point-of-care ultrasound-guided percutaneous cannulation of extracorporeal membrane oxygenation: make it simple. J Emerg Med. 2018;54(4):507–13.
48. Voicu S, Henry P, Malissin I, Dillinger JG, Koumoulidis A, Magkoutis N, et al. Improving cannulation time for extracorporeal life support in refractory cardiac arrest of presumed cardiac cause—comparison of two percutaneous cannulation techniques in the catheterization laboratory in a center without on-site cardiovascular surgery. Resuscitation. 2018;122:69–75.
49. Adedipe AA, Fly DL, Schwitz SD, Jorgenson DB, Duric H, Sayre MR, et al. Carotid Doppler blood flow measurement during cardiopulmonary resuscitation is feasible: a first in man study. Resuscitation. 2015;96:121–5.
50. Nolan JP, Soar J, Cariou A, Cronberg T, Moulaert VR, Deakin CD, et al. European Resuscitation Council and European Society of Intensive Care Medicine 2015 guidelines for post-resuscitation care. Intensive Care Med. 2015;41(12):2039–56.
51. Via G, Hussain A, Wells M, Reardon R, ElBarbary M, Noble VE, et al. International evidence-based recommendations for focused cardiac ultrasound. J Am Soc Echocardiogr. 2014;27(7):683. e1-e33
52. Volpicelli G, Elbarbary M, Blaivas M, Lichtenstein DA, Mathis G, Kirkpatrick AW, et al. International evidence-based recommendations for point-of-care lung ultrasound. Intensive Care Med. 2012;38(4):577–91.
53. Smereczynski A, Kolaczyk K, Bernatowicz E. Chest wall—underappreciated structure in sonography. Part II: non-cancerous lesions. J Ultrason. 2017;17(71):275–80.
54. Stengel D, Rademacher G, Ekkernkamp A, Guthoff C, Mutze S. Emergency ultrasound-based algorithms for diagnosing blunt abdominal trauma. Cochrane Database Syst Rev. 2015;(9):CD004446.
55. O'Dochartaigh D, Douma M. Prehospital ultrasound of the abdomen and thorax changes trauma patient management: a systematic review. Injury. 2015;46(11):2093–102.
56. Ertl M, Weber S, Hammel G, Schroeder C, Krogias C. Transorbital sonography for early prognostication of hypoxic-ischemic encephalopathy after cardiac arrest. J Neuroimaging. 2018;28(5):542–8.
57. Ueda T, Ishida E, Kojima Y, Yoshikawa S, Yonemoto H. Sonographic optic nerve sheath diameter: a simple and rapid tool to assess the neurologic prognosis after cardiac arrest. J Neuroimaging. 2015;25(6): 927–30.
58. You Y, Park J, Min J, Yoo I, Jeong W, Cho Y, et al. Relationship between time related serum albumin concentration, optic nerve sheath diameter, cerebrospinal fluid pressure, and neurological prognosis in cardiac arrest survivors. Resuscitation. 2018;131: 42–7.

59. Sundgreen C, Larsen FS, Herzog TM, Knudsen GM, Boesgaard S, Aldershvile J. Autoregulation of cerebral blood flow in patients resuscitated from cardiac arrest. Stroke. 2001;32(1):128–32.
60. Fischer M, Bottiger BW, Popov-Cenic S, Hossmann KA. Thrombolysis using plasminogen activator and heparin reduces cerebral no-reflow after resuscitation from cardiac arrest: an experimental study in the cat. Intensive Care Med. 1996;22(11):1214–23.
61. Mullner M, Sterz F, Binder M, Hellwagner K, Meron G, Herkner H, et al. Arterial blood pressure after human cardiac arrest and neurological recovery. Stroke. 1996;27(1):59–62.
62. Wolfson SK Jr, Safar P, Reich H, Clark JM, Gur D, Stezoski W, et al. Dynamic heterogeneity of cerebral hypoperfusion after prolonged cardiac arrest in dogs measured by the stable xenon/CT technique: a preliminary study. Resuscitation. 1992;23(1):1–20.
63. Hoedemaekers CW, Ainslie PN, Hinssen S, Aries MJ, Bisschops LL, Hofmeijer J, et al. Low cerebral blood flow after cardiac arrest is not associated with anaerobic cerebral metabolism. Resuscitation. 2017;120:45–50.
64. van den Brule JM, Vinke E, van Loon LM, van der Hoeven JG, Hoedemaekers CW. Middle cerebral artery flow, the critical closing pressure, and the optimal mean arterial pressure in comatose cardiac arrest survivors—an observational study. Resuscitation. 2017;110:85–9.
65. Wessels T, Harrer JU, Jacke C, Janssens U, Klotzsch C. The prognostic value of early transcranial Doppler ultrasound following cardiopulmonary resuscitation. Ultrasound Med Biol. 2006;32(12):1845–51.
66. Lemiale V, Huet O, Vigue B, Mathonnet A, Spaulding C, Mira JP, et al. Changes in cerebral blood flow and oxygen extraction during post-resuscitation syndrome. Resuscitation. 2008;76(1):17–24.
67. Doepp Connolly F, Reitemeier J, Storm C, Hasper D, Schreiber SJ. Duplex sonography of cerebral blood flow after cardiac arrest—a prospective observational study. Resuscitation. 2014;85(4):516–21.
68. Heimburger D, Durand M, Gaide-Chevronnay L, Dessertaine G, Moury PH, Bouzat P, et al. Quantitative pupillometry and transcranial Doppler measurements in patients treated with hypothermia after cardiac arrest. Resuscitation. 2016;103:88–93.
69. Bisschops LL, van der Hoeven JG, Hoedemaekers CW. Effects of prolonged mild hypothermia on cerebral blood flow after cardiac arrest. Crit Care Med. 2012;40(8):2362–7.
70. van den Brule JM, Vinke EJ, van Loon LM, van der Hoeven JG, Hoedemaekers CW. Low spontaneous variability in cerebral blood flow velocity in non-survivors after cardiac arrest. Resuscitation. 2017;111:110–5.
71. Carbutti G, Romand JA, Carballo JS, Bendjelid SM, Suter PM, Bendjelid K. Transcranial Doppler: an early predictor of ischemic stroke after cardiac arrest? Anesth Analg. 2003;97(5):1262–5.
72. Reynolds JC, Elmer J. The adventure of the dying detective: commentary on "quantitative pupillometry and transcranial Doppler measurements in patients treated with hypothermia after cardiac arrest" by Heimberger et al. Resuscitation. 2016;103:A1–2.
73. Lockey DJ. Prehospital trauma management. Resuscitation. 2001;48(1):5–15.
74. Scalea TM, Rodriguez A, Chiu WC, Brenneman FD, Fallon WF Jr, Kato K, et al. Focused assessment with sonography for trauma (FAST): results from an international consensus conference. J Trauma. 1999;46(3):466–72.
75. Neri L, Storti E, Lichtenstein D. Toward an ultrasound curriculum for critical care medicine. Crit Care Med. 2007;35(5 Suppl):S290–304.
76. Montoya J, Stawicki SP, Evans DC, Bahner DP, Sparks S, Sharpe RP, et al. From FAST to E-FAST: an overview of the evolution of ultrasound-based traumatic injury assessment. Eur J Trauma Emerg Surg. 2016;42(2):119–26.
77. Subcommittee A, American College of Surgeons' Committee on T, International Awg. Advanced trauma life support (ATLS(R)): the ninth edition. J Trauma Acute Care Surg. 2013;74(5):1363–6.
78. Ketelaars R, Reijnders G, van Geffen GJ, Scheffer GJ, Hoogerwerf N. ABCDE of prehospital ultrasonography: a narrative review. Crit Ultrasound J. 2018;10(1):17.
79. Kim SE, Hong EP, Kim HC, Lee SU, Jeon JP. Ultrasonographic optic nerve sheath diameter to detect increased intracranial pressure in adults: a meta-analysis. Acta Radiol. 2019;60(2):221–9.
80. Liao CC, Chen YF, Xiao F. Brain midline shift measurement and its automation: a review of techniques and algorithms. Int J Biomed Imaging. 2018;2018:4303161.
81. Motuel J, Biette I, Srairi M, Mrozek S, Kurrek MM, Chaynes P, et al. Assessment of brain midline shift using sonography in neurosurgical ICU patients. Crit Care. 2014;18(6):676.
82. Llompart Pou JA, Abadal Centellas JM, Palmer Sans M, Perez Barcena J, Casares Vivas M, Homar Ramirez J, et al. Monitoring midline shift by transcranial color-coded sonography in traumatic brain injury. A comparison with cranial computerized tomography. Intensive Care Med. 2004;30(8):1672–5.
83. Ract C, Le Moigno S, Bruder N, Vigue B. Transcranial Doppler ultrasound goal-directed therapy for the early management of severe traumatic brain injury. Intensive Care Med. 2007;33(4):645–51.
84. Tazarourte K, Atchabahian A, Tourtier JP, David JS, Ract C, Savary D, et al. Pre-hospital transcranial Doppler in severe traumatic brain injury: a pilot study. Acta Anaesthesiol Scand. 2011;55(4):422–8.
85. Rasulo FA, Bertuetti R, Robba C, Lusenti F, Cantoni A, Bernini M, et al. The accuracy of transcranial Doppler in excluding intracranial hypertension following acute brain injury: a multicenter prospective pilot study. Crit Care. 2017;21(1):44.

Part IV

Pathology and Clinical Applications: General ICU

Sepsis, Liver Failure

11

Giovanni Volpicelli

Contents

11.1 Introduction

Some life-threatening conditions and some chronic conditions, like sepsis, and metabolic and liver diseases, may severely impair the function of the brain and determine associated brain disorders. These disorders may not be linked to a direct mechanism of damage of the brain. Rather, they are often related to an indirect effect on the vascularization and blood inflow to the brain [1]. The pathophysiology of these disorders is usually multifactorial and is due to the effect of neuroinflammation factors, dysfunction of neurotransmitters, and ischemic processes, but it is also linked to alteration of cerebral perfusion and increase in intracranial pressure [1–4]. The development of related brain disorders during the time course of sepsis and metabolic diseases may severely affect prognosis and is associated with higher mortality but also lower quality of life in survivors, who may develop long-term neurological sequelae. Brain dysfunction may also be linked to alteration of the blood flow that may reach the point of ischemia in the absence of obstruction. Systemic arterial hypotension may determine impaired blood flow, but even in the absence of hemodynamic impairment a change in cerebral autoregulation determined by pathologic metabolic and inflammatory factors may become the main determinant of the brain damage [1, 5]. Thus, in severe multiorgan conditions like sepsis but also in metabolic and acute liver diseases the early diagnosis of altered brain blood flow represents an important clue to predict the cerebral involvement. Cerebral blood flow may be evaluated by advanced and invasive technological tools, but also noninvasively at bedside by the application of cerebral ultrasound. This chapter describes the role of transcranial Doppler ultrasound in related brain disorders in sepsis and

G. Volpicelli (✉)
Department of Emergency Medicine, San Luigi Gonzaga University Hospital, Torino, Italy

C. Robba, G. Citerio (eds.), *Echography and Doppler of the Brain*,
https://doi.org/10.1007/978-3-030-48202-2_11

acute liver diseases and describes the state of the art of the application of cerebral ultrasound to the study of blood flow and its alteration during the time course of these disorders.

11.2 Sepsis

Sepsis is a condition of infection with multiorgan involvement and dysfunction caused by a dysregulated host response, which may become life threatening when severe [6]. The majority of septic patients in the intensive care unit develop sepsis-associated brain dysfunction and often manifest delirium as a consequence [7]. This condition is also associated with high mortality. Quite rarely, involvement of the brain may be due to diffusion of the infection through the hemato-encephalic barrier. Indeed, in most cases, impairment of brain function may also be observed in the absence of a central nervous system infection, effect of drug overdose, and other mechanisms of direct damage. Brain dysfunction is considered the most frequent sepsis-related organ dysfunction in a disease that for definition is multiorgan affecting. Not only dysfunction of the brain is highly frequent, but also usually manifests very early during the time course of severe sepsis and often precedes involvement of other organs [8]. For these reasons, awareness of the presence of even minimal signs of brain dysfunction becomes crucial in the early diagnostic process of sepsis. Sometimes, the evidence of brain dysfunction based on the observation of presenting symptoms and a few bedside instrumental diagnostic tools may even become the main and unique clue orientating the clinician to the diagnosis of severe sepsis, giving also important prognostic information.

Causes of sepsis-related brain dysfunction are mainly linked to mechanisms owing to ischemic cerebral damage. The vascular dysfunction may be due to a condition of shock and hypotension but more frequently, in the absence of hemodynamic instability, it can be the result of impairment in the homeostatic mechanism that physiologically regulates the blood inflow to compensate hypo- or hyper-perfusion [9, 10]. The mechanism of cerebral autoregulation is largely and actively compensatory in conditions of altered perfusion, but during sepsis its function may be severely depressed. This may create a loss of control in the cerebral blood flow due to the lack of adaptation of the caliber of the small cerebral arterioles [11].

Cerebral autoregulation may be assessed by using transcranial Doppler ultrasound at bedside [8]. The mean flow index assessed at Doppler ultrasound can be used as a measure of autoregulation of the cerebral blood flow [12]. By transcranial Doppler it is possible to measure the blood flow velocity in intracranial vessels and relate it to the variations in arterial blood pressure, a surrogate of cerebral perfusion pressure (see Table 11.1) [12]. The technique for the measurement of the cerebral mean flow index consists of the insonation of the middle cerebral artery by placing the probe in the transtemporal window and maintaining at a constant angle of insonation to allow monitoring of the cerebral blood velocity in time. Variation of the cerebral blood velocity is correlated to the contemporary change in arterial blood pressure. The mean flow is a continuous index that ranges from positive +1 when there is a positive perfect relationship between mean arterial pressure and cerebral flow velocity, which means totally inhibited capacity of cerebral autoregulation and passive dependence on systemic pressure, to −1 when there is full independence of the cerebral vessels from the arterial pressure, which means intact power of autoregulation [12].

In a study performed on critically ill septic patients during the time course of intensive care, it was demonstrated that the patients with significantly impaired cerebral autoregulation based on the assessment of increased mean flow index were those showing clear neurologic signs of sepsis-associated brain dysfunction [12]. Patients with brain dysfunction were also those with a worst prognosis in terms of increased length of stay in the ICU and high mortality. Data showing the correlation between impaired autoregulation and brain dysfunction demonstrate that cerebral functional hypoxia can be the main mechanism involved to explain cerebral involvement in severe

Table 11.1 List of the main transcranial Doppler methods used to assess associated brain dysfunction in sepsis and acute liver failure (ALF). Doppler is applied to the middle cerebral artery through the transtemporal window

Disease	Method	Main ref.	Formula	Description	Values
Sepsis	Mean flow index	Crippa et al. Ref. [12]	Pearson's correlation coefficient between MAP and FV	Time domain index of CAR; MAP is a surrogate of CPP and FV a surrogate of CBF	> 0.18 (predictive of CAR dysfunction)
Sepsis	Pulsatility index (PI)	Pierrakos et al. Ref. [14]	$\frac{(\text{VelSyst} - \text{VelDiast})}{\text{MBV}}$	Initial (24 h) static evaluation of the resistance in the cerebral microcirculation	>1.3 (predictive of delirium)
Sepsis	CV reactivity	Szatmári et al. Ref. [15]	$\frac{(\text{MBV}_{\text{ACZ}} - \text{MBV}_{\text{rest}})}{\text{MBV}_{\text{rest}}}$	Assessment of vasomotor reactivity to vasodilatory stimulus (acetazolamide)	Reduced reactivity as a sign of brain dysfunction
ALF	MBV and PI	Abdo et al. Ref. [24]	Pattern MBV vs PI	Relationship between low flow and high resistance as signs of brain dysfunction	Low flow (low values of MBV); high resistance (normal MBV high PI)
ALF	Windkessel notch	Aggarwal et al. Ref. [31]	Slopes ($\Delta V/\Delta t$; cm S^{-2}) Angles (°) Systolic upstroke; Windkessel upstroke and downstroke	The second systolic peak of the linearized waveform corresponds to the arterial compliance	Impaired compliance is a sign of high ICP
ALF	Estimated ICP	Rajajee et al. Ref. [35]	MAP – CPP where CPP = MAP * EDV/ TAPV	Estimation of the ICP by correlating MAP and flow velocities obtained at transcranial Doppler	High negative predictive value for excluding ICP >20 mmHg

MAP mean arterial pressure, *FV* flow velocity, *CAR* cerebral autoregulation, *CPP* cerebral perfusion pressure, *CBF* cerebral blood flow, *VelSyst* velocity systolic, *VelDiast* velocity diastolic, *MBV* mean blood velocity, *CV* cerebrovascular, MBV_{ACZ} mean blood velocity after acetazolamide stimulus, MBV_{rest} mean blood velocity at rest, *ICP* intracranial pressure, *CPP* cerebral perfusion pressure, *EDV* end diastolic velocity, *TAPV* time-averaged peak velocity

sepsis. It is known that even the mildest reduction in the regional cerebral blood flow during a compromised condition, such as in septic patients, may justify significant impairment of superior cognitive functions [13]. When autoregulation of cerebral blood flow is impaired, mechanisms of cerebral injury may be even independent from the hemodynamic state of the patient and from a stable unresponsive systemic hypotension. Thus, a combination of cognitive impairment due to brain dysfunction and normal hemodynamic in initial sepsis may represent a condition of difficult diagnosis and management, especially in emergency. In hemodynamically stable patients showing brain dysfunction, mechanisms causing impaired cerebral autoregulation may be various and mainly correlated to accumulation of factors favoring the breakdown of the blood-brain barrier, like nitric oxide and neuro-inflammation mediators. In these patients, bedside evaluation and monitoring of cerebral blood velocity at the level of the middle cerebral artery may become crucial in the future to help define the diagnosis and allow a prognostic framework.

Another study on critically ill septic patients assessed the possibility to characterize the associated brain dysfunction by measuring a static parameter obtained by Doppler ultrasound of the middle cerebral artery [14]. Cerebral endothelial cells are involved in the process of general inflammation that characterizes sepsis and are activated early during the first phase of the disease. This activation causes the release of pro-inflammatory cytokines and nitric monoxide in the brain, as already said, but also edema, platelet accumulation, and other mechanisms, all together causing impairment of microcirculation. Hypoxia is the final result of these phenomena and represents the main mechanism of brain damage. These alterations are characterized by the decrease in density of the microvessels regularly perfused, the main determinant of inadequate oxygen supply. Hypoxia is mechanically the result of the increase in the distance between the neurons and the capillaries [11]. The increase in vascular resistance of the capillary bed explains the decrease of density of perfused capillaries. Ultrasound has the power to assess the cerebral vascular resistance by measuring the pulsatility index, obtained by measuring the blood velocity at the level of the middle cerebral artery by transcranial Doppler. The measurement of blood velocity at this level by transcranial Doppler can be considered an open window on the evaluation of cerebral blood flow and changes in time of this velocity represent a surrogate to predict the regional hemodynamic changes mediated by cerebral microcirculation [15]. It is largely demonstrated that an increase in the resistance to the blood flow distal to the site of insonation is characterized by an increase in blood flow pulsatility [16]. Thus, pulsatility positively correlated to change in vascular resistance due to the change in tone and caliber of the peripheral small arteries. To obtain the pulsatility index, the middle cerebral artery is visualized by scanning through the temporal bone window and measuring the blood velocity for 10 s [14]. Measurements can be done on both sides of the skull and the highest mean velocity is considered valid. The pulsatility index is calculated as (Systolic velocity − Diastolic velocity)/Mean velocity (see Table 11.1). It is a static parameter that, when increased, demonstrates microcirculation disturbances that are significantly related to clear clinical signs of sepsis-associated brain dysfunction. High values of pulsatility index over 1.3 measured at the very first approach (within 24 h) after the initial symptoms of sepsis indicate the impending damage and occurrence of brain dysfunction [14]. Indeed, increased static pulsatility index as a sign of diffuse intracranial microcirculation disease may be found even in patients with stable hemodynamics. In sepsis however, only the increase in the very early phase was correlated and considered predictive of functional cerebral alterations and severe prognosis [14]. This observation paves the way to the possibility that an early evaluation of the vascular resistance at the level of the cerebral microcirculation, via the calculation of the pulsatility index obtained by Doppler ultrasound of the middle cerebral artery, may make more efficient the initial diagnostic assessment and serve as a good prognostic indicator in severe sepsis. Furthermore, because sepsis is a dynamic state and has a systemic multifaceted characteristic, using the assessment of the pulsatility index during the time course of the disease may have the power to predict the response to treatment and be used as a sign of worsening, independent even from the assessment of the hemodynamic state. Increase of the pulsatility index may be a sign of increase in the cerebrovascular resistance and onset of autoregulatory disturbances, which may lead to exposure of the brain of the septic patient to reduction of cerebral blood flow. Thus, in clinical practice, the initial assessment and monitoring of the pulsatility index may become a first-line bedside technique in the early diagnosis and follow-up of critically ill septic patients.

Other studies analyzed the effect of different stimuli on the cerebral microcirculation to demonstrate the anomalies in cerebral autoregulation [15, 17, 18]. These stimuli may be drugs like acetazolamide or gases like increase of partial pressure of carbon dioxide. The pulsatility index can be used to assess variations during different phases when the cerebral circulation is exposed to the stimulus. These experimental models proved that in patients with sepsis and established symptoms of associated brain dysfunction involving superior cognitive functions, the autoregulated vasomotor reactivity was significantly impaired. The reaction to the stimulus is lower in magnitude and is also of slower adaptation in patients with signs of brain dysfunction (see Table 11.1) [15]. Thus, the impairment in the cerebral autoregulation can be demonstrated not only as a maximal capacity in a fixed moment but also during the time course of the exposure to the stimulus.

In conclusion, both dynamic and static indexes measured by Doppler ultrasound of the middle cerebral artery are useful parameters to assess and monitor alteration of the cerebral blood flow and onset of sepsis-associated brain dysfunction. The pulsatility index and the mean flow index have been demonstrated to correlate with symptoms of brain disfunction in septic patients and represent signs of alteration of the cerebral autoregulation of blood flow and increased microvascular resistance, causing diffuse hypoxia and consequent overt superior cognitive abnormalities.

There are limitations to the conclusion of studies on transcranial Doppler ultrasound in sepsis. First, the techniques of transcranial Doppler ultrasound here described consider the evaluation of blood flow at the level of a large intracranial artery, that is, the middle cerebral artery. Even if the assessment of blood flow at this level represents a predictor of the condition of the microcirculation, it is only an indirect evaluation and cannot be fully representative of the real impairment of microcirculation that may lead to regional isolated and not diffuse ischemia consequences. Indeed, the mean flow index and the pulsatility index are mathematical simplification of the complex biological phenomenon, that is, cerebral vascular autoregulation.

Second, it is well known that chronic renal disease negatively affects the function of microcirculation in the brain, giving similar alterations than those described in the pathophysiology of sepsis-associated brain dysfunction. Indeed, advanced renal failure favors endothelial dysfunction and inflammation, and determines accumulation of urea and other vasoactive factors altering the sympathetic system control. All these alterations cause increase in the vascular resistance and impairment in the cerebral autoregulation. Thus, in septic critically ill patients the effect on brain microcirculation of acute or chronic kidney diseases may become a confounding effect not necessarily linked only to the evolution of severe sepsis. The negative effects of acute and chronic uremia on the cerebral vasculature in critically ill patients should be separated to conclude about the pure effects of sepsis [12]. Not always in studies differentiation of renal failure is an easy task to be accomplished, also in consideration of the complexity of a multiorgan model of disease like sepsis. For this reason, it is crucial to study a very high number of patients, not yet sufficiently done in the existing literature. Indeed, all the studies published so far enrolled a limited number of patients and they were on a monocenter basis. Thus, new studies are needed to consolidate what was already tested and find the real correlation between the transcranial Doppler patterns and brain dysfunction at the onset of sepsis and during its evolution. Finally, another potential significant limitation is the inadequacy of a transtemporal acoustic window, which is reported to be in as many as 10–20% of patients in some studies [18].

11.3 Liver Failure

Liver diseases and brain dysfunction have a tight correlation [19]. Like for sepsis and renal failure, also acute and chronic liver diseases, when characterized by consolidated failure of the organ function, usually result in brain microcirculatory dysfunction related to inflammatory and endothelial biomarkers [19]. Increased microvascular resistance and loss of cerebral vascular autoregulation are the two main mechanisms leading to cerebral hypoxia and encephalopathy. In the most severe conditions, loss of autoregulation determines increased cerebral blood flow that can lead to raised intracranial pressure. Circulating neurotoxins including ammonia and other factors causing neuroinflammation all have a vasoactive effect and reduce the physiologic function of cerebral blood flow autoregulation [20]. Also, ammonia accumulating in the glial cells creates an osmotic gradient and favors cellular edema that, together with vasodilation, determines increase of the intracranial pressure [20, 21]. These changes are observed in a significant percentage of cases of acute severe liver failure. In these patients, encephalopathy is characterized by intracranial hypertension, a condition that worsens the prognosis because it increases the morbidity and predisposes to herniation and death [20–22]. Thus, intracranial hypertension needs to be diagnosed and monitored in critically ill liver failure patients to orientate treatment and prevent neurological injuries and death.

A promising bedside noninvasive tool to monitor brain dysfunction in liver failure is the transcranial Doppler. Intracranial pressure influences the pattern of the cerebral blood flow velocity waveform assessed by ultrasound at the level of the middle cerebral artery [23]. In literature, only very few original studies demonstrated the power of transcranial Doppler in the prediction of intracranial hypertension in acute liver failure. Some of the evidence we may extract from literature is based on case series. The mean cerebral blood flow was reduced and the pulsatility index increased in a series of patients with acute failure from viral hepatitis [24–26]. In these studies, the transcranial Doppler pattern was demonstrative of hypoperfusion when compared to normal patterns. Thus, from this experience it seems that hypoperfusion of the cerebral vascular bed is the main factor that should be corrected by increasing cerebral perfusion and treating hypoxia. This data was confirmed by a specifically designed original study on acute-onset end-stage liver failure patients who were examined by transcranial Doppler of the middle cerebral artery to measure systolic, diastolic, and mean blood flow velocities and pulsatility index [27]. This small study confirmed that the most frequent pattern in these patients was low flow and high resistance with high pulsatility index (see Table 11.1). This combination was more significant in the subgroup of patients who died. The high pulsatility index is considered a marker of increased intracranial pressure, in agreement with previous literature produced by studying other diseases [28–30]. In patients with acute liver failure this data is confirmed, and high pulsatility index can be used as a sign of intracranial hypertension and worse prognosis.

Another study examined retrospectively more in detail the change in the Doppler waveform with respect to change in cerebral perfusion in acute liver failure [31]. This study demonstrated that the correlation between the blood flow and the condition of acute liver failure is time dependent and evolves concomitantly with the progression of the disease. The shape of the waveform at the transcranial Doppler indicating initial increase in the blood flow and cerebral vasodilation may justify the progressive increase in the intracranial pressure. From the moment cerebral vasodilation is first detected onwards, the cerebral hemodynamics continue to deteriorate, and this is demonstrated by a progressive increase of intracranial pressure, concomitant signs of vasoparalysis of the cerebral vessels, and loss of autoregulation. In a condition of intracranial hypertension, vasoparalysis is due to the increase in the extramural pressure due to cerebral swelling that, at the final stage, may bring to Doppler evidence of sharp systolic peak and retrograde flow [32]. However, even if this detailed analysis of the waveform was find to correlate with the evolution of the increase of intracranial pressure and changes in the hemodynamics of the cerebral vessels, it should also be considered that the intracranial hemodynamics is subjected to complex interactions, including the effect of temperature, systemic arterial pressure, and $PaCO_2$ and their fluctuations [33]. Thus, such a detailed quantitative analysis of the waveform may oversimplify a complex phenomenon that needs the consideration of a more complex model to be read and interpreted. The consideration of pulsatility index simplifies the assessment. It is an index easy to calculate, less influenced by the correct angle of insonation, and is more accurate in expressing the combination of many factors affecting the cerebral blood flow. However, this index represents a good picture of the resistance of the cerebral microcirculation but is not enough detailed to allow the analysis of the dynamic changes in the compliance of arterial vessels under the effect of the cerebral swelling and progressive increase of the intracranial pressure [33, 34]. A combination of the simple pulsatility index, which looks at the extrema in flow velocities, and a rough analysis of a few features of the linearized Doppler flow waveform may be more promising [31]. These latter analyses may be centered to the evaluation of the Windkessel effect, that is, the reduced blood vessel elasticity demonstrated by reduced elastic rebound of the cerebral vasculature (see Table 11.1) [31, 32].

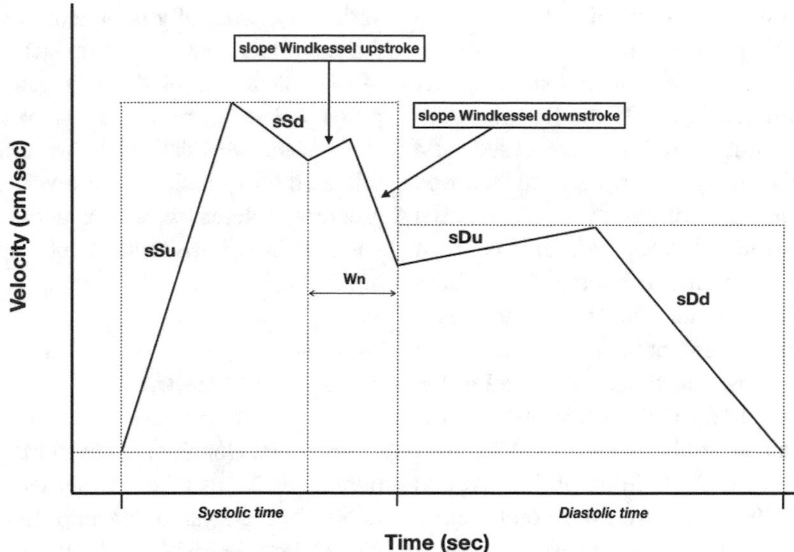

Fig. 11.1 The simplified linearized Doppler flow waveform [31]. The analysis of the waveform allows to distinguish systolic and diastolic phases (upstroke and downstroke). The Windkessel notch corresponds to the second peak during the systolic phase. This latter is the effect of the compliance of the arterial wall after receiving the first peak due to the myocardial contractility. The Windkessel notch is also divided into upstroke and downstroke slopes. The analysis of the slopes and angles indicates the vascular resistance in the distal vessels. *sSu* slope systolic upstroke, *sSd* slope systolic downstroke, *sDu* slope diastolic upstroke, *sDd* slope diastolic downstroke, *Wn* Windkessel notch

These are demonstrated in the linearized waveform by the change in the notches corresponding to the angles of adjacent slopes (see Fig. 11.1). Indeed, the changes in these angles of the linearized waveform reflect the effect of raising intracranial pressure and fall in the cerebral perfusion pressure typical of deterioration of the brain function in acute liver failure. In these cases, the waveform shows the increase in systolic velocity and loss in arterial compliance as that Windkessel notch angle becomes more obtuse while the Windkessel slope lessens. In a more advanced condition, when intracranial pressure further increases and cerebral perfusion decreases, the Windkessel phenomenon disappears [31]. This detailed analysis of the waveform may be useful to assign patients into categories with different combinations of two parameters, intracranial pressure and cerebral flow pressure, tightly linked by a physiological equation. However, not necessarily these arbitrary categories may reflect factual differentiation of practical medical interventions. Also, the analysis of velocity slopes and time points of a linearized transcranial Doppler waveform is based on a visual identification, which for definition is somewhat subjective and, as such, reflecting interoperator variability. Thus, further studies are needed to define the methodology based on the detailed reading of the blood flow waveform.

Another retrospective study evaluated the ability of transcranial Doppler and also optic nerve sheath diameter, assessed by trans-ocular ultrasound, to predict elevated intracranial pressure measured invasively in acute liver failure patients admitted to the ICU [35]. Surprisingly, both the optic nerve measure and the pulsatility index, calculated by transcranial Doppler of the middle cerebral artery, resulted to be not accurate enough to predict intracranial hypertension superior to 20 mmHg and not significantly associated to mortality. Only the Doppler estimation of the intracranial pressure based on a method published by Czosnyka et al. showed high negative predictivity for intracranial hypertension, thus allowing safe exclusion of the condition in patients with acute liver failure. This method allows the estimation of the cerebral perfusion pressure through measurement of cerebral blood flow velocities at the level of the middle cerebral artery and consideration of the systemic mean arterial pressure (MAP), thus indirectly indicating the level of intracranial pressure [36]. It is based on the combination of two formulae: the first to estimate the cerebral perfusion pressure (CPPe): MAP x (EDV/TAPV), where EDV is the end diastolic velocity and TAPV is the time-averaged peak velocity; the second to calculate the intracranial pressure: MAP – CPPe (see Table 11.1). Based on these evidences, it is possible to hypothesize a role of the Doppler-estimated intracranial pressure as a practical bedside tool to rule out significant intracranial hypertension in patients with acute liver failure.

The data showing inaccuracy of ultrasound of the optic nerve and pulsatility index for the prediction of intracranial hypertension may be considered surprising because it is not in agreement with the previous literature [30, 37–40]. However, the pathophysiology of intracranial hypertension in acute liver failure is strikingly different from the other models well studied in literature, such us hydrocephalus, stroke, and trauma [35]. In liver failure the brain involvement is characterized by both cerebral edema and vasodilation, thus representing a peculiar model. This difference may explain the discrepancy found in the study of Rajajee et al. [35]. The formula used to calculate the surrogate of intracranial pressure has a great limitation as it is tightly linked to the measured value of the systemic mean arterial pressure. This latter is subjected to variability, especially in patients with acute liver failure, which can deeply impact the variability of the calculation of the surrogated intracranial pressure. For this reason, the same authors of the study were skeptical on the possibility of using this method to indicate the level of intracranial pressure, whereas a simple application to rule out sustained intracranial hypertension is more promising [35].

11.4 Conclusion

Transcranial Doppler is of usefulness in the study of brain disorders related to sepsis and acute liver failure. The analysis of the blood flow velocities at the level of the middle cerebral artery represents an open window on the evaluation of cerebral blood inflow, resistance in the microcirculation, and state of the cerebral vascular autoregulation. In sepsis the loss of autoregulation and increase in vascular resistance represent the main determinants of sepsis-related brain dysfunction, which may be detected at the first examination by bedside transcranial Doppler through the analysis of the pulsatility and the mean flow indexes. In acute liver failure the main determinant of related brain dysfunction is intracranial hypertension due mainly to cerebral edema and swelling. A combination of pulsatility index and analysis of the linearized blood flow waveform may be useful to predict the alterations in microcirculatory resistance and cerebral blood flow that causes intracranial hypertension and brain damage. Also, the use of a surrogate of the intracranial pressure calculated by combining the transcranial Doppler measures of blood flow velocities and the mean arterial pressure may be of great value to rule out the condition of intracranial hypertension. However, even if data published in the existing literature are promising, further studies testing transcranial Doppler in a high number of patients are needed to standardize a method to extend its use to the practical approach to sepsis and acute liver failure.

References

1. Heming N, Mazeraud A, Verdonk F, Bozza FA, Chrétien F, Sharshar T. Neuroanatomy of sepsis-associated encephalopathy. Crit Care. 2017;21:65.
2. Stravitz RT, Kramer AH, Davern T, Shaikh AO, Caldwell SH, Mehta RL, Blei AT, Fontana RJ, McGuire BM, Rossaro L, Smith AD, Lee WM. Acute Liver Failure Study Group. Intensive care of patients with acute liver failure: recommendations of the U.S. Acute Liver Failure Study Group. Crit Care Med. 2007;35:2498–508.
3. Bunchorntavakul C, Reddy KR. Acute liver failure. Clin Liver Dis. 2017;21:769–92.
4. Butterworth RF. The concept of "the inflamed brain" in acute liver failure: mechanisms and new therapeutic opportunities. Metab Brain Dis. 2016;31:1283–7.
5. Brito-Azevedo A, Perez RM, Maranhão PA, Coelho HS, Fernandes ESM, Castiglione RC, de Souza MD, Villela-Nogueira CA, Bouskela E. Organ dysfunction in cirrhosis: a mechanism involving the microcirculation. Eur J Gastroenterol Hepatol. 2019;31:618–25.
6. Singer M, Deutschman CS, Seymour CW, Shankar-Hari M, Annane D, Bauer M, Bellomo R, Bernard GR, Chiche JD, Coopersmith CM, Hotchkiss RS, Levy MM, Marshall JC, Martin GS, Opal SM, Rubenfeld GD, van der Poll T, Vincent JL, Angus DC. The third international consensus definitions for sepsis and septic shock (sepsis-3). JAMA. 2016;315:801–10.
7. Piva S, McCreadie VA, Latronico N. Neuroinflammation in sepsis: sepsis associated delirium. Cardiovasc Hematol Disord Drug Targets. 2015;15:10–8.
8. de Azevedo DS, Salinet ASM, de Lima OM, Teixeira MJ, Bor-Seng-Shu E, de Carvalho Nogueira R. Cerebral hemodynamics in sepsis assessed by transcranial Doppler: a systematic review and meta-analysis. J Clin Monit Comput. 2017;31:1123–32.
9. Peterson EC, Wang Z, Britz G. Regulation of cerebral blood flow. Int J Vasc Med. 2011;2011:823525.
10. Taccone FS, Su F, De Deyne C, Abdellhai A, Pierrakos C, He X, Donadello K, Dewitte O, Vincent JL, De Backer D. Sepsis is associated with altered cerebral microcirculation and tissue hypoxia in experimental peritonitis. Crit Care Med. 2014;42:e114–22.
11. Taccone FS, Su F, Pierrakos C, He X, James S, Dewitte O, Vincent JL, De Backer D. Cerebral microcirculation is impaired during sepsis: an experimental study. Crit Care. 2010;14:R140.
12. Crippa IA, Subirà C, Vincent JL, Fernandez RF, Hernandez SC, Cavicchi FZ, Creteur J, Taccone FS. Impaired cerebral autoregulation is associated with brain dysfunction in patients with sepsis. Crit Care. 2018;22:327.
13. Bowton DL, Bertels NH, Prough DS, Stump DA. Cerebral blood flow is reduced in patients with sepsis syndrome. Crit Care Med. 1989;17:399–403.
14. Pierrakos C, Attou R, Decorte L, Kolyviras A, Malinverni S, Gottignies P, Devriendt J, De Bels D. Transcranial Doppler to assess sepsis-associated encephalopathy in critically ill patients. BMC Anesthesiol. 2014;14:45.
15. Szatmári S, Végh T, Csomós A, Hallay J, Takács I, Molnár C, Fülesdi B. Impaired cerebrovascular reactivity in sepsis-associated encephalopathy studied by acetazolamide test. Crit Care. 2010;14:R50.
16. Taylor KJ, Holland S. Doppler US: Part I. Basic principles, instrumentation, and pitfalls. Radiology. 1990;174:297–307.
17. Kadoi Y, Saito S, Kawauchi C, Hinohara H, Kunimoto F. Comparative effects of propofol vs dexmedetomidine on cerebrovascular carbon dioxide reactivity in patients with septic shock. Br J Anaesth. 2008;100:224–9.
18. Naqvi J, Yap KH, Ahmad G, Ghosh J. Transcranial Doppler ultrasound: a review of the physical principles and major applications in critical care. Int J Vasc Med. 2013;2013:629378.
19. D'Mello C, Swain MG. Liver-brain inflammation axis. Am J Physiol Gastrointest Liver Physiol. 2011;301:G749–61.
20. Sheikh MF, Unni N, Agarwal B. Neurological Monitoring in Acute Liver Failure. J Clin Exp Hepatol. 2018;8:441–7.
21. Reynolds AS, Brush B, Schiano TD, Reilly KJ, Dangayach NS. Neurological Monitoring in Acute Liver Failure. Hepatology. 2019;70:1830–5.
22. Datar S, Wijdicks EF. Neurologic manifestations of acute liver failure. Handb Clin Neurol. 2014;120:645–59.
23. Cardim D, Robba C, Bohdanowicz M, Donnelly J, Cabella B, Liu X, Cabeleira M, Smielewski P, Schmidt B, Czosnyka M. Non-invasive monitoring of intracranial pressure using transcranial Doppler ultrasonography: is it possible? Neurocrit Care. 2016;25:473–91.
24. Abdo A, López O, Fernández A, Santos J, Castillo J, Castellanos R, González L, Gómez F, Limonta D. Transcranial Doppler sonography in fulminant hepatic failure. Transplant Proc. 2003;35:1859–60.
25. Kawakami M, Koda M, Murawaki Y. Cerebral pulsatility index by transcranial Doppler sonography predicts the prognosis of patients with fulminant hepatic failure. Clin Imaging. 2010;34:327–31.
26. Bindi ML, Biancofiore G, Esposito M, Meacci L, Bisà M, Mozzo R, Urbani L, Catalano G, Montin U, Filipponi F. Transcranial Doppler sonography is useful for the decision-making at the point of care in patients with acute hepatic failure: a single centre's experience. J Clin Monit Comput. 2008;22:449–52.
27. Abdo A, Pérez-Bernal J, Hinojosa R, Porras F, Castellanos R, Gómez F, Gutiérrez J, Castellanos A, Leal G, Espinosa N, Gómez-Bravo M. Cerebral hemodynamics patterns by transcranial doppler in

patients with acute liver failure. Transplant Proc. 2015;47:2647–9.
28. Cardim D, Robba C, Donnelly J, Bohdanowicz M, Schmidt B, Damian M, Varsos GV, Liu X, Cabeleira M, Frigieri G, Cabella B, Smielewski P, Mascarenhas S, Czosnyka M. Prospective study on noninvasive assessment of intracranial pressure in traumatic brain-injured patients: comparison of four methods. J Neurotrauma. 2016;33:792–802.
29. Cardim D, Czosnyka M, Donnelly J, et al. Assessment of noninvasive ICP during CSF infusion test: an approach with transcranial Doppler. Acta Neurochir. 2016;158:279–87.
30. Bellner J, Romner B, Reinstrup P, Kristiansson KA, Ryding E, Brandt L. Transcranial Doppler sonography pulsatility index (PI) reflects intracranial pressure (ICP). Surg Neurol. 2004;62:45–51.
31. Aggarwal S, Brooks DM, Kang Y, Linden PK, Patzer JF 2nd. Noninvasive monitoring of cerebral perfusion pressure in patients with acute liver failure using transcranial doppler ultrasonography. Liver Transpl. 2008;14:1048–57.
32. Larsen FS, Strauss G, Moller K, Hansen BA. Regional cerebral blood flow autoregulation in patients with fulminant hepatic failure. Liver Transpl. 2000;6:795–800.
33. de Riva N, Budohoski KP, Smielewski P, Kasprowicz M, Zweifel C, Steiner LA, Reinhard M, Fábregas N, Pickard JD, Czosnyka M. Transcranial Doppler pulsatility index: what it is and what it isn't. Neurocrit Care. 2012;17:58–66.
34. Schmidt B, Klingelhofer J, Schwarze JJ, Sander D, Wittich I. Noninvasive prediction of intracranial pressure curves using transcranial Doppler ultrasonography and blood pressure curves. Stroke. 1997;28:2465–72.
35. Rajajee V, Williamson CA, Fontana RJ, Courey AJ, Patil PG. Noninvasive intracranial pressure assessment in acute liver failure. Neurocrit Care. 2018;29:280–90.
36. Czosnyka M, Matta BF, Smielewski P, Kirkpatrick PJ, Pickard JD. Cerebral perfusion pressure in head-injured patients: a noninvasive assessment using transcranial Doppler ultrasonography. J Neurosurg. 1998;88:802–8.
37. Strumwasser A, Kwan RO, Yeung L, Miraflor E, Ereso A, Castro-Moure F, Patel A, Sadjadi J, Victorino GP. Sonographic optic nerve sheath diameter as an estimate of intracranial pressure in adult trauma. J Surg Res. 2011;170:265–71.
38. Dubourg J, Javouhey E, Geeraerts T, Messerer M, Kassai B. Ultrasonography of optic nerve sheath diameter for detection of raised intracranial pressure: a systematic review and meta-analysis. Intensive Care Med. 2011;37:1059–68.
39. Robba C, Cardim D, Tajsic T, Pietersen J, Bulman M, Donnelly J, Lavinio A, Gupta A, Menon DK, Hutchinson PJA, Czosnyka M. Ultrasound non-invasive measurement of intracranial pressure in neurointensive care: a prospective observational study. PLoS Med. 2017;14:e1002356.
40. Rajajee V, Vanaman M, Fletcher JJ, Jacobs TL. Optic nerve ultrasound for the detection of raised intracranial pressure. Neurocrit Care. 2011;15:506–15.

Stroke

12

Victoria A. McCredie

Contents

12.1 Introduction

Brain ultrasonography (BUS) is an important monitoring modality in stroke due to its portability, rapid performance, reduced need for sedation, real-time image acquisition, and, most importantly, lack of ionizing radiation, and non-invasive nature of the technique. Various imaging modalities have been employed to diagnose cerebral blood flow disturbances in acute neurological illness, including xenon inhalation computed tomography (CT) scanning, perfusion CT, magnetic resonance imaging (MRI) perfusion and angiography, single-photon emission tomography, and positron-emission tomography. These methods all have value, but unfortunately are limited to a single point in time, whereas most acute conditions like acute ischemic stroke are dynamic. Continuous methods for monitoring aspects of brain anatomy, perfusion, and autoregulation are important concepts in the management of these neurocritically ill patients. The noninvasive and repeatable bedside method of BUS may augment conventional neuroradiologic

V. A. McCredie (✉)
Division of Critical Care Medicine, Department of Medicine, University Health Network, Toronto, Ontario, Canada

Interdepartmental Division of Critical Care Medicine, Department of Medicine, University of Toronto, Toronto, Ontario, Canada

Krembil Research Institute, Toronto Western Hospital, Toronto, Ontario, Canada
e-mail: victoria.mccredie@mail.utoronto.ca

C. Robba, G. Citerio (eds.), *Echography and Doppler of the Brain*,
https://doi.org/10.1007/978-3-030-48202-2_12

imaging. The aim of this review is to provide an overview of the potential clinical applications of BUS in acute ischemic stroke.

12.2 Acute Ischemic Stroke

This section specifically discusses the indications for BUS in acute ischemic stroke (AIS). Intracerebral hematomas and subarachnoid hemorrhage will be covered in further chapters. BUS can be used in the acute setting as a minimally invasive way of determining vascular patency, identifying large vessel occlusions and monitoring the response to stroke treatment. When performed by trained personnel, according to a standardized and validated protocol, neurosonological evaluation does not result in any delay in the AIS management [1].

12.2.1 Diagnosis of Stroke Etiology

Contrast-enhanced BUS can assist in the workup for a possible cardioembolic source of cryptogenic stroke by diagnosing paradoxical emboli in the cerebral arterial circulation. Using agitated saline as a contrast medium, the patient is asked to perform a Valsalva maneuver to potentially reverse the normal flow through the PFO and create a right-to-left shunt (RLS). As the agitated saline is injected, the ultrasound probe is placed over the temporal acoustic window to insonate the MCA. If a shunt is present the air microbubbles will pass directly from venous to systemic circulation and then visualized as microbubbles, or micro-embolic signals (MES), in the anterior cerebral vessels [2]. The finding of a single microbubble in cerebral arterial circulation is considered diagnostic of RLS. The use of contrast-enhanced BUS also permits a semiquantitative estimate of the severity of RLS [2, 3]. The International Consensus Criteria four-level MES grading score uses unilateral MCA monitoring to classify the following: no shunt if no MES is seen; low-grade shunt includes 1–10 MES; moderate-grade shunt with 11–25 MES; and high-grade shunt where MES is greater than 25 (shower) or uncountable (curtain effect) [2]. Both the International Consensus Criteria and Spencer Logarithmic Scale are 100% sensitive for detection of large PFO [4].

A meta-analysis by Katsanos and colleagues compared the diagnostic value of transthoracic echocardiography (TTE) in the detection of PFO in patients with cryptogenic ischemic stroke with that of contrast-enhanced BUS [5]. The authors found that BUS is more sensitive (96% vs. 92%), but less specific (45% vs. 100%) compared to TTE for the detection of PFO and RLS. As the overall diagnostic yield of BUS appears to be higher than that of TTE (area under the curve (AUC) 0.98 vs. 0.86, $p < 0.001$), it may be reasonable to use contrast-enhanced BUS as an initial screening method for RLS detection in patients with cryptogenic stroke. Another meta-analysis conducted by Mojadidi and colleagues found contrast-enhanced BUS to be similarly sensitive (97%) but with higher specificity (93%) in the detection of RLS, when compared to the gold standard, transesophageal echocardiography (TEE) [6]. In a subgroup analysis, increasing the number of microbubbles needed for a positive BUS from 1 to 10 resulted in a predictable significant improvement in specificity (89–100%, $p = 0.04$). Overall, BUS does not allow identification of the anatomic position of the RLS; it cannot distinguish between a PFO, an atrial septal defect, or a pulmonary arteriovenous fistula. The time window of MES crossing into the systemic circulation and subsequently detection with BUS cannot differentiate between RLS at the atrial level and RLS at different sites of the vascular system [2]. TEE may therefore be needed to determine the anatomical lesion responsible for the shunt as it remains the gold standard for detection of a patent foramen ovale or an atrial septum defect. TTE has a low yield in distinguishing between PFO and atrial septal defect and management options may depend on the TEE clarification.

12.2.2 Diagnosis of Large Vessel Occlusion

Although BUS is a low-cost, convenient, and rapidly repeatable bedside test compared to other imaging modalities, it is limited by its reduced ability to visualize the posterior circulation and dependence on operator experience requiring considerable skill and experience for accurate interpretation. Consequently, CT angiography and magnetic resonance (MR) angiography remain the preferred first-line imaging techniques in acute ischemic stroke. It would appear reasonable to correlate BUS with the initial imaging, CT or MRI, as a baseline and to use BUS for repeated monitoring throughout the acute admission period. A study conducted by Demchuk and colleagues evaluated the frequency and accuracy of specific BUS flow findings in patients with angiographically proven arterial occlusion [7]. In a cohort of 190 patients with symptoms of cerebral ischemia, BUS had an overall sensitivity of 83%, specificity of 94%, positive predictive value of 83%, negative predictive value of 94%, and accuracy of 92% to identify all sites of occlusion. Using a standardized intracranial insonation protocol [8–11], and detailed diagnostic criteria, BUS was highly sensitive for proximal internal carotid artery (ICA) (94%) and MCA occlusions (93%). The sensitivity for posterior circulation occlusions was significantly less, with 56% for the terminal vertebral artery and 60% for the basilar artery. The specificity was 96–98% for all arterial segments. The accuracy of BUS to detect anterior cerebral artery (ACA) and posterior cerebral artery (PCA) occlusions was not analyzed because of the small numbers of both types of occlusion. Neurosonological characteristics useful to localize anterior circulation occlusion include collaterals, abnormal waveforms or velocities, and flow diversion to perforators. To detect and differentiate the level of arterial occlusion the pathophysiologic changes of collateralization, increased resistance, and delayed flow acceleration must be taken into consideration. These specific BUS findings are common with large vessel occlusion and can be applied to improve the accuracy of noninvasive monitoring in AIS patients [10]. These results, along with similar studies, highlight the need to standardize insonation protocols, establish skill recommendations for operators, and implement specific diagnostic criteria to improve operator dependency and interrater reliability, which currently impede the accuracy and advancement of this imaging modality [12–16].

12.2.3 Monitoring of Recanalization

Considering that hyperacute stroke represents a dynamic cerebrovascular state and reocclusion can occur post-intervention, the potential role of BUS in stroke expands to include continuous monitoring of residual flow grades and recanalization after endovascular and thrombolytic therapy. By performing serial BUS examinations, hemodynamic changes following stroke that would otherwise go undetected by a single static CT or MR scan can be elicited. However, implementation of operator training for the neurointensivist is a necessary step if these extended applications are to be further developed and refined in the neurocritical care environment [15]. The BUS characteristics of flow provide information not only about occlusion, but also about recanalization and reperfusion following thrombus dissolution, and reocclusion. To monitor these critical changes, several grading systems have been developed to classify residual flow status in AIS patients [17, 18].

Demchuk and colleagues developed a BUS grading system for residual flow within intracranial vessels, similar to the thrombolysis in myocardial ischemia (TIMI) flow grades used to assess perfusion or residual flow around coronary arteries [17]. They created a systematic classification called thrombolysis in brain ischemia (TIBI) and subsequently evaluated in 94 AIS patients with BUS performed during the initial stroke evaluation and on day 2. TIBI flows were measured at the distal MCA, via the transtemporal approach at a depth of less than 54 mm, and basilar artery, through a transforaminal window at a depth of 80–100 mm, depending on the site of occlusion. TIBI waveforms were graded as follows: 0, absent; 1, minimal; 2, blunted; 3, dampened; 4, stenotic; and 5, normal. Nedelmann and colleagues developed a TCCS-based grading system named the Consensus on Grading Intracranial Flow Obstruction (COGIF) score

[18]. This scoring system is based on known hemodynamic changes of the Doppler spectrum that can be observed in the acute stage of stroke (see Table 12.1 for descriptions of TIBI and the COGIF classifications) [17, 18]. Both scores can be used for the initial assessment of cerebral hemodynamics and follow-up assessment of the recanalization process. Care should be taken to perform follow-up measurements at exactly the same localization as baseline measurements, i.e., insonation depth and angle correction. Using the COGIF classification, cerebral hemodynamic alterations at follow-up compared to baseline can be classed as reflow (partial or complete recanalization), no change, or deterioration (see Table 12.2) [18]. Both scoring systems correlate well with the initial stroke severity (National Institutes of Health Stroke Scale (NIHSS) scores), likelihood of reperfusion, clinical recovery (based on modified Rankin scale (mRS)), and mortality [17, 19].

The time to recanalization identified on BUS is also associated with stroke severity, clinical improvement, and overall mortality [20, 21]. A meta-analysis by Stolz and colleagues evaluated the prognostic value of full recanalization detected by bedside BUS within 6 h after AIS onset [22]. Combining data from 11 studies and 620 patients with initially occluded MCA, full recanalization is associated with a greater than fivefold chance for clinical improvement at 48 h (odds ratio (OR) 5.64, 95% confidence intervals (CI) 3.82–8.31). However, this finding is affected by significant clinical and statistical heterogeneity due to the quality of the studies and publication bias. Full recanalization identified with BUS is also significantly associated with a higher chance of functional independence 3 months

Table 12.2 Hemodynamic changes at follow-up assessment compared to baseline

Hemodynamic change	COGIF grade
Reflow: Partial recanalization	Improvement by ≥1 grade
Reflow: Complete recanalization	Improvement to COGIF grade 4
No change	Baseline COGIF grade persists
Worsening	Deterioration by ≥1 grade

COGIF Consensus on Grading Intracranial Flow Obstruction

Table 12.1 Description of TIBI and COGIF scores (adapted from Demchuk and colleagues, and Nedelmann and colleagues [17, 18])

Grade	Description	Grade	Description
TIBI 0	Absent: Absent flow signals are defined by the lack of regular pulsatile flow signals despite varying degrees of background noise.	COGIF 1	Occlusion: No flow
TIBI 1	Minimal: Systolic spikes of variable velocity and duration. Absent diastolic flow during all cardiac cycles based on a visual interpretation of periods of no flow during end diastole. Reverberating flow is a type of minimal flow.	COGIF 2	Partial recanalization Low flow velocities without diastolic flow
TIBI 2	Blunted: Flattened systolic flow acceleration of variable duration compared to control. Positive end diastolic flow and pulsatility index <1.2.	COGIF 3	Low flow velocities with diastolic flow
TIBI 3	Dampened: Normal systolic flow acceleration. Positive end diastolic flow. Decreased MFV by >30% compared to control.	COGIF 3	
TIBI 4	Stenotic: MFV >80 cm/s and >30% compared to control side OR if both sides affected and MFVs <80 cm/s due to low end diastolic velocities, MFV >30% compared to control side and signs of turbulence.	COGIF 4c	Hyperperfusion: High segmental flow velocities
TIBI 4		COGIF 4b	Stenosis: High focal flow velocities
TIBI 5	Normal: <30% MFV difference compared to control. Similar waveform shapes compared to controls.	COGIF 4a	Flow velocities equal to contralateral side

TIBI thrombolysis in brain ischemia, *COGIF* consensus on grading intracranial flow obstruction, *MFV* mean flow velocity

after stroke (OR 6.07, 95% CI 3.94–9.35, 972 patients). Therefore, it appears important to obtain knowledge on the vascular status, with regard to recanalization, as it carries important information on the clinical prognosis of AIS patients.

More recent work has sought to evaluate the diagnostic accuracy of TIBI criteria to monitor recanalization with BUS during reperfusion procedures [23]. Tsivgoulis and colleagues assessed recanalization simultaneously by digital subtraction angiography (DSA) using TIMI classification and BUS using TIBI criteria during 96 intra-arterial reperfusion procedures. Independent assessors blinded to DSA estimated the TIBI flow grades to facilitate the assessment of the interrater reliability of TIBI grades. The interrater reliability for the assessment of recanalization and estimation of TIBI grades was good (Cohen κ: 0.838 and 0.874, respectively; $p < 0.001$). The accuracy of BUS (combined grades 4 and 5) compared to DSA (TIMI grade 3) for diagnosis of complete recanalization is as follows: sensitivity of 88%; specificity of 89%; positive predictive value of 81%; negative predictive value of 93%; and overall accuracy of 89%. The most common cause of TCD false-negative results was suboptimal angle of insonation caused by head movements during the reperfusion procedure resulting in BUS headframe displacement. Overall, taking into consideration the interrater reliability within centers, applying the TIBI criteria appears to accurately identify brain recanalization in real time when compared with TIMI angiographic scores.

12.2.4 Cerebral Autoregulation

Cerebral autoregulation (CA) is the ability to maintain a constant cerebral blood flow (CBF) despite fluctuations in systemic arterial blood pressure (ABP). Existing data suggest that CA is frequently compromised in the early phase of AIS leaving the brain tissue at risk of hypo- or hyper-perfusion when faced with alterations in ABP, resulting in further brain insults and a deterioration in overall neurocognitive outcome [24–27]. Thus, the importance of CA in acute stroke care is becoming increasingly recognized. A better understanding of CA and its response to pathological derangements may help guide management decisions, assess response to interventions, and possibly provide prognostic information. Classically, studies focused on measures of static autoregulation, in which regional changes in CBF were assessed at a single time point after ABP manipulation. However, recent focus has shifted toward dynamic autoregulation using techniques to track instantaneous changes in cerebral blood flow in response to ABP fluctuation [28]. With high temporal resolution, BUS can provide continuous measurements of CBF velocity in the basal cerebral arteries and although no gold standard for measuring CA has been defined, BUS is the most commonly utilized tool to study dynamic CA in AIS [29, 30]. The advanced monitoring of dynamic autoregulation with BUS is covered in detail in another chapter of this book; readers are referred to this for an in-depth discussion on the different methods and parameters.

In one of the largest studies looking at CA in AIS, Ma and colleagues studied CA in 67 AIS patients, primarily small-artery occlusions, within 3 days of symptom onset [31]. Serial measurements were performed on days 1–3 and days 7–10. MCA blood flow velocities and simultaneous ABP were recorded continuously with BUS combined with a servo-controlled finger plethysmograph. Transfer function analysis was used to derive CA parameters, and phase shift (PS) in the low-frequency range (0.06–0.12 Hz). Bilateral PS was significantly lower (indicating impaired CA) in AIS patients at both time points when compared with healthy controls ($p < 0.001$). PS did not differ between the ipsilateral and contralateral hemispheres (34.3 ± 17.8° versus 34.2 ± 16.7°, $p = 0.93$). In comparison, Peterson and colleagues assessed 28 patients within 48 h of MCA stroke onset and found that PS was lower in the affected cerebral hemisphere, compared to the contralateral side. Although the utility of BUS in the assessment of CA after stroke has been considerably studied, wide differences in autoregulation capability among AIS patients have been noted. The discrepancy between these results may be partially explained by the different underlying neuropathologic mechanisms and effect on cerebral hemodynamics. Within stroke subtypes, CA appears to be impaired in both hemispheres for patients with unilateral small-artery occlusions [32, 33]. This finding is consistent with the hypothesis of lacunar infarcts occurring on the background of bilateral small vessel disease, inducing a global cerebral pattern of impaired CA. In large-artery atherosclerotic strokes appears CA impairment limited to the affected cerebral hemisphere. In these latter patients, impaired CA also looks to be predictive of secondary complications such as cerebral edema and hemorrhagic transformation, and consequently worse functional outcome. Castro and colleagues evaluated the relationship between CA status within 6 h of stroke onset and risk of developing hemorrhagic transformation and cerebral edema at 24 h poststroke in 46 patients [24]. These secondary complications were significantly higher in those with early impairment of CA; lower PS (impaired CA) was associated with hemorrhagic transformation (7 ± 30° vs. 45 ± 38°; $p = 0.033$) and with cerebral edema (10 ± 30° vs. 41 ± 38°; $p = 0.002$) at 24 h. Progression to edema was also associated with cerebral vasodilatation (i.e., lower cerebrovascular resistance index, calculated by mean ABP divided by mean flow velocity) and increased mean flow velocities on admission to hospital, implying that breakthrough hyper-perfusion and microvascular injury may contribute to the development of malignant cerebral edema.

Although studies of static autoregulation show that CA is often preserved in AIS, recent studies have revealed that dynamic autoregulation derangement detected by BUS may follow a temporal course remaining abnormal for several weeks after presentation [34–36]. Patients who receive rt-PA thrombolysis also tend to have less impaired CA during the acute phase [31]. The relationship between rt-PA thrombolysis and CA has not been frequently studied. Theoretically, rt-PA thrombolysis may have beneficial effects on autoregulation by effectively recanalizing and minimizing the ischemic core to salvage the penumbra region where autoregulation is often proven to be disturbed. Monitoring of dynamic CA at the bedside is becoming increasingly more accessible in the neurocritical care environment and may possibly provide potential therapeutic targets in the future for AIS patients. However, literature shows considerable variation in the implementation of dynamic CA measurement practices, which has limited comparisons between studies and hindered progress toward clinical application. Efforts are ongoing to improve the standardization of data collection and methods adopted for the measurement of dynamic cerebral autoregulation [37]. Further studies are also needed to understand the mechanisms underlying impaired autoregulation in AIS patients and whether this measure can help guide hemodynamic management and reliably predict secondary complications, potentially improving the care of these patients in the acute care setting.

12.2.5 Hemorrhagic Transformation

During the acute phase of AIS, BUS imaging may be helpful to monitor for complications such as hemorrhagic conversion of an ischemic lesion which negatively impact clinical outcome. BUS can identify and differentiate between intracranial hematomas and ischemic strokes, with hematomas being hyperechogenic and ischemic lesions hypoechogenic. On grayscale B-mode, acute intracranial hematomas can be detected as hyperechoic masses within the first 5 days of presentation, differentiating them from hypoechogenic ischemic lesions [38–41]. After 5 days, the hematomas become hypoechoic with a peripheral hyperechoic halo [42]. The main differential diagnoses of hematomas on BUS are arteriovenous malformations and cerebral tumors, which are also hyperechoic; consequently confirmation of new hematomas detected on BUS by CT scan is mandatory [43]. The initial detection of intracranial hematomas with BUS primarily depends on the location more than size of the hematoma. Deep hematomas, such as hypertensive bleeds in the basal ganglia, are more likely to be detected compared with lobar hematomas, such as parietal or frontal lobe hematomas. In a cohort of 133 patients admitted with acute neurological deficits and adequate acoustic windows, the sensitivity and specificity of BUS compared with CT to differentiate intracranial hematomas from ischemic lesions are 94% and 95%, respectively, with a positive predictive value of 91% and negative predictive value of 95% [38]. In this study by Maurer and colleagues, BUS missed three atypical bleedings (two upper parietal hemorrhages). The findings for four patients were incorrectly classified as intracerebral hemorrhage where BUS detected a diffuse increase in the echo density of the white matter in the setting of ischemic stroke and marked microangiopathy. BUS may therefore represent an interesting tool for also monitoring intracerebral hemorrhage expansion at the bedside, and recommendations to perform daily measurements of the cerebral hematoma volume for early detection of intracranial hemorrhage expansion have been suggested [44]. In addition to transtemporal axial planes, coronal views are also needed for the calculation of hematoma volume. The anteroposterior and transverse dimensions (measured in centimeters) are obtained in the axial planes and the height (centimeters) by switching to the coronal insonation plane. Using the same CT equation for estimation of intracranial hematoma volume, the formula $(A \times B \times C)/2$ is applied for the calculation of hematoma volume (in cubic centimeters) by BUS, where A corresponds to anteroposterior diameter, B to transverse diameter, and C to height. Prior studies have found a good correlation, and more importantly agreement, between BUS and CT for height, sagittal and coronal diameters, and hematoma volume [45, 46].

12.2.6 Midline Shift

AIS may be complicated by hemorrhagic transformation or malignant MCA infarction syndrome leading to the evolution of mass effect and midline shift (MLS). The supratentorial mass effect primarily causes horizontal displacement of the midbrain, aqueduct, pineal gland, and septum pellucidum, with the degree of MLS on CT scan directly proportional to the level of consciousness [47]. The resulting MLS is considered a major predictor of outcome for stroke patients requiring urgent diagnosis and treatment. A MLS threshold greater than 3 mm on CT scan within 48 h of stroke, rather than lesion volume, is independently associated with 14-day mortality [48]. Although CT head is considered to be the gold standard to detect MLS, serial CT scan is time consuming, requires transportation, and is associated with significant secondary brain insults [49, 50]. MLS assessment using brain ultrasound at the bedside may facilitate early identification of patients at high risk of death from mass effect, assist patient management decisions, and expedite neurosurgical interventions for the rapidly deteriorating patient.

In 1996, Seidel and colleagues were the first to measure the dislocation of the third ventricle by brain duplex sonography in patients with space-occupying ischemic stroke [51]. This study describes a simple method for estimating the degree of MLS compared with the measured distance between the center of the third ventricle and the tabula externa of the skull on CT brain scans matching the sonographic plane. They were able to identify the third ventricle in 45 of 52 participants using a 2.5 MHz probe through the temporal window. The dislocation of the third ventricle from the suspected midline on ultrasound was calculated using the following formula $MLS = (A - B)/2$, where A is the distance between the skull and the third ventricle on the side of the stroke and B is the same distance on the contralateral side. Ultrasound MLS correlated well with findings on CT (Pearson's correlation coefficient 0.87; $p < 0.001$). Subsequent studies have also been able to reproduce these findings showing good correlation between BUS and CT MLS measurements [52–54]. Significant third ventricular dilation was found subsequently in most patients with infratentorial mass effect, and midline shift occurred in all patients with supratentorial space-occupying lesions.

In one study by Bertram and colleagues, BUS was performed in 21 patients with space-occupying ischemic middle cerebral infarction and brain hemorrhage 2 h before and after follow-up cranial CT scans. They measured third ventricular width as a parameter for infratentorial and third ventricular MLS for supratentorial mass effect. Using the temporal acoustic bone window, the probe is placed on the orbitomeatal line in the axial insonation plane, similar to Seidel and colleagues [51], and scanning depth adjusted to visualize the hyperechoic inner border of the contralateral skull at the mesencephalic level. After identifying the butterfly-shaped midbrain, the probe is fanned 10° upwards in order to detect the third ventricle with its hyperechoic margins. The oblique diameter of the third ventricle at its maximal width is measured as the distance between the inner border of the margins and should be less than 10 mm apart. The mean difference between BUS and cranial CT measurements was 0.8 mm for ventricular width (SD 1 mm, Pearson's correlation coefficient $r = 0.97$) and 1.1 mm for MLS (SD 1.46 mm, Pearson's correlation coefficient $r = 0.94$) with a tendency for parameters to be underestimated at higher values using BUS [54]. The small difference between BUS and CT measurements may be due to small deviations in the examination planes and insonation of the third ventricle may not occur at a right angle to its longitudinal axis on BUS.

The time course and extent of MLS development may serve as early biomarkers of outcome. In one study by Gerriets and colleagues, all patients with MLS <4 mm at 32 h survived, whereas patients with MLS >4 mm died as a result of cerebral herniation, with the exception of one patient who underwent decompressive hemicraniectomy [55]. Further studies evaluating the prognostic significance of repeated BUS examination are needed to confirm these preliminary results. Overall, BUS may detect MLS with reasonable accuracy in stroke patients and may be a useful bedside tool to detect early cerebral complications and the need for further imaging or neurosurgical intervention. However, these preliminary results support the use of BUS to assess MLS as a relative value, rather than an absolute number, and trended over time. The time course of MLS may be even more important than the maximal value of MLS; therefore repeated BUS examinations might be helpful in the management of these patients.

12.2.7 Multimodal Neuromonitoring Approach

Another interesting area of development is the additional information that BUS may provide as part of a multimodal imaging stroke protocol in the setting of hyperacute strokes. Brunser and colleagues evaluated the complementary information BUS provided to non-contrast CT, CTA, and diffusion-weighted MRI in 86 patients with AIS [56]. Optimal temporal sonographic windows were not found in 20% of patients. However, BUS provided additional information on collateral flow, active microemboli, detection of occlusion missed on CTA (CT perfusion not performed), and vessel patency in 57% (49/86) of cases. This additional information changed the management in 17% of cases: eight patients required endovascular rescue therapy after failure of intravenous thrombolysis with recombinant tissue plasminogen activator (r-tPA); five patients did not receive angiography because reperfusion was demonstrated on BUS; and neurocritical care medical therapies were increased in two patients who had contraindications for reperfusion management. These two cases presented with distal branch occlusions in the MCA and good collateral flow on BUS, flow velocity in the affected MCA increased, and collateral pathways improved with flat head of bed positioning, induced hypertension, and volume expansion. Both patients had a final mRS of 2 on day 90. These preliminary results demonstrate that BUS may provide additional useful information in half of the patients in centers not utilizing advanced imaging modes such as CT perfusion. Although changes in management occurred in one out of six cases, further studies are needed to evaluate whether a tailored approach to hyperacute stroke management using BUS improves neurocognitive outcomes. A multicenter study from the Neurosonology in Acute Ischemic Stroke (NAIS) Group assessed the supplementary value of BUS within the first 6 h after AIS to provide additional prognostic information in the hyperacute stage of stroke [57]. The sonographic status of MCA within 6 h after stroke can help to identify patients with a high risk for poor functional outcome; occlusion of the MCA main stem within 6 h after stroke is an independent predictor for poor outcome.

12.2.8 Sonothrombolysis

Access to endovascular reperfusion therapies is not readily available in many stroke centers around the world, and therefore methods to amplify the effectiveness of alteplase in thrombus dissolution remain an important goal for medical stroke treatment development. Sonothrombolysis is an evolving ultrasound method with the therapeutic potential to augment clot lysis using ultrasound aimed at the residual flow and thrombus interface to increase the chances of early recanalization. Recent meta-analyses found that sonothrombolysis can significantly increase the rate of recanalization in patients with AIS compared with non-sonothrombolysis, but found no significant effect on neurological functional recovery and complication rates [58, 59]. The details of these therapeutic modalities are beyond the scope of this chapter, and readers are referred to the relevant literature [58–60].

12.3 Conclusions

The portability, repeatability, noninvasiveness, and high temporal resolution of BUS have promoted its use for critically ill patients, especially for the bedside monitoring of cerebrovascular dynamics and complications associated with AIS. The information from this imaging modality may be particularly helpful when neurological assessment is limited. The role of BUS will likely continue to expand in the future as standardization of measurements is adopted, advancements are seen in technology, and training criteria are defined for the inclusion of BUS into point-of-care ultrasound core competencies. Noninvasive BUS imaging may facilitate an individualized physiology-based approach in the management of AIS aimed at reducing the risk of secondary brain injury. Carefully designed studies are needed to better determine quality standards in autoregulatory testing and to evaluate the benefit of autoregulation-oriented therapy in AIS. Furthermore, operator dependency is a significant limitation to its clinical utility. However, the temporal resolution and convenience of BUS make it a vital asset in observing the evolution of blood flow changes in the critically ill patient.

References

1. Schlachetzki F, Herzberg M, Holscher T, Ertl M, Zimmermann M, Ittner KP, et al. Transcranial ultrasound from diagnosis to early stroke treatment: part 2: prehospital neurosonography in patients with acute stroke: the Regensburg stroke mobile project. Cerebrovasc Dis. 2012;33(3):262–71.
2. Jauss M, Zanette E. Detection of right-to-left shunt with ultrasound contrast agent and transcranial Doppler sonography. Cerebrovasc Dis. 2000;10(6):490–6.
3. Serena J, Segura T, Perez-Ayuso MJ, Bassaganyas J, Molins A, Davalos A. The need to quantify right-to-left shunt in acute ischemic stroke: a case-control study. Stroke. 1998;29(7):1322–8.
4. Lao AY, Sharma VK, Tsivgoulis G, Frey JL, Malkoff MD, Navarro JC, et al. Detection of right-to-left shunts: comparison between the international consensus and Spencer logarithmic scale criteria. J Neuroimaging. 2008;18(4):402–6.
5. Katsanos AH, Psaltopoulou T, Sergentanis TN, Frogoudaki A, Vrettou AR, Ikonomidis I, et al. Transcranial Doppler versus transthoracic echocardiography for the detection of patent foramen ovale in patients with cryptogenic cerebral ischemia: a systematic review and diagnostic test accuracy meta-analysis. Ann Neurol. 2016;79(4):625–35.
6. Mojadidi MK, Roberts SC, Winoker JS, Romero J, Goodman-Meza D, Gevorgyan R, et al. Accuracy of transcranial Doppler for the diagnosis of intracardiac right-to-left shunt: a bivariate meta-analysis of prospective studies. JACC Cardiovasc Imaging. 2014;7(3):236–50.
7. Demchuk AM, Christou I, Wein TH, Felberg RA, Malkoff M, Grotta JC, et al. Accuracy and criteria for localizing arterial occlusion with transcranial Doppler. J Neuroimaging. 2000;10(1):1–12.
8. Grolimund P, Seiler RW, Aaslid R, Huber P, Zurbruegg H. Evaluation of cerebrovascular disease by combined extracranial and transcranial Doppler

sonography. Experience in 1,039 patients. Stroke. 1987;18(6):1018–24.

9. Lindegaard KF, Bakke SJ, Aaslid R, Nornes H. Doppler diagnosis of intracranial artery occlusive disorders. J Neurol Neurosurg Psychiatry. 1986;49(5):510–8.
10. Demchuk AM, Christou I, Wein TH, Felberg RA, Malkoff M, Grotta JC, et al. Specific transcranial Doppler flow findings related to the presence and site of arterial occlusion. Stroke. 2000;31(1):140–6.
11. Aaslid R, Markwalder TM, Nornes H. Noninvasive transcranial Doppler ultrasound recording of flow velocity in basal cerebral arteries. J Neurosurg. 1982;57(6):769–74.
12. Saqqur M, Hill MD, Alexandrov AV, Roy J, Schebel M, Krol A, et al. Derivation of power M-mode transcranial Doppler criteria for angiographic proven MCA occlusion. J Neuroimaging. 2006;16(4):323–8.
13. Tsivgoulis G, Sharma VK, Hoover SL, Lao AY, Ardelt AA, Malkoff MD, et al. Applications and advantages of power motion-mode Doppler in acute posterior circulation cerebral ischemia. Stroke. 2008;39(4):1197–204.
14. Gomez CR, Brass LM, Tegeler CH, Babikian VL, Sloan MA, Feldmann E, et al. The transcranial Doppler standardization project. Phase 1 results. The TCD Study Group, American Society of Neuroimaging. J Neuroimaging. 1993;3(3):190–2.
15. Robba C, Poole D, Citerio G, Taccone FS, Rasulo FA. Brain ultrasonography consensus on skill recommendations and competence levels within the critical care setting. Neurocrit Care. 2020;32(2):502–11.
16. Sloan MA, Alexandrov AV, Tegeler CH, Spencer MP, Caplan LR, Feldmann E, et al. Assessment: transcranial Doppler ultrasonography: report of the Therapeutics and Technology Assessment Subcommittee of the American Academy of Neurology. Neurology. 2004;62(9):1468–81.
17. Demchuk AM, Burgin WS, Christou I, Felberg RA, Barber PA, Hill MD, et al. Thrombolysis in brain ischemia (TIBI) transcranial Doppler flow grades predict clinical severity, early recovery, and mortality in patients treated with intravenous tissue plasminogen activator. Stroke. 2001;32(1):89–93.
18. Nedelmann M, Stolz E, Gerriets T, Baumgartner RW, Malferrari G, Seidel G, et al. Consensus recommendations for transcranial color-coded duplex sonography for the assessment of intracranial arteries in clinical trials on acute stroke. Stroke. 2009;40(10): 3238–44.
19. Sobrino-Garcia P, Garcia-Pastor A, Garcia-Arratibel A, Dominguez-Rubio R, Rodriguez-Cruz PM, Iglesias-Mohedano AM, et al. Diagnostic, prognostic and therapeutic implications of transcranial color-coded duplex sonography in acute ischemic stroke: TIBI and COGIF scores validation. Rev Neurol. 2016;63(8):351–7.
20. Alexandrov AV, Burgin WS, Demchuk AM, El-Mitwalli A, Grotta JC. Speed of intracranial clot lysis with intravenous tissue plasminogen activator therapy: sonographic classification and short-term improvement. Circulation. 2001;103(24):2897–902.
21. Christou I, Alexandrov AV, Burgin WS, Wojner AW, Felberg RA, Malkoff M, et al. Timing of recanalization after tissue plasminogen activator therapy determined by transcranial doppler correlates with clinical recovery from ischemic stroke. Stroke. 2000;31(8):1812–6.
22. Stolz E, Cioli F, Allendoerfer J, Gerriets T, Del Sette M, Kaps M. Can early neurosonology predict outcome in acute stroke? A meta-analysis of prognostic clinical effect sizes related to the vascular status. Stroke. 2008;39(12):3255–61.
23. Tsivgoulis G, Ribo M, Rubiera M, Vasdekis SN, Barlinn K, Athanasiadis D, et al. Real-time validation of transcranial Doppler criteria in assessing recanalization during intra-arterial procedures for acute ischemic stroke: an international, multicenter study. Stroke. 2013;44(2):394–400.
24. Castro P, Azevedo E, Serrador J, Rocha I, Sorond F. Hemorrhagic transformation and cerebral edema in acute ischemic stroke: link to cerebral autoregulation. J Neurol Sci. 2017;372:256–61.
25. Castro P, Serrador JM, Rocha I, Sorond F, Azevedo E. Efficacy of cerebral autoregulation in early ischemic stroke predicts smaller infarcts and better outcome. Front Neurol. 2017;8:113.
26. Dohmen C, Bosche B, Graf R, Reithmeier T, Ernestus RI, Brinker G, et al. Identification and clinical impact of impaired cerebrovascular autoregulation in patients with malignant middle cerebral artery infarction. Stroke. 2007;38(1):56–61.
27. Reinhard M, Rutsch S, Lambeck J, Wihler C, Czosnyka M, Weiller C, et al. Dynamic cerebral autoregulation associates with infarct size and outcome after ischemic stroke. Acta Neurol Scand. 2012;125(3):156–62.
28. Xiong L, Liu X, Shang T, Smielewski P, Donnelly J, Guo ZN, et al. Impaired cerebral autoregulation: measurement and application to stroke. J Neurol Neurosurg Psychiatry. 2017;88(6):520–31.
29. Intharakham K, Beishon L, Panerai RB, Haunton VJ, Robinson TG. Assessment of cerebral autoregulation in stroke: a systematic review and meta-analysis of studies at rest. J Cereb Blood Flow Metab. 2019;39(11):2105–16.
30. Rivera-Lara L, Zorrilla-Vaca A, Geocadin R, Ziai W, Healy R, Thompson R, et al. Predictors of outcome with cerebral autoregulation monitoring: a systematic review and meta-analysis. Crit Care Med. 2017;45(4):695–704.
31. Ma H, Guo ZN, Jin H, Yan X, Liu J, Lv S, et al. Preliminary study of dynamic cerebral autoregulation in acute ischemic stroke: association with clinical factors. Front Neurol. 2018;9:1006.

32. Guo ZN, Liu J, Xing Y, Yan S, Lv C, Jin H, et al. Dynamic cerebral autoregulation is heterogeneous in different subtypes of acute ischemic stroke. PLoS One. 2014;9(3):e93213.
33. Immink RV, van Montfrans GA, Stam J, Karemaker JM, Diamant M, van Lieshout JJ. Dynamic cerebral autoregulation in acute lacunar and middle cerebral artery territory ischemic stroke. Stroke. 2005;36(12):2595–600.
34. Dawson SL, Panerai RB, Potter JF. Serial changes in static and dynamic cerebral autoregulation after acute ischaemic stroke. Cerebrovasc Dis. 2003;16(1):69–75.
35. Petersen NH, Ortega-Gutierrez S, Reccius A, Masurkar A, Huang A, Marshall RS. Dynamic cerebral autoregulation is transiently impaired for one week after large-vessel acute ischemic stroke. Cerebrovasc Dis. 2015;39(2):144–50.
36. Reinhard M, Roth M, Guschlbauer B, Harloff A, Timmer J, Czosnyka M, et al. Dynamic cerebral autoregulation in acute ischemic stroke assessed from spontaneous blood pressure fluctuations. Stroke. 2005;36(8):1684–9.
37. Claassen JA, Meel-van den Abeelen AS, Simpson DM, Panerai RB. Transfer function analysis of dynamic cerebral autoregulation: a white paper from the International Cerebral Autoregulation Research Network. J Cereb Blood Flow Metab. 2016;36(4):665–80.
38. Maurer M, Shambal S, Berg D, Woydt M, Hofmann E, Georgiadis D, et al. Differentiation between intracerebral hemorrhage and ischemic stroke by transcranial color-coded duplex-sonography. Stroke. 1998;29(12):2563–7.
39. Blanco P, Matteoda M. Images in emergency medicine. Extra-axial intracranial hematoma, midline shift, and severe intracranial hypertension detected by transcranial color-coded duplex sonography. Ann Emerg Med. 2015;65(2):e1–2.
40. Kukulska-Pawluczuk B, Ksiazkiewicz B, Nowaczewska M. Imaging of spontaneous intracerebral hemorrhages by means of transcranial color-coded sonography. Eur J Radiol. 2012;81(6):1253–8.
41. Caricato A, Mignani V, Sandroni C, Pietrini D. Bedside detection of acute epidural hematoma by transcranial sonography in a head-injured patient. Intensive Care Med. 2010;36(6):1091–2.
42. Blanco P, Blaivas M. Applications of transcranial color-coded sonography in the emergency department. J Ultrasound Med. 2017;36(6):1251–66.
43. Blanco P, Abdo-Cuza A. Transcranial Doppler ultrasound in neurocritical care. J Ultrasound. 2018;21(1):1–16.
44. Robba C, Goffi A, Geeraerts T, Cardim D, Via G, Czosnyka M, et al. Brain ultrasonography: methodology, basic and advanced principles and clinical applications. A narrative review. Intensive Care Med. 2019;45(7):913–27.
45. Matsumoto N, Kimura K, Iguchi Y, Aoki J. Evaluation of cerebral hemorrhage volume using transcranial color-coded duplex sonography. J Neuroimaging. 2011;21(4):355–8.
46. Perez ES, Delgado-Mederos R, Rubiera M, Delgado P, Ribo M, Maisterra O, et al. Transcranial duplex sonography for monitoring hyperacute intracerebral hemorrhage. Stroke. 2009;40(3):987–90.
47. Ropper AH. Lateral displacement of the brain and level of consciousness in patients with an acute hemispheral mass. N Engl J Med. 1986;314(15):953–8.
48. Pullicino PM, Alexandrov AV, Shelton JA, Alexandrova NA, Smurawska LT, Norris JW. Mass effect and death from severe acute stroke. Neurology. 1997;49(4):1090–5.
49. Andrews PJ, Piper IR, Dearden NM, Miller JD. Secondary insults during intrahospital transport of head-injured patients. Lancet. 1990;335(8685):327–30.
50. Bekar A, Ipekoglu Z, Tureyen K, Bilgin H, Korfali G, Korfali E. Secondary insults during intrahospital transport of neurosurgical intensive care patients. Neurosurg Rev. 1998;21(2–3):98–101.
51. Seidel G, Gerriets T, Kaps M, Missler U. Dislocation of the third ventricle due to space-occupying stroke evaluated by transcranial duplex sonography. J Neuroimaging. 1996;6(4):227–30.
52. Stolz E, Gerriets T, Fiss I, Babacan SS, Seidel G, Kaps M. Comparison of transcranial color-coded duplex sonography and cranial CT measurements for determining third ventricle midline shift in space-occupying stroke. AJNR Am J Neuroradiol. 1999;20(8):1567–71.
53. Horstmann S, Koziol JA, Martinez-Torres F, Nagel S, Gardner H, Wagner S. Sonographic monitoring of mass effect in stroke patients treated with hypothermia. Correlation with intracranial pressure and matrix metalloproteinase 2 and 9 expression. J Neurol Sci. 2009;276(1–2):75–8.
54. Bertram M, Khoja W, Ringleb P, Schwab S. Transcranial colour-coded sonography for the bedside evaluation of mass effect after stroke. Eur J Neurol. 2000;7(6):639–46.
55. Gerriets T, Stolz E, Konig S, Babacan S, Fiss I, Jauss M, et al. Sonographic monitoring of midline shift in space-occupying stroke: an early outcome predictor. Stroke. 2001;32(2):442–7.
56. Brunser AM, Mansilla E, Hoppe A, Olavarria V, Sujima E, Lavados PM. The role of TCD in the evaluation of acute stroke. J Neuroimaging. 2016;26(4):420–5.
57. Allendoerfer J, Goertler M, von Reutern GM. Prognostic relevance of ultra-early doppler sonography in acute ischaemic stroke: a prospective multicentre study. Lancet Neurol. 2006;5(10):835–40.
58. Chen Z, Xue T, Huang H, Xu J, Shankar S, Yu H, et al. Efficacy and safety of sonothrombolysis versus

non-sonothrombolysis in patients with acute ischemic stroke: a meta-analysis of randomized controlled trials. PLoS One. 2019;14(1):e0210516.
59. Zafar M, Memon RS, Mussa M, Merchant R, Khurshid A, Khosa F. Does the administration of sonothrombolysis along with tissue plasminogen activator improve outcomes in acute ischemic stroke? A systematic review and meta-analysis. J Thromb Thrombolysis. 2019;48(2):203–8.
60. Alexandrov AV, Kohrmann M, Soinne L, Tsivgoulis G, Barreto AD, Demchuk AM, et al. Safety and efficacy of sonothrombolysis for acute ischaemic stroke: a multicentre, double-blind, phase 3, randomised controlled trial. Lancet Neurol. 2019;18(4):338–47.

13 Cardiac Arrest

Ilaria Alice Crippa and Fabio Silvio Taccone

Contents

13.1 Introduction

Cardiac arrest, especially out-of-hospital cardiac arrest, is a major cause of morbidity and mortality worldwide [1, 2]. Thanks to recent advances, in-hospital survival after cardiac arrest has increased over recent years in different countries [3, 4]. Despite this, only about one out of ten patients is discharged alive from hospital after having suffered from postanoxic injury [5, 6]. Heart and brain recovery determines the ultimate prognosis of patients resuscitated from cardiac arrest. Neurologic failure is the main cause of death, especially in case of out-of-hospital cardiac arrest [7, 8], and is associated with significant disability in survivors, ranging from psychiatric complications [9] to mild cognitive deficits or vegetative state [10]. Substantial neuronal loss occurs during circulatory arrest: oxygen and energetic substrate deprivation determines a metabolic crisis with depletion of adenosine triphosphate [11] and cellular death by necrosis occurs within minutes. Furthermore, excitatory neurotransmitter release activates apoptosis in cerebral cells [11, 12]. No-flow time (time from collapse to the beginning of resuscitation) and low-flow time (time from beginning of resuscitation to return of spontaneous circulation) are strong outcome predictors [13]. However, hypoxic-ischemic encephalopathy persists and evolves after return of spontaneous circulation (ROSC). Secondary brain injury involves different pathophysiological processes, such as cerebral vasogenic and cytotoxic edema and endothelial and microvascular dysfunction [14]. Prevention and control of secondary brain injury is the focus of post-resuscitation care [15]. Assuring adequate brain perfusion is of utmost importance to prevent neurological damage progression after cardiac arrest. Unfortunately,

I. A. Crippa (✉) · F. S. Taccone
Department of Intensive Care, Hôpital Erasme, Université Libre de Bruxelles, Brussels, Belgium
e-mail: ftaccone@ulb.ac.be

C. Robba, G. Citerio (eds.), *Echography and Doppler of the Brain*,
https://doi.org/10.1007/978-3-030-48202-2_13

various pathological processes affect cerebral perfusion after cardiac arrest. Spotty vascular changes occur within minutes from interruption of cerebral blood flow (CBF). Such vascular changes interfere with the re-establishment of normal CBF, so that they are referred to as "no-reflow" phenomenon [16]. Within the first 30 min from ROSC, coexisting or superimposing on local perfusion deficits, transient, heterogeneous areas of vasoparalysis with subsequent hyperemia are seen [17]. This results in a combination characterized by local areas of no flow interspersed with areas of either low flow or increased flow, determining early global post-resuscitation perfusion defects [16–20]. Duration of primary ischemic insult is associated to the amount of brain interested by hemodynamic disturbances [17, 19] and most likely contributes to secondary brain injury. Furthermore, hypotension often occurs early after ROSC because of cardiac and vascular failure [21] and, especially in case cerebral autoregulation is deranged, global cerebral blood flow (CBF) decrease superimposes on local perfusion deficits, to the point that stroke may occur [22]. On the opposite, whether early after ROSC hyperemia is detrimental to ischemia-reperfusion injury is uncertain [10]. This may explain why higher blood pressure was not beneficial on outcome when it occurred within minutes form cardiac arrest [23], while correlated with better outcome when observed in the first few hours [23, 24]. Later on, increased vascular tone determines a delayed and protracted global hypoperfusion with CBF decreased to 50% or less than normal [19]. Whether such reduction is disproportionate compared to cerebral metabolic needs or not is debated, with some studies showing that metabolic coupling of CBF is preserved after cardiac arrest [25, 26] and some other data that is uncertain or supporting the idea that global hypoperfusion does not correspond to a decreased metabolic activity and brain suffers a secondary ischemic injury during this period [27–31]. Multiple mechanisms are implicated in the development of delayed hypoperfusion, including endothelial cell damage, local vasodilator/vasoconstrictor activity imbalance, and impaired autoregulation in the setting of decreased blood pressure [14]. After 72 h, either vascular tone has returned to normal and so has the CBF, or vascular tone is lost and has CBF passively increased [32, 33]. Late hyperemia is possibly related to extensive loss of functional brain tissue with decrease in cerebral oxygen consumption together with loss of vascular tone [27, 34] and seems to be associated with negative outcome [35].

Cerebral blood flow direct measurement is difficult to obtain in clinical setting. It is usually invasive and expensive and requires moving the patients outside the intensive care unit. Transcranial Doppler (TCD) is a noninvasive, non-expensive bedside technique that can provide serial assessment of cerebral perfusion without interfering with clinical care. Although it does not assess cerebral perfusion directly, as explained elsewhere in this textbook, it can be used to assess modifications in cerebral blood flow and cerebral autoregulation, in addition to inferring functional status of cerebral microcirculation.

13.2 TCD During Cardiopulmonary Resuscitation

A noninvasive method for cerebral perfusion assessment during cardiopulmonary resuscitation (CPR) is beneficial for at least two reasons. First, in light of the impact of neurological failure on the prognosis of cardiac arrest patient, the possibility of a real-time assessment and optimization of cerebral perfusion during CPR may have a relevant impact on patients' management [36]. Second, cerebral perfusion assessment during CPR could help in early prognostication, for example in case of enduring absence or very low cerebral perfusion despite resuscitation attempts. The gold standard to assess cerebral perfusion would require an arterial catheter as well as an intracerebral probe to measure intracranial pressure (ICP) and, therefore, cerebral perfusion pressure (CPP). End-tidal carbon dioxide ($EtCO_2$) levels during CPR are easily available and are usually monitored as an index of quality of chest compression [36]. However, despite being a reliable tool to estimate systemic circulation in this setting [37], $EtCO_2$ does not give any information on target organ perfusion, in particular the brain. Lewis et al. investigated the use of TCD to assess cerebral circulation during CPR on animal model [38] and human subjects [39] and concluded that TCD can provide real-time information about cerebral perfusion. During CPR, cerebral perfusion is produced during chest compressions and maximum systolic velocity in intracranial arteries reflects cerebral perfusion during each compression. Data showed that optimal cerebral blood flow is maintained for no longer than 3 min during CPR on human subjects, despite the rescuer not complaining of any fatigue [39]. Successfully resuscitated patients showed recovery of cerebral blood flow immediately before return of spontaneous circulation was noted, while patients without ROSC showed progressive deterioration in cerebral blood flow velocities over time during CPR, until absence of net forward blood flow was seen [39]. Similarly, de Wilde et al. observed return of spontaneous cerebral blood flow before arterial pressure was recorded on invasive monitoring in a male patient who suffered from cardiac arrest during ICU stay [40]. Carmona-Jimenez et al. compared intracranial blood flow velocities during manual and mechanical chest compression by LUCAS® device in four patients affected by nontraumatic, witnessed cardiac arrest. They found mean maximum flow velocity during manual chest compression to be 31.6 ± 8.32 cm/s compared to 50.6 ± 27.1 cm/s during mechanical chest compression, thus supporting the hypothesis that mechanical chest compressions are more effective than manual compressions in maintaining adequate brain perfusion [41]. Blumestein et al. reported a case of incidental use of TCD during cardiopulmonary resuscitation in a female patient undergoing minimally invasive transcatheter aortic valve implantation under general anesthesia. The authors expanded intravascular volume and increased depth of chest compression in order to obtain continuously positive diastolic blood flow. The authors were also able to evaluate the effect of different therapeutic interventions to ameliorate cerebral blood flow, among which administration of sodium bicarbonate seemed to be most effective. The patient eventually recovered with no neurological deficits [42]. However, artifacts are frequent and may interfere with interpretation of signal. Lewis et al. reported insonation of both middle cerebral artery through temporal window and ophthalmic artery to be unsuccessful or to result in damped or to be concealed by artifact signal. However, insonation of the internal carotid artery by transorbital approach was successful and resulted in a good-quality and stable signal.

Despite looking a promising technique, for the time being TCD is not part of routine cardiopulmonary resuscitation monitoring (Table 13.1, Fig. 13.1). Moreover, whether TCD can help in

Table 13.1 Potential uses of TCD in cardiac arrest patients: actual = supported by published studies and future = to be evaluated

During CPR	After ROSC
Actual	***Actual***
– Monitoring of brain hemodynamics during CPR – Early achievement of ROSC	– Monitoring of cerebral autoregulation – Assess the critical closing pressure of the brain vasculature – Brain hypoperfusion – Estimation of cerebral perfusion pressure – Early prognostication through serial assessment of intracranial hemodynamic pattern
Future	***Future***
– Optimization of cerebral perfusion pressure via different therapeutic interventions (i.e., increasing depth of chest compression, fluid administration) – Early termination of CPR in case of persistently low cerebral blood flow velocities – Quantify the extent of the anoxic injury	– Estimation of intracranial pressure – Prognostication of postanoxic injury – Individualized arterial pressure targets – Individualized respiratory parameters (i.e., $PaCO_2$)

CPR cardiopulmonary resuscitation, *ROSC* return of spontaneous circulation

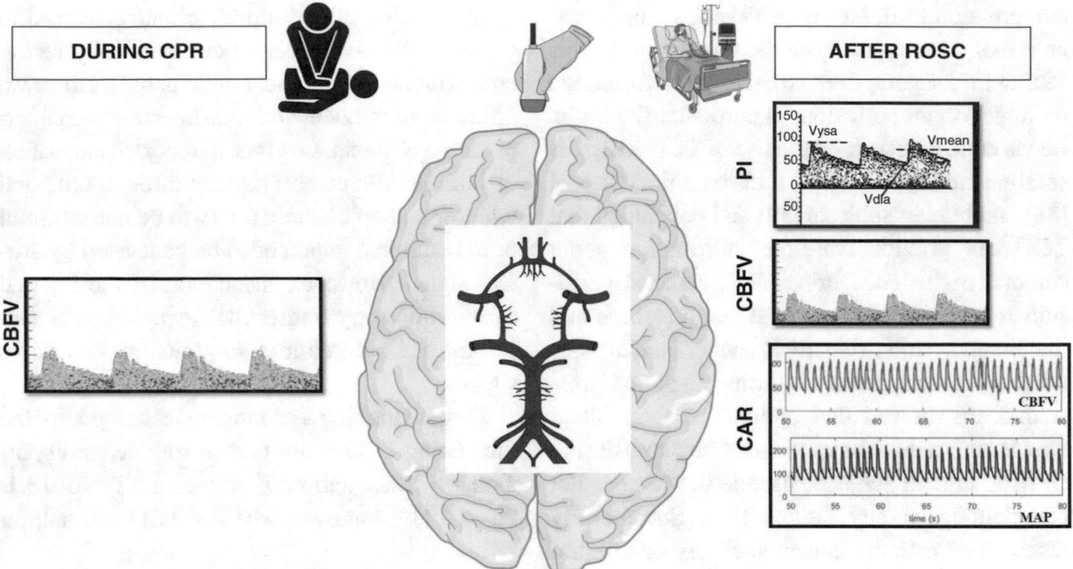

Fig. 13.1 Application of TCD during cardiopulmonary resuscitation (CPR) or after the return of spontaneous circulation (ROSC). *CBFV* cerebral blood flow velocities, *PI* pulsatility index, *CAR* cerebral autoregulation

optimizing cerebral perfusion pressure via different therapeutic interventions (i.e., increasing depth of chest compression), in identifying patients with extremely low brain perfusion during CPR for resuscitation termination, or in assessing the extent of the anoxic injury should be further evaluated.

13.3 Post-resuscitation Care and Neuro-Prognostication

The main focus of post-resuscitation care is limitation of secondary brain injury [43]. Cerebral oxygen delivery is dependent on cerebral blood flow, which in turn depends on mean systemic arterial pressure, cerebrovascular resistances (CVR), and intracranial pressure (ICP). Although being considered as a rare event, elevated ICP can occur because of the hypoxic-ischemic insult induced by the reperfusion into the brain tissue [13]. At the time being, ICP monitoring is not recommended in post-CA patients, unless cranial CT scan shows abnormalities (i.e., subarachnoid hemorrhage) [44], and maintaining MAP ≥65 mmHg and systolic blood pressure ≥90 mmHg after ROSC is recommended as a measure to avoid brain hypoperfusion [15]. However, the "one-size-fits-all" approach has been questioned by several authors [45, 46] and TCD might help to assess brain hemodynamics in this setting.

Cerebral autoregulation is the intrinsic ability of cerebral vasculature to maintain a stable CBF over a wide range of MAP with constant $PaCO_2$ and cerebral oxygen consumption. The effective MAP ranges within such mechanism have been reported to be between 50 and 150 mmHg [47]; however, substantial variability between subjects exists [48, 49] and several chronic (i.e., arterial hypertension [50] or diabetes [51]) and acute (acute brain injury of different origin [52]) diseases have been shown to impair cerebral autoregulation. This is why achieving recommended blood pressure targets in post-cardiac arrest care may not guarantee adequate brain perfusion in case of impaired autoregulation. In a landmark study, Sundgreen et al. showed that CBF autoregulation was altered in the majority of patients within 24 h from cardiac arrest. They investigated static cerebral autoregulation by stepwise increasing mean arterial blood pressure with vasopressors and they concluded that 5 patients out of 18 (28%) had normal autoregulation, 8 patients

(45%) had impaired autoregulation, and 5 patients (28%) had preserved but right-shifted autoregulation, with the lower limit of autoregulation around 114 (80–120) mmHg [53]. Importantly, this study was conducted before the era of targeted temperature management (TTM). Several studies, conducted with different techniques, showed a correlation between deranged autoregulation and outcome after cardiac arrest [35, 45, 54]. Since hypotension after cardiac arrest was shown to be deleterious and higher blood pressure after cardiac arrest was associated with favorable outcome [46, 55]; maintaining the blood pressure within effective autoregulation is advisable. Despite being promising, limitations exist for the use of cerebral autoregulation monitoring to titrate MAP after cardiac arrest. Manipulation of MAP by vasopressors can affect other organs, especially the heart, which may not be able to tolerate the increased afterload. Furthermore, use of vasopressors is not without side effects such as digital or mesenteric ischemia or arrhythmias. Therefore, the risks associated with increased MAP targets must be weighed against the potential benefits of improved cerebral perfusion.

The critical closing pressure (CrCP) is defined as the lower limit of arterial blood pressure below which vessels collapse and flow ceases [56, 57]. It is a function of cerebral artery smooth muscle tone and ICP; CrCP was investigated in 11 comatose, post-cardiac arrest patients; CrCP decreased from ROSC to 48 h after ROSC and was higher in patients who survived compared to those who did not [35]. CrCP was most likely elevated immediately after cardiac arrest because of vasoconstriction, while it decreased because of loss of vasoactive tone in patients with unfavorable outcome, resulting in reduced cerebrovascular resistance and increased CBF. Furthermore, spontaneous variability of mean flow velocity in intracranial arteries was low early after cardiac arrest and increased to normal values in survivors whereas it further decreased in non-survivors [54].

Another potential mechanism leading to brain hypoperfusion after cardiac arrest is probably related to the development of microthrombi and severe endothelial dysfunction. Alvarez-Fernandez et al. summarized the evolution of mean blood flow velocity (FV) and pulsatility index (PI) on middle cerebral artery after recovery from cardiac arrest [58]. In general, PI between 0.6 and 1.1 is considered to be associated with normal intracranial hemodynamics; PI below 0.6 may indicate hyperemia; PI between 1.2 and 1.6 indicates high resistance, such as during mild intracranial hypertension or microvascular alterations; PI above 1.6 indicates very high resistance, such as in severe intracranial hypertension or impelling circulatory arrest [58]. Early after ROSC, low FV and high PI is the predominant pattern; values are usually back to normal in 72 h and poor neurological prognosis is more likely in case of this persistent hypodynamic pattern [33, 58, 59]. In 17 children investigated during targeted temperature management after cardiac arrest, normal FV and PI during rewarming were associated to better outcome than low FV and high PI [60]. In another study, a hyperemic pattern characterized by high FV, medium-to-low PI, and Lindegaard ratio <3 was observed [61]. Persistence of hyperemia beyond 30 min was associated with unfavorable neurological outcome because of development of intracranial hypertension [62]. After this initial phase and during the first 12 h after resuscitation, hypoperfusion (i.e., low FV and high PI) became more frequent, followed by normalization of FV and PI 24 h later and increased FV and low PI 48–72 h later [33]. Wessels et al. aimed at determining the prognostic value of transcranial Doppler in cardiac arrest patients [59]. They performed serial TCD within 72 h from CPR on 39 patients. They found that both early (4 h) and late (72 h) systolic flow velocities in the middle cerebral artery were significantly lower in non-survivors than survivors. Furthermore, the resistance index (RI), which is very similar to pulsatility index, on anterior and posterior cerebral arteries was higher in non-survivors. Similarly, autoregulation seemed to be disrupted early (i.e., 4–16 h after resuscitation) in non-survivors compared to survivors, who showed intact cerebral autoregulation. Similar results came from a recent study by Rafi et al. [63]; the authors investigated 42 out-of-hospital cardiac arrest patients about 5 h after return of spontaneous circulation. In their study, PI was higher in patients who had worse neurological outcome compared to patients who had better neurological outcome at 3 months (1.49 vs. 1.12). Consistently, patients with worse neurological function had lower diastolic flow velocity compared to patients with better outcome at 3 months. In both cases the authors suggested that using serial TCD examinations, patients with severely disabling or fatal outcome could be identified within the first 24 h. On the opposite, a recent study that investigated CBF in 53 patients after cardiac arrest failed to show any correlations between TCD parameters and outcome. In this study, CBF was calculated as the product of cross-sectional area and the time-averaged blood flow velocity of the internal carotid artery at the time points: within 48 h from cardiac arrest, at 3–5 and 6–10 days post-resuscitation [64].

The cerebrovascular reactivity to modifications in arterial carbon dioxide tension (CO_2 reactivity) appears to be maintained after cardiac arrest. Bisschops et al. showed preserved cerebrovascular reactivity to fluctuations in arterial tension of carbon dioxide ($PaCO_2$) during mild therapeutic hypothermia after cardiac arrest [25]. Previously, Yenari et al. had demonstrated a preserved cerebrovascular reactivity to changes in $PaCO_2$ under normothermic conditions in patients after ROSC [65]. Thus, hyperventilation after cardiac arrest might induce cerebral vasoconstriction and a secondary ischemic insult and should, therefore, be avoided. Another interesting, although still in its early stage, application of transcranial Doppler is the estimate of cerebral perfusion pressure. TCD has proven useful in excluding elevated ICP in acute brain injury patients through estimation of CPP (eCPP) [66]. Taccone et al. successfully applied the same technique to assess eCPP in cardiac arrest patients and showed an association between low eCPP and negative outcome in those patients [67] (Table 13.1, Fig. 13.1).

Unfortunately, comparisons of results of different studies are limited by differences in study protocols. Core temperature may have an influence on cerebral blood flow and its regulation [68] and hypothermia showed some benefits on CAR in the animal model of TBI [69]. However, clinical management differs from center to center and to date few studies have been published enrolling patients treated by targeted temperature management, showing opposite results [64, 70, 71]. Furthermore, population may differ in baseline or cardiac arrest characteristics (e.g., in-hospital or out-of-hospital cardiac arrest). Patients who died for non-neurological reason were alternatively included in survivor group [59] or excluded [63] when neurological outcome was assessed. TCD measurements differed, ranging from static cerebral autoregulation [53] to pulsatility index [72], and to resistance index [63]. Also insonated intracranial arteries differed: while the middle cerebral artery is most commonly used, some authors investigated the whole intracranial circulation, with inconsistent results [59]. Also, arterial pressure or respiratory setting manipulation in study protocol must be carefully considered when interpreting results [72, 73]. Such heterogeneity in study methods may explain conflicting results in outcome studies, with some showing an association between TCD measurements and outcome after cardiac arrest [59, 62], and some others not [64, 71].

13.4 Conclusions

Transcranial Doppler may have several applications in cardiac arrest patients' care. There is a growing interest in the clinical application of TCD for early or late prognostication and therapeutic management of patients suffering from hypoxic/anoxic injury, both during and after cardiopulmonary resuscitation. During the last decades, the number of publications related to the subject has increased almost tenfold. Most studies investigate physiological mechanisms and alterations of cerebral blood flow, cerebral blood flow autoregulation, or microcirculation, in basal conditions or after manipulation of physiological variables such as mean arterial pressure or arterial carbon dioxide tension. Few pioneering studies investigated the use of TCD during cardiopulmonary resuscitation. TCD was able to detect suboptimal cerebral blood flow during external cardiac massage as well as early recovery of cerebral perfusion, before any other sign of ROSC was noted, in a small cohort of human subjects [39], but any other consideration on the clinical use of TCD during resuscitation efforts is anecdotal [42]. A larger body of literature is available on the use of TCD in post-resuscitation care. TCD has been extensively applied to monitor the evolution of cerebral blood flow after resuscitation from cardiac arrest [33, 58–62]. With certain limitations, monitoring of cerebral autoregulation by TCD may be applicable in titrating MAP after cardiac arrest, so as to avoid hypo- or hyper-perfusion and limit secondary brain injury after cardiac arrest. Alteration of TCD parameters, such as indexes related to blood flow or vascular resistance in intracranial arteries after cardiac arrest, may also be of prognostic values [35, 45, 53, 54, 64, 72]. Unfortunately, comparisons of results of different studies are limited by differences in study protocols and a definite result on association between alterations in TCD parameters and outcome in patients resuscitated from cardiac arrest is still lacking. At the time being, despite its many potential applications and despite being recommended as a part of multi-modality monitoring in the intensive care unit [74], more studies are needed to implement TCD in cardiac arrest survivors as part of routine practice in hospital centers.

References

1. Mozaffarian D, Benjamin EJ, Go AS, Arnett DK, Blaha MJ, Cushman M, et al. Heart disease and stroke Statistics-2016 update: a report from the American Heart Association. Circulation. 2016;133(4):e38–360.
2. Berdowski J, Berg RA, Tijssen JG, Koster RW. Global incidences of out-of-hospital cardiac arrest and survival rates: systematic review of 67 prospective studies. Resuscitation. 2010;81(11):1479–87.
3. Fugate JE, Brinjikji W, Mandrekar JN, Cloft HJ, White RD, Wijdicks EF, et al. Post-cardiac arrest mortality is declining: a study of the US National Inpatient Sample 2001 to 2009. Circulation. 2012;126(5):546–50.
4. Iwami T, Nichol G, Hiraide A, Hayashi Y, Nishiuchi T, Kajino K, et al. Continuous improvements in "chain of survival" increased survival after out-of-hospital cardiac arrests: a large-scale population-based study. Circulation. 2009;119(5):728–34.
5. Girotra S, Nallamothu BK, Spertus JA, Li Y, Krumholz HM, Chan PS, et al. Trends in survival after in-hospital cardiac arrest. N Engl J Med. 2012;367(20):1912–20.
6. Bossaert LL, Perkins GD, Askitopoulou H, Raffay VI, Greif R, Haywood KL, et al. European Resuscitation Council Guidelines for Resuscitation 2015: Section 11. The ethics of resuscitation and end-of-life decisions. Resuscitation. 2015;95:302–11.
7. Laver S, Farrow C, Turner D, Nolan J. Mode of death after admission to an intensive care unit following cardiac arrest. Intensive Care Med. 2004;30(11):2126–8.
8. Mongardon N, Dumas F, Ricome S, Grimaldi D, Hissem T, Pène F, et al. Postcardiac arrest syndrome: from immediate resuscitation to long-term outcome. Ann Intensive Care. 2011;1(1):45.
9. Wilder Schaaf KP, Artman LK, Peberdy MA, Walker WC, Ornato JP, Gossip MR, et al. Anxiety, depression, and PTSD following cardiac arrest: a systematic review of the literature. Resuscitation. 2013;84(7):873–7.
10. Nolan JP, Neumar RW, Adrie C, Aibiki M, Berg RA, Bbttiger BW, et al. Post-cardiac arrest syndrome: epidemiology, pathophysiology, treatment, and prognostication: a scientific statement from the International Liaison Committee on Resuscitation; the American Heart Association Emergency Cardiovascular Care Committee; the Council on Cardiovascular Surgery and Anesthesia; the Council on Cardiopulmonary, Perioperative, and Critical Care; the Council on Clinical Cardiology; the Council on Stroke (Part II). Int Emerg Nurs. 2010;18(1):8–28.
11. Xiong W, Hoesch RE, Geocadin RG. Post-cardiac arrest encephalopathy. Semin Neurol. 2011;31(2):216–25.
12. Kiessling M, Stumm G, Xie Y, Herdegen T, Aguzzi A, Bravo R, et al. Differential transcription and translation of immediate early genes in the gerbil hippocampus after transient global ischemia. J Cereb Blood Flow Metab. 1993;13(6):914–24.
13. Adnet F, Triba MN, Borron SW, Lapostolle F, Hubert H, Gueugniaud PY, et al. Cardiopulmonary resuscitation duration and survival in out-of-hospital cardiac arrest patients. Resuscitation. 2017;111:74–81.
14. Sekhon MS, Ainslie PN, Griesdale DE. Clinical pathophysiology of hypoxic ischemic brain injury after cardiac arrest: a "two-hit" model. Crit Care. 2017;21(1):90.
15. Peberdy MA, Callaway CW, Neumar RW, Geocadin RG, Zimmerman JL, Donnino M, et al. Part 9: post-cardiac arrest care: 2010 American Heart Association Guidelines for Cardiopulmonary Resuscitation and Emergency Cardiovascular Care. Circulation. 2010;122(18 Suppl 3):S768–86.

16. Ames A, Wright RL, Kowada M, Thurston JM, Majno G. Cerebral ischemia. II. The no-reflow phenomenon. Am J Pathol. 1968;52(2):437–53.
17. Hossmann KA. Reperfusion of the brain after global ischemia: hemodynamic disturbances. Shock. 1997;8(2):95–101. discussion 2-3
18. Li L, Poloyac SM, Watkins SC, St Croix CM, Alexander H, Gibson GA, et al. Cerebral microcirculatory alterations and the no-reflow phenomenon in vivo after experimental pediatric cardiac arrest. J Cereb Blood Flow Metab. 2019;39(5):913–25.
19. Kågström E, Smith ML, Siesjö BK. Local cerebral blood flow in the recovery period following complete cerebral ischemia in the rat. J Cereb Blood Flow Metab. 1983;3(2):170–82.
20. Wolfson SK, Safar P, Reich H, Clark JM, Gur D, Stezoski W, et al. Dynamic heterogeneity of cerebral hypoperfusion after prolonged cardiac arrest in dogs measured by the stable xenon/CT technique: a preliminary study. Resuscitation. 1992;23(1):1–20.
21. Kilgannon JH, Roberts BW, Reihl LR, Chansky ME, Jones AE, Dellinger RP, et al. Early arterial hypotension is common in the post-cardiac arrest syndrome and associated with increased in-hospital mortality. Resuscitation. 2008;79(3):410–6.
22. Carbutti G, Romand JA, Carballo JS, Bendjelid SM, Suter PM, Bendjelid K. Transcranial Doppler: an early predictor of ischemic stroke after cardiac arrest? Anesth Analg. 2003;97(5):1262–5.
23. Müllner M, Sterz F, Binder M, Hellwagner K, Meron G, Herkner H, et al. Arterial blood pressure after human cardiac arrest and neurological recovery. Stroke. 1996;27(1):59–62.
24. Roberts BW, Kilgannon JH, Hunter BR, Puskarich MA, Shea L, Donnino M, et al. Association between elevated mean arterial blood pressure and neurologic outcome after resuscitation from cardiac arrest: results from a multicenter prospective cohort study. Crit Care Med. 2019;47(1):93–100.
25. Bisschops LL, Hoedemaekers CW, Simons KS, van der Hoeven JG. Preserved metabolic coupling and cerebrovascular reactivity during mild hypothermia after cardiac arrest. Crit Care Med. 2010;38(7):1542–7.
26. Michenfelder JD, Milde JH. Postischemic canine cerebral blood flow appears to be determined by cerebral metabolic needs. J Cereb Blood Flow Metab. 1990;10(1):71–6.
27. Buunk G, van der Hoeven JG, Meinders AE. Prognostic significance of the difference between mixed venous and jugular bulb oxygen saturation in comatose patients resuscitated from a cardiac arrest. Resuscitation. 1999;41(3):257–62.
28. Singh NC, Kochanek PM, Schiding JK, Melick JA, Nemoto EM. Uncoupled cerebral blood flow and metabolism after severe global ischemia in rats. J Cereb Blood Flow Metab. 1992;12(5):802–8.
29. Lassen NA. The luxury-perfusion syndrome and its possible relation to acute metabolic acidosis localised within the brain. Lancet. 1966;2(7473):1113–5.
30. Crouzet C, Wilson RH, Bazrafkan A, Farahabadi MH, Lee D, Alcocer J, et al. Cerebral blood flow is decoupled from blood pressure and linked to EEG bursting after resuscitation from cardiac arrest. Biomed Opt Express. 2016;7(11):4660–73.
31. Manole MD, Kochanek PM, Bayır H, Alexander H, Dezfulian C, Fink EL, et al. Brain tissue oxygen monitoring identifies cortical hypoxia and thalamic hyperoxia after experimental cardiac arrest in rats. Pediatr Res. 2014;75(2):295–301.
32. Buunk G, van der Hoeven JG, Frölich M, Meinders AE. Cerebral vasoconstriction in comatose patients resuscitated from a cardiac arrest? Intensive Care Med. 1996;22(11):1191–6.
33. Lemiale V, Huet O, Vigué B, Mathonnet A, Spaulding C, Mira JP, et al. Changes in cerebral blood flow and oxygen extraction during post-resuscitation syndrome. Resuscitation. 2008;76(1):17–24.
34. Buunk G, van der Hoeven JG, Meinders AE. Cerebral blood flow after cardiac arrest. Neth J Med. 2000;57(3):106–12.
35. van den Brule JM, Vinke E, van Loon LM, van der Hoeven JG, Hoedemaekers CW. Middle cerebral artery flow, the critical closing pressure, and the optimal mean arterial pressure in comatose cardiac arrest survivors - an observational study. Resuscitation. 2017;110:85–9.
36. Meaney PA, Bobrow BJ, Mancini ME, Christenson J, de Caen AR, Bhanji F, et al. Cardiopulmonary resuscitation quality: [corrected] improving cardiac resuscitation outcomes both inside and outside the hospital: a consensus statement from the American Heart Association. Circulation. 2013;128(4):417–35.
37. Kodali BS, Urman RD. Capnography during cardiopulmonary resuscitation: current evidence and future directions. J Emerg Trauma Shock. 2014;7(4):332–40.
38. Lewis LM, Stothert JC, Gomez CR, Ruoff BE, Hall IS, Chandel B, et al. A noninvasive method for monitoring cerebral perfusion during cardiopulmonary resuscitation. J Crit Care. 1994;9(3):169–74.
39. Lewis LM, Gomez CR, Ruoff BE, Gomez SM, Hall IS, Gasirowski B. Transcranial Doppler determination of cerebral perfusion in patients undergoing CPR: methodology and preliminary findings. Ann Emerg Med. 1990;19(10):1148–51.
40. de Wilde RBP, Helmerhorst HJF, van Westerloo DJ. Cerebral blood flow velocity during chest compressions in cardiac arrest. Netherlands J Crit Care. 2017;25(4):3.41.
41. Carmona Jiménez F, Palma Padró P, Soto García MA, Rodríguez Venegas JC. Cerebral blood flow measured by transcranial doppler ultrasound during manual chest wall or automated LUCAS-2 compressions during cardiopulmonary resuscitation. Emergencias. 2012;24:47–9.
42. Blumenstein J, Kempfert J, Walther T, Van Linden A, Fassl J, Borger M, et al. Cerebral flow pattern monitoring by transcranial Doppler during cardiopulmonary resuscitation. Anaesth Intensive Care. 2010;38(2):376–80.

43. Callaway CW, Donnino MW, Fink EL, Geocadin RG, Golan E, Kern KB, et al. Part 8: post-cardiac arrest care: 2015 American Heart Association Guidelines Update for Cardiopulmonary Resuscitation and Emergency Cardiovascular Care. Circulation. 2015;132(18 Suppl 2):S465–82.
44. Reis C, Akyol O, Araujo C, Huang L, Enkhjargal B, Malaguit J, et al. Pathophysiology and the monitoring methods for cardiac arrest associated brain injury. Int J Mol Sci. 2017;18(1):129.
45. Sekhon MS, Griesdale DE. Individualized perfusion targets in hypoxic ischemic brain injury after cardiac arrest. Crit Care. 2017;21(1):259.
46. Bhate TD, McDonald B, Sekhon MS, Griesdale DE. Association between blood pressure and outcomes in patients after cardiac arrest: a systematic review. Resuscitation. 2015;97:1–6.
47. Lassen NA. Cerebral blood flow and oxygen consumption in man. Physiol Rev. 1959;39(2):183–238.
48. Liu J, Tseng BY, Khan MA, Tarumi T, Hill C, Mirshams N, et al. Individual variability of cerebral autoregulation, posterior cerebral circulation and white matter hyperintensity. J Physiol. 2016;594(11):3141–55.
49. Gröschel K, Terborg C, Schnaudigel S, Ringer T, Riecker A, Witte OW, et al. Effects of physiological aging and cerebrovascular risk factors on the hemodynamic response to brain activation: a functional transcranial Doppler study. Eur J Neurol. 2007;14(2):125–31.
50. Strandgaard S, Olesen J, Skinhoj E, Lassen NA. Autoregulation of brain circulation in severe arterial hypertension. Br Med J. 1973;1(5852):507–10.
51. Kim YS, Immink RV, Stok WJ, Karemaker JM, Secher NH, van Lieshout JJ. Dynamic cerebral autoregulatory capacity is affected early in type 2 diabetes. Clin Sci (Lond). 2008;115(8):255–62.
52. Calviello LA, Donnelly J, Zeiler FA, Thelin EP, Smielewski P, Czosnyka M. Cerebral autoregulation monitoring in acute traumatic brain injury: what's the evidence? Minerva Anestesiol. 2017;83(8):844–57.
53. Sundgreen C, Larsen FS, Herzog TM, Knudsen GM, Boesgaard S, Aldershvile J. Autoregulation of cerebral blood flow in patients resuscitated from cardiac arrest. Stroke. 2001;32(1):128–32.
54. van den Brule JM, Vinke EJ, van Loon LM, van der Hoeven JG, Hoedemaekers CW. Low spontaneous variability in cerebral blood flow velocity in non-survivors after cardiac arrest. Resuscitation. 2017;111:110–5.
55. Janiczek JA, Winger DG, Coppler P, Sabedra AR, Murray H, Pinsky MR, et al. Hemodynamic resuscitation characteristics associated with improved survival and shock resolution after cardiac arrest. Shock. 2016;45(6):613–9.
56. Burton AC. On the physical equilibrium of small blood vessels. Am J Phys. 1951;164(2):319–29.
57. Dewey RC, Pieper HP, Hunt WE. Experimental cerebral hemodynamics. Vasomotor tone, critical closing pressure, and vascular bed resistance. J Neurosurg. 1974;41(5):597–606.
58. Alvarez-Fernández JA, Pérez-Quintero R. Use of transcranial Doppler ultrasound in the management of post-cardiac arrest syndrome. Resuscitation. 2009;80(11):1321–2.
59. Wessels T, Harrer JU, Jacke C, Janssens U, Klötzsch C. The prognostic value of early transcranial Doppler ultrasound following cardiopulmonary resuscitation. Ultrasound Med Biol. 2006;32(12):1845–51.
60. Gomez CR, McLaughlin JR, Njemanze PC, Nashed A. Effect of cardiac dysfunction upon diastolic cerebral blood flow. Angiology. 1992;43(8):625–30.
61. Nebra Puertas AC, Virgós Señor B, Suárez Pinilla MA, Munárriz Hinojosa J, Ridruejo Sáez R, Sánchez Miret JI, et al. Changes in cerebral flow velocity measured by transcranial Doppler after advanced life support maneuvers. Med Intensiva. 2003;27:5.
62. Iida K, Satoh H, Arita K, Nakahara T, Kurisu K, Ohtani M. Delayed hyperemia causing intracranial hypertension after cardiopulmonary resuscitation. Crit Care Med. 1997;25(6):971–6.
63. Rafi S, Tadie JM, Gacouin A, Leurent G, Bedossa M, Le Tulzo Y, et al. Doppler sonography of cerebral blood flow for early prognostication after out-of-hospital cardiac arrest: DOTAC study. Resuscitation. 2019;141:188.
64. Doepp Connolly F, Reitemeier J, Storm C, Hasper D, Schreiber SJ. Duplex sonography of cerebral blood flow after cardiac arrest—a prospective observational study. Resuscitation. 2014;85(4):516–21.
65. Yenari M, Kitagawa K, Lyden P, Perez-Pinzon M. Metabolic downregulation: a key to successful neuroprotection? Stroke. 2008;39(10):2910–7.
66. Rasulo FA, Bertuetti R, Robba C, Lusenti F, Cantoni A, Bernini M, et al. The accuracy of transcranial Doppler in excluding intracranial hypertension following acute brain injury: a multicenter prospective pilot study. Crit Care. 2017;21(1):44.
67. Taccone FS, Crippa IA, Creteur J, Rasulo F. Estimated cerebral perfusion pressure among post-cardiac arrest survivors. Intensive Care Med. 2018;44(6):966–7.
68. Doering TJ, Aaslid R, Steuernagel B, Brix J, Niederstadt C, Breull A, et al. Cerebral autoregulation during whole-body hypothermia and hyperthermia stimulus. Am J Phys Med Rehabil. 1999;78(1):33–8.
69. Fujita M, Wei EP, Povlishock JT. Effects of hypothermia on cerebral autoregulatory vascular responses in two rodent models of traumatic brain injury. J Neurotrauma. 2012;29(7):1491–8.
70. Lin JJ, Hsia SH, Wang HS, Chiang MC, Lin KL. Transcranial Doppler ultrasound in therapeutic hypothermia for children after resuscitation. Resuscitation. 2015;89:182–7.

71. Heimburger D, Durand M, Gaide-Chevronnay L, Dessertaine G, Moury PH, Bouzat P, et al. Quantitative pupillometry and transcranial Doppler measurements in patients treated with hypothermia after cardiac arrest. Resuscitation. 2016;103:88–93.
72. Buunk G, van der Hoeven JG, Meinders AE. Cerebrovascular reactivity in comatose patients resuscitated from a cardiac arrest. Stroke. 1997;28(8):1569–73.
73. van den Brule JMD, van Kaam CR, van der Hoeven JG, Claassen JAHR, Hoedemaekers CWE. Influence of induced blood pressure variability on the assessment of cerebral autoregulation in patients after cardiac arrest. Biomed Res Int. 2018;2018:8153241.
74. Citerio G, Oddo M, Taccone FS. Recommendations for the use of multimodal monitoring in the neurointensive care unit. Curr Opin Crit Care. 2015;21(2):113–9.

Severe Respiratory Failure: ARDS and ECMO

14

Alberto Goffi,
Airton Leonardo de Oliveira Manoel,
and Chiara Robba

Contents

14.1 Introduction

Respiratory complications are common in patients with acute brain injury [1–3]. In three different prospective cohort studies and including patients receiving mechanical ventilation from approximately 900 ICUs in 40 countries, neurologic and neuromuscular disorders represented a significant percentage of conditions requiring respiratory support. Approximately 20% of patients on mechanical ventilation are affected by a neurological disease. Moreover, common conditions affecting critically ill neurological patients, such as pneumonia, sepsis, and aspiration, represent another large group of conditions that may require the institution of mechanical ventilation [3]. Acute respiratory

A. Goffi (✉)
Interdepartmental Division of Critical Care Medicine and Department of Medicine, University of Toronto, Toronto, ON, Canada

Department of Medicine, Division of Critical Care Medicine, St. Michael's Hospital, Toronto, ON, Canada
e-mail: alberto.goffi@unityhealth.to

A. L. de Oliveira Manoel
Neurocritical Care Unit, Hospital Santa Paula, São Paulo, Brazil

C. Robba
Anesthesia and Intensive Care, Policlinico San Martino, IRCCS for Oncology and Neuroscience, Genoa, Italy

C. Robba, G. Citerio (eds.), *Echography and Doppler of the Brain*,
https://doi.org/10.1007/978-3-030-48202-2_14

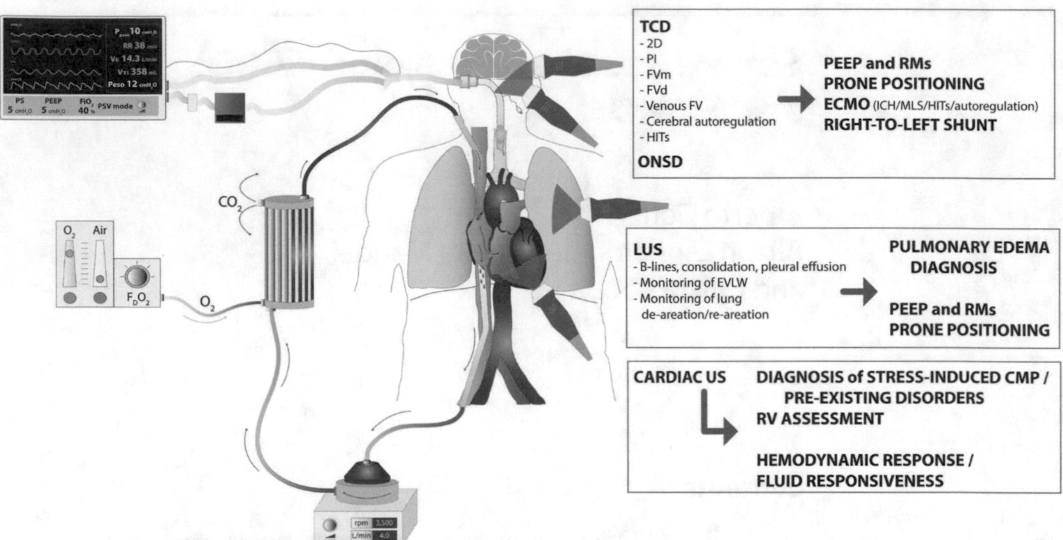

Fig. 14.1 Applications of brain and general ultrasonography for the management of patients with respiratory failure. Legend: PI: *ECMO* extra corporeal membrane oxygenation, *EVLW* extravascular lung water, *FVd* diastolic flow velocity, *FVm* mean flow velocity, *HITs* high-intensity transient signals, *ICH* intracranial hemorrhage, *LUS* lung ultrasound, *MLS* midline shift, *ONSD* optic nerve sheath diameter, *PEEP* positive end expiratory pressure, pulsatility index, *RM* recruitment maneuver, *TCD* transcranial Doppler

distress syndrome (ARDS) affects approximately 20% of patients admitted with traumatic brain injury (TBI) [1] and up to 35% of patients with aneurysmal subarachnoid hemorrhage (SAH) [2], which is associated with increased risk of unfavorable outcomes, with an estimated mortality of 28–33% and 61–75%, respectively. Additionally, survivors are frequently left with cognitive impairment after ARDS, being present in 70–100% of patients at hospital discharge and in 20% at 5 years [4]. Furthermore, commonly used ventilatory (e.g., high positive end-expiratory pressure—PEEP; recruitment maneuvers; lung-protective ventilation with permissive hypercapnia) and non-ventilatory strategies (e.g., prone positioning) may lead to increased intracranial pressure (ICP) and may also affect cerebral perfusion and cerebral oxygen delivery [5–8].

Therefore, the use of ultrasound techniques aimed at monitoring cerebral perfusion at the bedside, and also the response to therapeutic interventions in this patient population, sounds appealing. A lung/neuroprotective ventilatory strategy may be critical not only for patients with acute brain injury, but also for patients without evidence of primary brain insult. In this chapter we discuss the potential role of brain and general ultrasonography for the management of patients with respiratory failure (Fig. 14.1).

14.2 Brain Ultrasonography

The effect of increased intrathoracic pressures, the changes in arterial partial pressure of oxygenation (PaO_2) and carbon dioxide ($PaCO_2$), and also the application of non-ventilatory strategies such as prone positioning and ECMO may be monitored at the bedside with brain ultrasonographic techniques [transcranial Doppler (TCD) and optic nerve sheath diameter (ONSD) measurement] [5–7].

14.2.1 PEEP and Recruitment Maneuvers

Increased intrathoracic pressures may decrease cerebral perfusion due to the reduction in venous return, with consequent fall in cardiac output. Therefore, traditionally lower levels of PEEP and avoidance of recruitment maneuvers have been suggested in patients with acute brain injury. However, several factors modulate the effect of intrathoracic pressure on cerebral perfusion, as respiratory system compliance [9], effect of PEEP on lung recruitment/alveolar hyperinflation [10], ICP [11], and mean arterial pressure (MAP) [12]. For example, in a cohort of 20 patients with TBI and ARDS, progressive increase in PEEP levels did not significantly affect cerebral perfusion pressure (CPP) and brain tissue oxygenation [13]. As discussed elsewhere in this book, TCD and ONSD can noninvasively detect ICP changes. The intracranial effect of increased intrathoracic pressure may be monitored by assessing specific ultrasound parameters such as the pulsatility index (PI) and diastolic cerebral arterial blood flow velocity (dFV) by TCD, or ONSD measurements. When considering recruitment maneuvers or increase in PEEP levels in this population, altered values suggesting elevated ICP (e.g., PI > 1.25, dFV <25 cm/s, and/or ONSD >6 mm) may be analyzed cautiously. An appropriate invasive monitoring and/or careful risk/benefit analysis might be required before the application of those strategies (Fig. 14.2) [6].

Venous cerebral blood flow at the level of the straight sinus is another parameter that could be monitored to estimate the cerebral response to increased intrathoracic pressures [6, 14]. Moreover, TCD allows to address the effect of changes in PEEP on cerebral perfusion and autoregulation, even when invasive neuromonitoring is not present. For example, Schramm et al. [7] demonstrated that more than 50% (11/20) of patients with ARDS, irrespective of changes in MAP or $PaCO_2$, display signs of impaired cerebral autoregulation. Interestingly, although increasing PEEP levels did not significantly affect cerebral autoregulation in the overall cohort, it deteriorated in some patients and improved in others [7], which highlights the possible role of brain ultrasound as a tool to individualize the ventilatory support also from a "brain protective" perspective.

14.2.2 Prone Positioning

Prone positioning (PP) represents the standard of care in patients with moderate-severe ARDS, being associated with a significant mortality benefit [15]. However, its use in patients with elevated ICP is usually considered contraindicated. Roth et al. [16] studied the effect of PP in 29 patients with acute brain injury (for a total of 119 PP sessions) and demonstrated a significant increase in ICP during PP sessions (9.5 ± 5.9 mmHg vs. 15.4 ± 6.2 mmHg; $p < 0.0001$). Moreover, during PP patients experienced more episodes of ICP >20 mmHg. Similarly, in another study exploring the effect of PP in 16 patients with SAH and ARDS, Reinprecht et al. [17] observed significant deterioration of ICP (from 9.6 ± 3.5 mmHg to 15.8 ± 3.5 mmHg; $p < 0.0001$) and CPP (from 74.4 ± 8.4 mmHg to 67.0 ± 7.1 mmHg; $p < 0.0001$), with more episodes of elevated ICP and low CPP (<60 mmHg) detected during PP. However, in this study PP was associated with significant increase of brain tissue oxygenation (from 27.2 ± 4.2 mmHg to 33.5 ± 5.3 mmHg; $p < 0.001$) and overall less episodes of brain tissue hypoxia (supine: 32.7% vs. prone: 10%; $p = 0.0473$). Limited data are currently available on the use of brain ultrasound in patients undergoing prone positioning. In the study by Reinprecht et al. [17], cerebral blood flow velocities measured by TCD did not significantly change during PP compared to the baseline values in supine position; however, in one patient a significant increase in the mean middle cerebral artery velocity was observed during one of the sessions of prone positioning, potentially suggesting worsening angiographic vasospasm. Recently, Robba et al. [18] demonstrated its feasibility, by measuring the effect of prone positioning on three different methods to estimate ICP noninvasively. Thirty-three patients undergoing elective spine surgery and with normal respiratory function were included. Changes in position from supine to prone were associated with an increase in noninvasive estimates of ICP, with ONSD being the most sensitive. Brain ultrasonography may therefore be used in patients

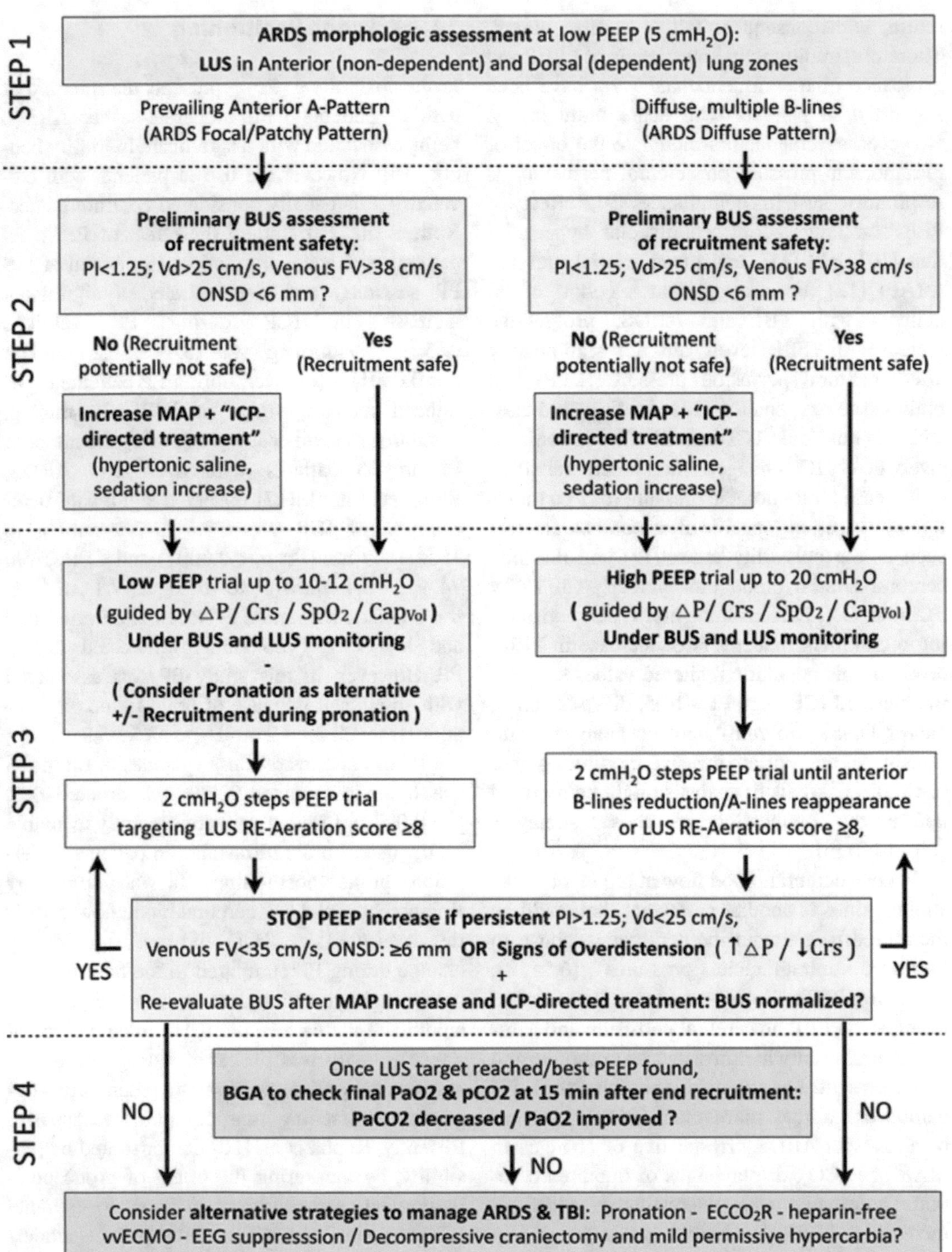

Fig. 14.2 Lung and brain ultrasound combined respiratory and neurological monitoring approach in patients with acute brain injury and severe respiratory failure. Reproduced from Corradi F, Robba C, Tavazzi G, Via G. Crit Ultrasound J 2018;10(1):24 (SpringerOpen) [6]; this figure is distributed under the terms of the Creative Commons Attribution 4.0 International License (http://creativecommons.org/licenses/by/4.0/), which permits unrestricted use, distribution, and reproduction in any medium

with indication for PP and lack of invasive neuromonitoring, both before institution of PP to identify patients at higher risk of developing critical reduction in cerebral perfusion and during PP to detect changes in ICP and cerebral perfusion pressure, which are concerning for secondary brain injury.

14.2.3 ECMO

Extracorporeal membrane oxygenation (ECMO), both V-V and V-A, is associated with several neurological complications that carry high mortality rates [19–22]. Conventional brain imaging (e.g., CT and MRI) is especially challenging in this patient population. Therefore, bedside point-of-care techniques represent an appealing alternative option, especially because the recognition of neurological changes by clinical exam in this population is often very limited due to the need for deep sedation and the use of neuromuscular blockade [23]. Brain ultrasonography may help to overcome these challenges, and it may be applied at the bedside for identification and monitoring of neurological complications during ECMO. Transcranial ultrasound can detect intra- and extra-axial intracranial hematomas, both supra- and infratentorial, although frontal and parietal lobe lesions are difficult to insonate due to limitation of acoustic windows [24–27]. It can also be used to measure midline shift (MLS) by identifying the third ventricle and the temporal bone as reference points [24, 28, 29]. Ischemic strokes are also non-infrequent complications during ECMO, due to hypoperfusion, anoxic injury, and embolism [19, 30]. Embolic strokes may be small (gaseous or thrombotic microemboli) or large, usually related to large clots [31], and they can be identified in real time with the use of TCD [32]. Microemboli are extremely frequent during ECMO (26% in V-V ECMO and 82% in V-A ECMO) [33] and their clinical significance is currently unknown, especially when considering long-term cognitive outcomes.

TCD analysis of cerebral blood flow velocities has also been proposed both for (early) identification of new cerebrovascular injuries during ECMO and as a tool for optimization of cerebral perfusion, especially in patients undergoing V-A ECMO but also for V-V ECMO [23, 34, 35]. In pediatric ECMO population, an increase in TCD velocities (especially if localized and asymmetric) has been associated with neurologic injury, and it seems to represent an early sign, anticipating by approximately 1–6 days of the clinical recognition [23, 35]. Reactive hyperemia secondary to uncoupling of cerebral metabolism and cerebral flow in the context of ischemic event may explain this finding, and it is associated with increased risk of intracranial hemorrhage (especially in the context of anticoagulation) [35]. Changes in pulsatility (PI) and/or resistivity (RI) indices have also been associated with increased risk of cerebrovascular complications in neonatal and pediatric ECMO patients [35, 36]. When analyzing TCD velocities, the type of ECMO, the site of cannulation, and the circuit flow rate are important parameters to take into consideration [35].

ARDS patients often present impaired cerebral autoregulation. Fanelli et al. [34] suggested that initiation of V-V ECMO may restore cerebral autoregulation in severe ARDS, as detected by TCD. Moreover, in a recent study conducted on patients undergoing V-V ECMO, intracranial bleeding was independently associated with the rapid $PaCO_2$ reduction at the initiation of ECMO [19]. A possible explanation of this finding could be related to ECMO-induced hypocapnia-related severe vasoconstriction, causing cerebral hypoperfusion and subsequent hemorrhagic transformation of an ischemic area [19, 37]. If confirmed in future studies, this observation could have a significant impact on how V-V ECMO is initiated, and TCD could further help identifying patients at higher risk of developing ECMO-induced hypoperfusion.

Finally, in jurisdictions where TCD is accepted as an ancillary test for neurological determination of death, it has been shown to be feasible and potentially useful in patients undergoing intra-aortic balloon pump or extracorporeal cardiorespiratory support; however, in patients on VA ECMO and non-pulsatile arterial flow, there is currently lack of data [38].

14.2.4 Identification of Right-to-Left Shunt with TCD

Patent foramen ovale (PFO) prevalence in general adult population is approximately 25% [39] but shunting through PFO is rare in healthy individuals as the foramen is usually kept closed by a flap when left atrial pressure is higher than right atrial pressure. However, in conditions associated with increased right atrial pressure (e.g., pulmonary hypertension, pulmonary embolism, ARDS), right-to-left shunting may occur, with possible worsening hypoxemia. For example, shunting through PFO has been observed in almost 20% of patients with ARDS and it is associated with poorer response to PEEP, greater use of adjunctive interventions, and longer ICU stay [40]. Intrapulmonary shunt is also recognized as a cause of worsening hypoxemia during ARDS, and it is observed in approximately 25% of patients affected by this condition [41]. Contrast transesophageal echocardiography (TEE) is considered the gold standard test for identification of right-to-left shunt. Contrast TCD represents an alternative method for the detection of right-to-left shunt. Identification of microembolic events [high-intensity transient signals (HITS)] in the cerebral circulation has been shown to be as accurate as cTEE (or even more) for detection of right-to-left shunting, especially at rest [42, 43]. Moreover, cTCD can be used as a semiquantitative method to estimate the volume of shunting. In the context of hypoxemia due to right-to-left shunting, different supportive treatment options aimed at reducing right ventricular load conditions and intrapulmonary shunt may be considered, as nitric oxide, alveolar recruitment, and prone positioning. Contrast TCD may also have a significant role in both detecting right-to-left shunting and assessing the response to these interventions [44].

14.3 General Ultrasonography

General ultrasound applications (i.e., lung, cardiac, and vascular ultrasound) also represent an important bedside tool for the management of acute brain injury patients with severe respiratory failure. A detailed description of findings, applications, and evidence of general ultrasonography use in respiratory failure is beyond the scope of this chapter, and is presented elsewhere [45–50].

14.3.1 Lung Ultrasound

Lung ultrasound (LUS) has emerged as an essential goal-directed diagnostic technique that can be applied in real time at the bedside for the assessment of patients with respiratory failure [46, 51]. LUS has been shown to outperform physical examination and chest radiography for the diagnosis and monitoring of many pulmonary and pleural conditions [46, 51–58]. LUS can be used in neurocritically ill patients to detect pulmonary edema (cardiogenic, neurogenic, and ARDS), to monitor extravascular lung water content, and to predict PEEP-induced lung recruitment [6, 59]. For example, in a study involving 59 patients with subarachnoid hemorrhage, LUS demonstrated good accuracy (sensitivity 90%, specificity 82%) for the detection of pulmonary edema [60]. Moreover, the integration of lung and brain ultrasound findings could be used to optimize ventilatory strategies (e.g., PEEP, minute ventilation, recruitment maneuvers, prone positioning) while concurrently monitoring the effect of these interventions on cerebrovascular physiology in patients at risk of significant deterioration (Fig. 14.2) [6].

14.3.2 Cardiac Ultrasound

Echocardiography plays an important role for both diagnosis of cardiac conditions (e.g., stress-induced cardiomyopathy or preexisting disorders potentially affecting the management of neurocritically ill patients) and monitoring the response to interventions (as fluid challenges and initiation or titration of vasoactive agents). Stress-induced cardiomyopathy is commonly encountered in brain-injured patients, especially in the presence of spontaneous intraparenchymal hemorrhage and aneurysmal subarachnoid hemorrhage, and it represents a significant risk factor for unfavorable outcome and death. An appropriate fluid management strategy is of great importance in neurocritically ill patients, due to the risks associated with both fluid overload and intravascular depletion. Fluid responsiveness can be estimated by echocardiography in both spontaneously breathing and mechanically ventilated patients, by the use of passive leg raising [61] and by the respiratory variations of maximal Doppler velocity in the left ventricular outflow tract [62] representing the most accurate indices, respectively.

14.4 Conclusion

Respiratory complications are common in patients with acute brain injury and represent a significant challenge. The concomitant use of brain and general critical care ultrasound techniques may offer a significant benefit in delivering both lung- and neuroprotective strategies in patients with complex ventilatory needs and deranged cerebrovascular physiology. However, current evidence is extremely limited, and more data are needed to support the routine use of this approach in clinical practice.

References

1. Rincon F, Ghosh S, Dey S, Maltenfort M, Vibbert M, Urtecho J, et al. Impact of acute lung injury and acute respiratory distress syndrome after traumatic brain injury in the United States. Neurosurgery. 2012;71(4):795–803.
2. Veeravagu A, Chen YR, Ludwig C, Rincon F, Maltenfort M, Jallo J, et al. Acute lung injury in patients with subarachnoid hemorrhage: a nationwide inpatient sample study. World Neurosurg. 2014;82(1):e235–41.
3. Esteban A, Frutos-Vivar F, Muriel A, Ferguson ND, Peñuelas O, Abraira V, et al. Evolution of mortality over time in patients receiving mechanical ventilation. Am J Respir Crit Care Med. 2013;188(2):220–30.
4. Wilcox ME, Brummel NE, Archer K, Ely EW, Jackson JC, Hopkins RO. Cognitive dysfunction in ICU patients: risk factors, predictors, and rehabilitation interventions. Crit Care Med. 2013;41(9 Suppl 1):S81–98.
5. Young N, Rhodes JKJ, Mascia L, Andrews PJD. Ventilatory strategies for patients with acute brain injury. Curr Opin Crit Care. 2010;16(1):45–52.
6. Corradi F, Robba C, Tavazzi G, Via G. Combined lung and brain ultrasonography for an individualized "brain-protective ventilation strategy" in neurocritical care patients with challenging ventilation needs. Crit Ultrasound J. 2018;10(1):24.
7. Schramm P, Closhen D, Felkel M, Berres M, Klein KU, David M, et al. Influence of PEEP on cerebral blood flow and cerebrovascular autoregulation in patients with acute respiratory distress syndrome. J Neurosurg Anesthesiol. 2013;25(2):162–7.
8. Frisvold SK, Robba C, Guérin C. What respiratory targets should be recommended in patients with brain injury and respiratory failure? Intensive Care Med. 2019;45(5):683–6.
9. Caricato A, Conti G, Della Corte F, Mancino A, Santilli F, Sandroni C, et al. Effects of PEEP on the intracranial system of patients with head injury and subarachnoid hemorrhage: the role of respiratory system compliance. J Trauma – Inj Infect Crit Care. 2005;58(3):571–6.
10. Mascia L, Grasso S, Fiore T, Bruno F, Berardino M, Ducati A. Cerebro-pulmonary interactions during the application of low levels of positive end-expiratory pressure. Intensive Care Med. 2005;31(3):373–9.
11. Mc Guire G, Crossley D, Richards J, Wong D. Effects of varying levels of positive end-expiratory pressure on intracranial pressure and cerebral perfusion pressure. Crit Care Med. 1997;25(6):1059–62.
12. Muench E, Bauhuf C, Roth H, Horn P, Phillips M, Marquetant N, et al. Effects of positive end-expiratory pressure on regional cerebral blood flow, intracranial pressure, and brain tissue oxygenation. Crit Care Med. 2005;33(10):2367–72.
13. Nemer SN, Caldeira JB, Santos RG, Guimarães BL, Garcia JM, Prado D, et al. Effects of positive end-expiratory pressure on brain tissue oxygen pressure of severe traumatic brain injury patients with acute respiratory distress syndrome: a pilot study. J Crit Care. 2015;30(6):1263–6.
14. Robba C, Cardim D, Tajsic T, Pietersen J, Bulman M, Donnelly J, et al. Ultrasound non-invasive measurement of intracranial pressure in neurointensive care: a prospective observational study. PLoS Med. 2017;14(7):e1002356.
15. Guérin C, Reignier J, Richard J-C, Beuret P, Gacouin A, Boulain T, et al. Prone positioning in severe acute respiratory distress syndrome. N Engl J Med. 2013;368(23):2159–68.
16. Roth C, Ferbert A, Deinsberger W, Kleffmann J, Kästner S, Godau J, et al. Does prone positioning increase intracranial pressure? A retrospective analysis of patients with acute brain injury and acute respiratory failure. Neurocrit Care. 2014;21(2):186–91.
17. Reinprecht A, Greher M, Wolfsberger S, Dietrich W, Illievich UM, Gruber A. Prone position in subarachnoid hemorrhage patients with acute respiratory distress syndrome: effects on cerebral tissue oxy-

genation and intracranial pressure. Crit Care Med. 2003;31(6):1831–8.
18. Robba C, Bragazzi NL, Bertuccio A, Cardim D, Donnelly J, Sekhon M, et al. Effects of prone position and positive end-expiratory pressure on noninvasive estimators of ICP: a pilot study. J Neurosurg Anesthesiol. 2017;29(3):243–50.
19. Luyt C-E, Bréchot N, Demondion P, Jovanovic T, Hékimian G, Lebreton G, et al. Brain injury during venovenous extracorporeal membrane oxygenation. Intensive Care Med. 2016;42(5):897–907.
20. Australia and New Zealand Extracorporeal Membrane Oxygenation (ANZ ECMO) Influenza Investigators, Davies A, Jones D, Bailey M, Beca J, Bellomo R, et al. Extracorporeal membrane oxygenation for 2009 influenza a(H1N1) acute respiratory distress syndrome. JAMA. 2009;302(17):1888–95.
21. Kasirajan V, Smedira NG, McCarthy JF, Casselman F, Boparai N, McCarthy PM. Risk factors for intracranial hemorrhage in adults on extracorporeal membrane oxygenation. Eur J Cardiothorac Surg. 1999;15(4):508–14.
22. Sutter R, Tisljar K, Marsch S. Acute neurologic complications during extracorporeal membrane oxygenation: a systematic review. Crit Care Med. 2018;46(9):1506–13.
23. Rilinger JF, Smith CM, deRegnier RAO, Goldstein JL, Mills MG, Reynolds M, et al. Transcranial Doppler identification of neurologic injury during pediatric extracorporeal membrane oxygenation therapy. J Stroke Cerebrovasc Dis. 2017;26(10):2336–45.
24. Blanco P, Blaivas M. Applications of transcranial color-coded sonography in the emergency department. J Ultrasound Med. 2017;36(6):1251–66.
25. Mäurer M, Shambal S, Berg D, Woydt M, Hofmann E, Georgiadis D, et al. Differentiation between intracerebral hemorrhage and ischemic stroke by transcranial color-coded duplex-sonography. Stroke. 1998;29(12):2563–7.
26. Kukulska-Pawluczuk B, Ksiazkiewicz B, Nowaczewska M. Imaging of spontaneous intracerebral hemorrhages by means of transcranial color-coded sonography. Eur J Radiol. 2012;81(6):1253–8.
27. Niesen WD, Burkhardt D, Hoeltje J, Rosenkranz M, Weiller C, Sliwka U. Transcranial grey-scale sonography of subdural haematoma in adults. Ultraschall der Medizin. 2006;27(3):251–5.
28. Llompart Pou JA, Abadal Centellas JM, Palmer Sans M, Pérez Bárcena J, Casares Vivas M, Homar Ramírez J, et al. Monitoring midline shift by transcranial color-coded sonography in traumatic brain injury: a comparison with cranial computerized tomography. Intensive Care Med. 2004;30(8):1672–5.
29. Tang SC, Huang SJ, Jeng JS, Yip PK. Third ventricle midline shift due to spontaneous supratentorial intracerebral hemorrhage evaluated by transcranial color-coded sonography. J Ultrasound Med. 2006;25(2):203–9.
30. Omar HR, Mirsaeidi M, Shumac J, Enten G, Mangar D, Camporesi EM. Incidence and predictors of ischemic cerebrovascular stroke among patients on extracorporeal membrane oxygenation support. J Crit Care. 2016;32:48–51.
31. Mehta A, Ibsen LM. Neurologic complications and neurodevelopmental outcome with extracorporeal life support. World J Crit Care Med. 2013;2(4):40–7.
32. Ringelstein EB, Droste DW, Babikian VL, Evans DH, Grosset DG, Kaps M, et al. Consensus on microembolus detection by TCD: international consensus group on microembolus detection. Stroke. 1998;29(3):725–9.
33. Marinoni M, Migliaccio ML, Trapani S, Bonizzoli M, Gucci L, Cianchi G, et al. Cerebral microemboli detected by transcranial doppler in patients treated with extracorporeal membrane oxygenation. Acta Anaesthesiol Scand. 2016;60(7):934–44.
34. Fanelli V, Mazzeo AT, Battaglini I, Caccia S, Boffini M, Ricci D, et al. Cerebral autoregulation in patients treated with V-V ECMO for severe ARDS. Intensive Care Med Exp. 2015;3(Suppl 1):A509–3.
35. O'Brien NF, Hall MW. Extracorporeal membrane oxygenation and cerebral blood flow velocity in children. Pediatr Crit Care Med. 2013;14(3):e126–34.
36. Zamora CA, Oshmyansky A, Bembea M, Berkowitz I, Alqahtani E, Liu S, et al. Resistive index variability in anterior cerebral artery measurements during daily transcranial duplex sonography: a predictor of cerebrovascular complications in infants undergoing extracorporeal membrane oxygenation? J Ultrasound Med. 2016;35(11):2459–65.
37. Kredel M, Lubnow M, Westermaier T, Müller T, Philipp A, Lotz C, et al. Cerebral tissue oxygenation during the initiation of venovenous ECMO. ASAIO J. 2014;60(6):694–700.
38. Marinoni M, Cianchi G, Trapani S, Migliaccio ML, Bonizzoli M, Gucci L, et al. Retrospective analysis of transcranial doppler patterns in veno-arterial extracorporeal membrane oxygenation patients: feasibility of cerebral circulatory arrest diagnosis. ASAIO J. 2018;62(2):175–82.
39. Hagen PT, Scholz DG, Edwards WD. Incidence and size of patent foramen ovale during the first 10 decades of life: an autopsy study of 965 normal hearts. Mayo Clin Proc. 1984;59(1):17–20.
40. Mekontso Dessap A, Boissier F, Leon R, Carreira S, Campo FR, Lemaire F, et al. Prevalence and prognosis of shunting across patent foramen ovale during acute respiratory distress syndrome. Crit Care Med. 2010;38(9):1786–92.
41. Boissier F, Razazi K, Thille AW, Roche-Campo F, Leon R, Vivier E, et al. Echocardiographic detection of transpulmonary bubble transit during acute respiratory distress syndrome. Ann Intensive Care. 2015;5:5.
42. Tobe J, Bogiatzi C, Munoz C, Tamayo A, Spence JD. Transcranial Doppler is complementary to echocardiography for detection and risk stratification of patent foramen ovale. Can J Cardiol. 2016;32(8):986.
43. Vuković-Cvetković V. Microembolus detection by transcranial Doppler sonography: review of the literature. Stroke Res Treat. 2012;2012:382361.

44. Legras A, Dequin PF, Hazouard E, Doucet O, Tranquart F, Perrotin D. Right-to-left interatrial shunt in ARDS: dramatic improvement in prone position. Intensive Care Med. 1999;25(4):412–4.
45. Lui JK, Banauch GI. Diagnostic bedside ultrasonography for acute respiratory failure and severe hypoxemia in the medical intensive care unit: basics and comprehensive approaches. J Intensive Care Med. 2016;32(6):355–72.
46. Goffi A, Kruisselbrink R, Volpicelli G. The sound of air: point-of-care lung ultrasound in perioperative medicine. Can J Anaesth. 2018;65(4):399–416.
47. Kruisselbrink R, Chan V, Cibinel GA, Abrahamson S, Goffi A. I-AIM (indication, acquisition, interpretation, medical decision-making) framework for point of care lung ultrasound. Anesthesiology. 2017;127(3):568–82.
48. Mayo PH, Copetti R, Feller-Kopman D, Mathis G, Maury E, Mongodi S, et al. Thoracic ultrasonography: a narrative review. Intensive Care Med. 2019;45(9):1200–11.
49. Vieillard-Baron A, Millington SJ, Sanfillipo F, Chew M, Diaz-Gomez J, McLean A, et al. A decade of progress in critical care echocardiography: a narrative review. Intensive Care Med. 2019;45(6):770–88.
50. Bilotta F, Dei Giudici L, Lam A, Rosa G. Ultrasound-based imaging in neurocritical care patients: a review of clinical applications. Neurol Res. 2013;35(2):149–58.
51. Volpicelli G, Elbarbary M, Blaivas M, Lichtenstein DA, Mathis G, Kirkpatrick AW, et al. International evidence-based recommendations for point-of-care lung ultrasound. Intensive Care Med. 2012;38(4):577–91.
52. Pivetta E, Goffi A, Lupia E, Tizzani M, Porrino G, Ferreri E, et al. Lung ultrasound-implemented diagnosis of acute decompensated heart failure in the ED: a SIMEU multicenter study. Chest. 2015;148(1):202–10.
53. Lichtenstein DA, Mezière GA. Relevance of lung ultrasound in the diagnosis of acute respiratory failure: the BLUE protocol. Chest. 2008;134(1):117–25.
54. Volpicelli G, Mussa A, Garofalo G, Cardinale L, Casoli G, Perotto F, et al. Bedside lung ultrasound in the assessment of alveolar-interstitial syndrome. Am J Emerg Med. 2006;24(6):689–96.
55. Yousefifard M, Baikpour M, Ghelichkhani P, Asady H, Shahsavari Nia K, Moghadas Jafari A, et al. Screening performance characteristic of ultrasonography and radiography in detection of pleural effusion, a meta-analysis. Emerg (Tehran, Iran). 2016;4(1):1–10.
56. Reissig A, Copetti R, Mathis G, Mempel C, Schuler A, Zechner P, et al. Lung ultrasound in the diagnosis and follow-up of community-acquired pneumonia: a prospective, multicenter, diagnostic accuracy study. Chest. 2012;142(4):965–72.
57. Alrajab S, Youssef A, Akkus N, Caldito G. Pleural ultrasonography versus chest radiography for the diagnosis of pneumothorax: review of the literature and meta-analysis. Crit Care. 2013;17(5):R208.
58. Pivetta E, Goffi A, Nazerian P, Castagno D, Tozzetti C, Tizzani P, et al. Lung ultrasound integrated with clinical assessment for the diagnosis of acute decompensated heart failure in the emergency department: a randomized controlled trial. Eur J Heart Fail. 2019;21(6):754–66.
59. Merenkov VV, Kovalev AN, Gorbunov VV. Bedside lung ultrasound: a case of neurogenic pulmonary edema. Neurocrit Care. 2013;18(3):391–4.
60. Williamson CA, Co I, Pandey AS, Gregory Thompson B, Rajajee V. Accuracy of daily lung ultrasound for the detection of pulmonary edema following subarachnoid hemorrhage. Neurocrit Care. 2016;24(2):189–96.
61. Bentzer P, Griesdale DE, Boyd J, MacLean K, Sirounis D, Ayas NT. Will this hemodynamically unstable patient respond to a bolus of intravenous fluids? JAMA. 2016;316(12):1298–309.
62. Vignon P, Repessé X, Begot E, Léger J, Jacob C, Bouferrache K, et al. Comparison of echocardiographic indices used to predict fluid responsiveness in ventilated patients. Am J Respir Crit Care Med. 2017;195(8):1022–32.

Part V

Pathology and Clinical Applications: Neuro-ICU

15 Intracerebral Hematomas, Midline Shift, Hydrocephalus

Pedro Kurtz, Daniel Paes de Almeida dos Santos, and Ivan Rocha Ferreira da Silva

Contents

15.1 Introduction

The clinical applications of transcranial doppler (TCD) and transcranial color-coded duplex ultrasonography (TCCD) in neurocritical care have been extensively studied. The TCCD method includes ultrasonographic 2-dimensional imaging of the brain and Doppler analysis of cerebral blood flow. It may be referred to in the literature with other nomenclatures such as transcranial duplex sonography (TDS), transcranial color-coded sonography (TCCS), and others. In this chapter we use TCCD. Although the use of both methods of brain ultrasound (US) in patients with intracerebral hemorrhage (ICH) is not as widespread as in those with subarachnoid hemorrhage (SAH) or brain death, interest and publications in TCD and TCCD monitoring have grown in recent years. Additionally, clinical indications and parameters monitored have expanded along with the increased interest in

P. Kurtz (✉) · D. P. de A. dos Santos
Department of Neurointensive Care, Hospital Copa Star, Rio de Janeiro, RJ, Brazil

I. R. F. da Silva
Department of Neurological Sciences, Rush University Medical Center (IRFS), Chicago, IL, USA

C. Robba, G. Citerio (eds.), *Echography and Doppler of the Brain*,
https://doi.org/10.1007/978-3-030-48202-2_15

general bedside ultrasonography and the advancements in US technology. This chapter describes the main clinical applications of TCD and TCCD in neurocritical patients with special focus on intracerebral hemorrhage (ICH) and intracranial hypertension.

Spontaneous ICH should be suspected in any patient presenting with an acute-onset headache, seizure, focal neurological deficit, and/or altered mental state. Timely assessment and urgent neuroimaging (computed tomography [CT] or magnetic resonance imaging [MRI]) are crucial to differentiate between ischemic and hemorrhagic strokes. Early ICH management will then include blood pressure control, reversal of coagulopathy, decision on whether surgical evacuation of the hematoma is indicated, and assessment/treatment of intracranial hypertension [1, 2]. TCD and TCCD may have specific roles as a noninvasive bedside tool in the diagnosis and management of supratentorial ICH. Structural abnormalities of brain parenchyma such as hematoma volume estimation and epiphenomena such as midline shift (MLS) can be detected by transcranial ultrasound (Fig. 15.1) [3, 4]. Moreover, TCD provides a functional approach to intracranial hemodynamics and may assist in predicting ICH growth and global intracranial pressure increase, as shown in Fig. 15.2 [5, 6]. New ultrasound technologies using ultrasound contrast agents may further allow the visualization of the cerebral microcirculation, expanding the applications of US in the near future [7]. Thus, TCD and TCCD-guided assessment of complications such as non-invasive monitoring of intracranial hypertension, detection of hematoma expansion, estimation of cerebral autoregulation, and sequential evaluation of signs of worsening mass effect can be

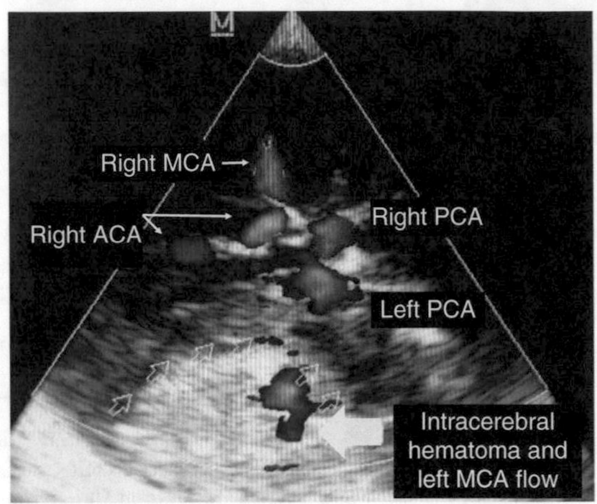

Fig. 15.2 Transcranial ultrasound with color-coded Doppler through right temporal window of a patient with left hemisphere intracerebral hematoma. Empty arrows delineate the intracerebral hematoma. *MCA* middle cerebral artery, *ACA* anterior cerebral artery, *PCA* posterior cerebral artery

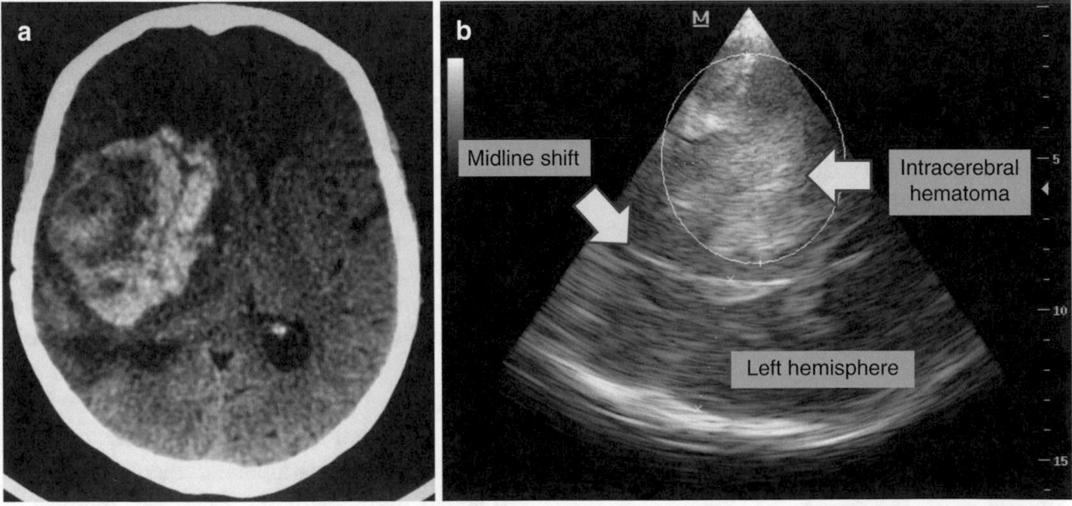

Fig. 15.1 (**a**) Right hemisphere large spontaneous intracerebral hemorrhage on CT scan. (**b**) Ultrasound image from left temporal window showing large intracerebral hematoma and midline shift

integrated in a multimodal approach to the critical care management of patients with ICH.

15.2 Cerebral Hemodynamics

15.2.1 Pulsatility Index, Blood Flow Velocities, and Cerebral Autoregulation

Transcranial Doppler has been applied in neurocritical and stroke patients for decades. The most common applications include the detection of intracranial artery occlusion and stenosis in ischemic stroke and the diagnosis and monitoring of vasospasm after subarachnoid hemorrhage [8, 9]. Although less studied than in the previous scenarios, several articles and reviews have evaluated the use of TCD-derived parameters for ICH patients. These parameters include the pulsatility index (PI); systolic, diastolic, and mean blood flow velocities (BFV); as well as various analyses of cerebral autoregulation, all measured in the middle cerebral arteries (MCA) through insonation of the temporal bone windows.

The PI was introduced in 1974 by Gosling and King and represents a parameter to describe and quantify the relationship between systolic and diastolic flow velocity [10]. Normal values range from 0.7 to 1.2 and elevated PIs may be associated with increased peripheral resistance to blood flow with consequent reductions in diastolic flow velocities. PI has been tested for more than 20 years as a noninvasive marker of reduced cerebral compliance, intracranial hypertension, and hence poor outcome [11]. Various prospective studies suggest that early evaluation of PI may correlate with CT findings (i.e., hematoma volume and midline shift) and intracranial hypertension and can also be associated with worse outcomes [5, 12, 13]. Although the clinical applicability of these findings remains controversial, the data suggest that early and follow-up TCD examinations during the first week may add value to the standard approach of repeated CT scans and clinical examination in the early detection of mental status deterioration and intracranial pressure development, especially in patients in the intermediate severity range without invasive ICP monitoring.

A more recent report evaluated a multimodal approach to ICH prognostication including TCD-derived parameters in combination with electroencephalography (EEG) as predictors of outcome. In this prospective study of 49 patients with ICH from China, quantitative EEG was assessed using different combinations of power, amplitude, and frequency analyses while TCD evaluated BFV and PIs. Results revealed that the relationship between slow and fast EEG frequencies (delta/alpha ratio—DAR) and TCD-derived PI were independent predictors of 6-month mortality and that the combination of both parameters demonstrated excellent discrimination of long-term survival with an area under the ROC curve of 0.95 [14]. As suggested by these findings, the multimodal noninvasive evaluation of patients with ICH may prove useful to determine those at high risk of death or long-term dependency, as early as during their ICU stay. More data is still needed to improve our knowledge of the temporal changes that individual patients present, potentially linked to worse outcomes.

Cerebral autoregulation (CA) is another TCD-derived functional parameter that adds to the information provided by flow velocities (especially Vd) and PIs after ICH [6]. The state of CA has potential implications in blood pressure management in the acute phase of ICH since aggressive BP reduction, aiming at limiting hematoma expansion, may or may not lead to hypoperfusion depending on the brain's capacity to autoregulate.

CA can be estimated in a variety of ways using TCD, both in its static and dynamic components. Static autoregulation is assessed by evaluating a baseline blood flow velocity on TCD and examining its response to induced changes in blood pressure. Dynamic CA (dCA) responds to instantaneous (over seconds) and spontaneous blood pressure fluctuations and associated cerebral perfusion pressure changes, as measured by TCD velocities. Dynamic CA has been estimated in clinical studies of ICH patients either through the correlation coefficient index Mx, which measures the correlation of blood pressure (BP) and MCA mean flow velocities, or by transfer function analysis parameters such as phase and gain. In summary, Mx is calculated as the moving average of 1-min Pearson correlation coefficients of BP and MCA mean BFV. Phase and gain, on the other hand, reflect the speed of the autoregulatory response and damping characteristics of dynamic regulation, respectively.

Most contemporary studies have focused on the evaluation of dCA in patients with ICH, with measures such as the Mx (the correlation coefficient between mean arterial blood pressure and MCA mean flow velocities) and phase/gain parameters. Repeatedly, data have shown that compromised CA is independently associated with larger hematoma volumes, intraventricular hemorrhage, systemic hypotension, and functional outcomes [15–18]. More recently, a systematic review identified 8 studies involving 293 patients with ICH where CA was evaluated. Results of the pooled analysis confirmed that higher Mx and lower phase (markers of impaired CA) are associated with hematoma volume and worse neurological status. In comparison with controls, meta-analysis also found that mean BFV in the MCAs is significantly lower following ICH [19]. Authors conclude that lower BFV and impaired CA may have implications for aggressive blood pressure treatment and should be taken into account in future studies of acute clinical management of patients with ICH.

15.3 Intracerebral Hematoma

Interest and experience in bedside ultrasonography have grown in recent years in general critical care. Although TCD has been integrated into the daily evaluation of some neurocritical care patients, additional ultrasound 2-D imaging of the brain has great potential to provide further important information to the clinician at the bedside, guiding management. One scenario where such clinical applications have been evaluated is the management of patients with ICH, specifically focused on hematoma expansion and signs of mass effect and intracranial hypertension (Figs. 15.1 and 15.2).

More than 20 years ago, authors have shown that TCCD is capable of reliably detecting intracerebral hematomas and differentiating hemorrhagic from ischemic stroke in patients that present with acute neurological signs [20, 21]. In this early report of 151 patients, despite the absence of a viable acoustic window in 12%, TCCD correctly diagnosed the etiology in 95% of acute strokes compared to CT scan results. Moreover, ultrasound was able to identify stroke-related complications such as midline shift and hemorrhagic transformation of ischemic stroke in 85% of patients. Although these results were interesting, the widespread availability of urgent CT scans probably prevented this specific indication of TCCD to be further studied and applied in clinical practice [20].

In a prospective study of 35 patients with spontaneous ICH, authors compared the volumes of hematomas measured by CT scans and TCCD. They found good agreement and excellent correlation of findings for volume estimation and midline shift ($r = 0.79$; $P < 0.001$ and $r = 0.83$; $P < 0.001$, respectively). TCCD-derived hematoma volume estimation was also independently associated with early neurological deterioration and mortality following ICH [22]. Similarly, another small cohort of 34 patients with ICH was studied with TCCD to estimate both the initial hematoma volume and early hematoma expansion. An excellent correlation was also found between TCCD and CT measurements. Hematoma growth was detected by TCCD in 26% of patients and correlation coefficient for all diameters evaluated—longitudinal, sagittal, and coronal—was 0.88 (95% CI 0.8–0.937) [23]. More recently, a similar pilot validation study was reported comparing sonographic estimation of supratentorial ICH volumetry with CT. In 40 patients assessed prospectively, they confirmed a good correlation between the two methodologies ($P = 0.79$) for hematoma volumetry, ICH score calculation, and outcome prognostication [24].

Few studies have evaluated TCCD's ability to detect hemorrhagic transformation of ischemic stroke. In a study that included 55 patients with large ischemic strokes, 20 had hemorrhagic transformation (HT) and TCCD demonstrated high sensitivity and specificity for HT detection (90% and 97.4%, respectively) [25]. More recently, a pilot study assessed the use of ultrasound perfusion imaging (UPI) to improve the ability to detect intracerebral hemorrhage and the capacity to differentiate spontaneous ICH from HT after ischemic stroke. A small group of 12 patients with parenchymal hematomas were analyzed twice during the first week after stroke and TCCD was performed before and after the administration of a sonographic contrast agent. Plain TCCD adequately identified hematomas but the volumes estimated were imprecise. The contrasted image allowed for an improved measurement of volumes and the calculation of a mismatch index, the relationship between the non-contrast echogenicity, and the contrasted perfusion deficit. Moreover, the mismatch index correctly differentiated spontaneous ICH from HT [7, 26].

As evidenced by the studies described above, the experience with TCCD for assessing patients with intracerebral hemorrhage is still limited to specialized centers and research groups. However, available data support the clinical application of TCCD as a reliable method of detecting intracerebral hemorrhage and possibly HT after ischemic stroke. Most of the available studies, although small, also confirm that volume estimation of hematomas is comparable to the one obtained by CT scans. Hence, we suggest that TCCD should be integrated into the multimodal clinical and imaging monitoring approach to patients with stroke. After the initial CT scan confirming an ICH, a baseline TCCD should be performed with analysis of hematoma volume and follow-up TCCD exams should be repeated in regular intervals during the acute phase of ICH. Although to date the time course of early expansion has remained poorly described, dynamic assessments can capture early hematoma expansion (EHE) in patients with intracerebral hematoma. In a small study, authors demonstrated that TCCD had good volume estimation for EHE as compared to the follow-up CT scan with a maximum absolute volume deviation within 7 mL [27]. Therefore, the authors concluded that sequential TCCD reliably detected hematoma expansion occurring in the first 8 h after symptom onset.

Finally, baseline and follow-up TCCD exams will not substitute CT scans but instead dynamic changes in the sonographic assessments should prompt an urgent neuroimaging assessment to evaluate hematoma expansion.

15.4 Midline Shift

Midline shift can be measured by TCCD by comparing the distances between each side of the skull and the center of the third ventricle, normally using a 2–4 MHz probe through the temporal window, as shown in Fig. 15.1. This method was initially described by Seidel et al. in 1995 and consisted of scanning with a depth of 16 cm, following the orbitomeatal line. The landmark for orientation is the butterfly-shaped brainstem. The largest transverse diameter of the third ventricle was acquired by tilting the duplex probe approximately 10° upward. To assess the middle part of the lateral ventricle at its maximum extension the ultrasound beam had to be angled on approximately 25° [28, 29].

A good correlation with CT has been demonstrated in several studies [30]. In a recent study previously cited above, TCCD-derived MLS showed a good correlation with CT-measured MLS ($r = 0.83$, $P < 0.001$) in patients with ICH [22]. A prospective single-center study (mostly comprised of patients with traumatic brain injuries) found that the correlation coefficient between TCCD and CT scan was 0.65 ($P < 0.001$), with an area under the ROC curve for detecting a significant (>5 mm) MLS with TCCD to be 0.86 (95% CI = 0.74–0.94). When applying a 0.35 cm as a cutoff, the disclosed sensitivity was 84.2%, with a specificity of 84.8% and a positive likelihood ratio of 5.56 [31]. A study involving ICH patients from a single center in Taiwan found also a good linear correlation between hematoma volume and MLS by TCCD (0.81; $P < 0.01$), as well as that MLS by TCCD was more sensitive and specific than the pulsatility index in detecting large-volume ICH (accuracy of 0.82 if MLS $\geq$ 2.5 mm) [32]. Moreover, similar correlation of CT imaging and TCCD for assessment of MLS was found in patients with acute ischemic stroke with malignant cerebral edema [33, 34].

TCCD assessment of the MLS might aid in the outcome prediction/prognostication of neurocritically ill patients. A large cohort of 68 ICH patients demonstrated that MLS measured by TCCD during the first 14 days of ictus correlated with other measures of severity (hematoma volume, NIHSS). Additionally, MLS on the range of 4.5 and 7.5 mm was associated with treatment failure and a cutoff of 12 mm discriminated survivors from nonsurvivors with an area under the ROC curve of 0.96, sensitivity of 69%, and specificity of 100% [3].

As well as for hematoma volume estimation and follow-up, we recommend that MLS should be monitored in patients with significant mass effect secondary to acute intracranial pathologies at high risk for neurological deterioration, cerebral edema, and intracranial hypertension. Repeated TCCD examinations can be a valuable noninvasive tool in patients with unchanged clinical exam. Dynamic changes in MLS should prompt an urgent CT scan that will guide decision on further clinical or surgical treatment, as well as more intensive and invasive monitoring.

15.5 Other Parameters and Applications

15.5.1 Hydrocephalus

The measurement of third ventricle dilation on TCCD has a good correlation with CT. For this application, a diencephalic plane or a ventricular plane is applied while the third ventricle is measured from inner border to inner border. Lateral ventricular dilation on TCCD does not seem to correlate well with CT. This is mainly because of the large inclination of the ultrasound beam needed to visualize this structure. However, repeated measurements in specific clinical situation can still be valuable. In a study of 37 patients with hemorrhagic stroke (ICH and SAH), authors evaluated lateral ventricle width before and after clamping of ventricular drains. They found a cutoff of 5.5 mm in TCCD-derived width and an area under the ROC curve of 0.97 to predict the need to reopen the drain [35]. Although more data is needed to guarantee safety, this approach may potentially substitute the need of repeated CT scans when managing extraventricular drains. The direct measurement of ventricular size using ultrasonography is a widespread practice in neonates and infants, as the ultrasound waves can penetrate the open fontanelles and provide high-quality imaging. In adults this practice is far more challenging, and the use of ultrasound for ventricular size measurement in patients with hydrocephalus is restricted to intraoperative use or in patients with postoperative surgical cranial defects. In a case series of 15 adult patients who underwent craniotomies for different indications (including tumors, aneurysms, abscesses, among others), in the immediate postoperative period the ventricles were visualized through cranial defects in 88% of the cases, aiding in the detection of hydrocephalus in four patients [36].

A study with 29 adults with hydrocephalus monitored with TCCD disclosed that pulsatility indexes were elevated preoperatively, with significant improvement after shunting, a finding that was even more pronounced in patients with ICP ≥35 mmHg [37]. Finally, in 23 children with shunted hydrocephalus, optic nerve sheath diameter measured sonographically was used to triage for high ICP secondary to shunt malfunction. Those patients with functioning ventriculoperitoneal shunts had a mean optic nerve sheath diameter of 2.9 (SD 0.5) mm; those with raised intracranial pressure had a mean optic nerve sheath diameter of 5.6 (0.6) mm ($P < 0.0001$) [38].

15.5.2 Subdural Hematomas

Measurement of the width and extension of a subdural hematoma (SDH) has been shown to be possible using ultrasonography. TCCD was used in 47 patients with either acute or chronic SDH previously confirmed by CT scans. A high correlation for the measurement of the SDH extent was found between TCCD and CT ($r = 0.962$). In patients requiring surgical evacuation, TCCD measurement yielded a sensitivity of roughly 91% and a specificity of 93.8% in predicting surgical intervention ($p < 0.001$) [39]. A prospective study involving 32 patients with chronic SDH measured the midline shift with TCCD pre- and postoperatively. Bland-Altman diagrams did not show any systematic bias of the data and linear regression showed a significant correlation between the measurements before and after surgery with CT scanning of the brain and TCCD [40].

15.5.3 Cerebral Venous Drainage Assessment

Some studies have demonstrated that cerebral venous outflow can be assessed by TCD and TCCD techniques. Also, venous hemodynamics may play an important role in the noninvasive evaluation of intracranial hypertension [41]. In a recent single-center study of 87 patients with primary ICH, venous outflow parameters of internal jugular veins, vertebral veins, basal veins of Rosenthal, straight sinus, and bilateral transverse sinuses were calculated to understand the relationship of venous hemodynamics with prognosis. Authors found in multivariate analysis that the time-averaged mean velocity and blood flow volume—based on a calculation that included vessel flow velocities and cross-sectional diameter measurements—of internal jugular veins were independently associated with worse outcomes. In addition, recently another group reported a study of 64 patients with various primary brain injuries requiring invasive ICP monitoring that underwent 445 ultrasound examinations. After extensive ultrasound assessment, the parameters that showed the best correlation with ICP were the optic nerve sheath diameter (ONSD) and the straight sinus systolic flow velocity (FVsv). The accuracy of these parameters was better as compared to the pulsatility index (PI) and the arterial diastolic flow velocity (FVd). In combination, ONSD and FVsv showed the best correlation with invasive ICP (P = 0.80) and an excellent ability to discriminate episodes of intracranial hypertension above 20 mmHg (area under the ROC curve 0.93, 95% CI 0.90–0.97, P = 0.0) [42]. Although data is still limited on venous drainage assessment by TCCD, measurements appear to be feasible and reproducible. More studies are needed to explore the clinical use of temporal changes of venous outflow monitoring as part of the noninvasive assessment of intracranial pressure.

15.6 Conclusions

TCD and TCCD are noninvasive bedside monitoring tools with important applications in neurocritical care (Table 15.1). However, both are still underutilized in patients with ICH. The

Table 15.1 Clinical applications of brain ultrasonography after intracerebral hemorrhage

TCD and TCCD-derived parameters		Comments	Practical applications
Hemodynamic findings	Pulsatility index (PI)	Elevated PI is a surrogate marker of cerebral hemodynamic compromise due to intracranial hypertension after ICH	Noninvasive ICP estimation in patients with ICH and altered consciousness, without ICP monitoring
	Cerebral autoregulation (CA)	Impaired CA is associated with larger hematoma volumes, signs of elevated ICP, and worse outcomes	Patients with impaired autoregulation are more likely to deteriorate and may require stricter blood pressure control CA may also inform prognostication
Ultrasound imaging	Hematoma volume estimation	Good reproducibility in comparison to CT scan early after ICH	Follow-up TCCD examinations may allow for bedside detection of early hematoma expansion
	Midline shift (MLS)	Good reproducibility in evaluating MLS in comparison to CT scan	Allows sequential evaluation of worsening cerebral edema or mass effect of large hematomas
	Hydrocephalus	Comparable to CT scan in the evaluation of the size of third and lateral ventricles	May allow follow-up examinations of ventricular size in patients with shunts or ventricular drains

ICP intracranial pressure, *TCD* transcranial Doppler, *TCCD* transcranial color duplex, *ICH* intracerebral hemorrhage

data available support the accuracy of ultrasound-based estimation of the hematoma volume and midline shift in comparison to the CT scan. Moreover, impaired autoregulation, low diastolic BFV, and PIs have been consistently associated with neurological deterioration and worse outcomes. Therefore, we believe that brain ultrasound should be incorporated into a multimodal neuromonitoring approach after spontaneous ICH. Sequential TCD/TCCD examinations may detect hematoma volume expansion, increasing PIs and worsening midline shift earlier than clinical changes or programmed follow-up CT scans. The structural and hemodynamic information obtained can lead to more invasive monitoring and earlier surgical interventions. More data is needed evaluating management changes after the implementation of such strategy and potential impact on outcomes. However, this should not discourage neurointensivists to expand their practice with brain ultrasound after ICH.

15.7 Future Directions

Brain ultrasonography is an evolving field. Technological advances and improvements in training will probably have a huge impact on clinical research and practical applications of TCD/TCCD in the near future. As an example, the use of contrast-enhanced US perfusion imaging will probably allow sophisticated hemodynamic and perfusion assessments in situations as different as mismatch in ischemic stroke and optimal blood pressure in traumatic brain injury. In the future, the combination of noninvasive tools such as pupillometry, noninvasive intracranial pressure waveform, quantitative EEG, and brain ultrasound may offer the ICU physician the information necessary to optimize brain function in all patients with acute brain injury, instead of depending on invasive monitoring only in the more severe comatose ones.

References

1. Gross BA, Jankowitz BT, Friedlander RM. Cerebral intraparenchymal hemorrhage: a review. JAMA. 2019;321(13):1295–303.
2. Claude Hemphill J 3rd, Lam A. Emergency neurological life support: intracerebral hemorrhage. Neurocrit Care. 2017;27(Suppl 1):89–101.
3. Kiphuth IC, Huttner HB, Breuer L, Schwab S, Kohrmann M. Sonographic monitoring of midline shift predicts outcome after intracerebral hemorrhage. Cerebrovasc Dis. 2012;34(4):297–304.
4. Meyer-Wiethe K, Sallustio F, Kern R. Diagnosis of intracerebral hemorrhage with transcranial ultrasound. Cerebrovasc Dis. 2009;27(Suppl 2):40–7.
5. Marti-Fabregas J, Belvis R, Guardia E, Cocho D, Munoz J, Marruecos L, et al. Prognostic value of pulsatility index in acute intracerebral hemorrhage. Neurology. 2003;61(8):1051–6.
6. Qureshi AI, Ottenlips JR, Colohan AR, Frankel MR. Loss of autoregulation in patients with intracerebral hemorrhage. J Stroke Cerebrovasc Dis. 1995;5(3):163–5.
7. Kern R, Kablau M, Sallustio F, Fatar M, Stroick M, Hennerici MG, et al. Improved detection of intracerebral hemorrhage with transcranial ultrasound perfusion imaging. Cerebrovasc Dis. 2008;26(3):277–83.
8. Sloan MA, Alexandrov AV, Tegeler CH, Spencer MP, Caplan LR, Feldmann E, et al. Assessment: transcranial Doppler ultrasonography: report of the Therapeutics and Technology Assessment Subcommittee of the American Academy of Neurology. Neurology. 2004;62(9):1468–81.
9. Seiler RW, Reulen HJ, Huber P, Grolimund P, Ebeling U, Steiger HJ. Outcome of aneurysmal subarachnoid hemorrhage in a hospital population: a prospective study including early operation, intravenous nimodipine, and transcranial Doppler ultrasound. Neurosurgery. 1988;23(5):598–604.
10. Gosling RG, King DH. Arterial assessment by Doppler-shift ultrasound. Proc R Soc Med. 1974;67(6 Pt 1):447–9.
11. Mayer SA, Thomas CE, Diamond BE. Asymmetry of intracranial hemodynamics as an indicator of mass effect in acute intracerebral hemorrhage. A transcranial Doppler study. Stroke. 1996;27(10):1788–92.
12. Wang W, Yang Z, Liu L, Dornbos D 3rd, Wang C, Song X, et al. Relationship between transcranial Doppler variables in acute stage and outcome of intracerebral hemorrhage. Neurol Res. 2011;33(5):487–93.
13. Kiphuth IC, Huttner HB, Dorfler A, Schwab S, Kohrmann M. Doppler pulsatility index in spontaneous intracerebral hemorrhage. Eur Neurol. 2013;70(3–4):133–8.
14. Chen Y, Xu W, Wang L, Yin X, Cao J, Deng F, et al. Transcranial Doppler combined with quantitative

EEG brain function monitoring and outcome prediction in patients with severe acute intracerebral hemorrhage. Crit Care. 2018;22(1):36.
15. Reinhard M, Neunhoeffer F, Gerds TA, Niesen WD, Buttler KJ, Timmer J, et al. Secondary decline of cerebral autoregulation is associated with worse outcome after intracerebral hemorrhage. Intensive Care Med. 2010;36(2):264–71.
16. Nakagawa K, Serrador JM, LaRose SL, Sorond FA. Dynamic cerebral autoregulation after intracerebral hemorrhage: a case-control study. BMC Neurol. 2011;11:108.
17. Oeinck M, Neunhoeffer F, Buttler KJ, Meckel S, Schmidt B, Czosnyka M, et al. Dynamic cerebral autoregulation in acute intracerebral hemorrhage. Stroke. 2013;44(10):2722–8.
18. Ma H, Guo ZN, Liu J, Xing Y, Zhao R, Yang Y. Temporal course of dynamic cerebral autoregulation in patients with intracerebral hemorrhage. Stroke. 2016;47(3):674–81.
19. Minhas JS, Panerai RB, Ghaly G, Divall P, Robinson TG. Cerebral autoregulation in hemorrhagic stroke: a systematic review and meta-analysis of transcranial Doppler ultrasonography studies. J Clin Ultrasound. 2019;47(1):14–21.
20. Maurer M, Shambal S, Berg D, Woydt M, Hofmann E, Georgiadis D, et al. Differentiation between intracerebral hemorrhage and ischemic stroke by transcranial color-coded duplex-sonography. Stroke. 1998;29(12):2563–7.
21. Seidel G, Kaps M, Dorndorf W. Transcranial color-coded duplex sonography of intracerebral hematomas in adults. Stroke. 1993;24(10):1519–27.
22. Camps-Renom P, Mendez J, Granell E, Casoni F, Prats-Sanchez L, Martinez-Domeno A, et al. Transcranial duplex sonography predicts outcome following an intracerebral hemorrhage. AJNR Am J Neuroradiol. 2017;38(8):1543–9.
23. Perez ES, Delgado-Mederos R, Rubiera M, Delgado P, Ribo M, Maisterra O, et al. Transcranial duplex sonography for monitoring hyperacute intracerebral hemorrhage. Stroke. 2009;40(3):987–90.
24. Niesen WD, Schlaeger A, Bardutzky J, Fuhrer H. Correct outcome prognostication via sonographic volumetry in supratentorial intracerebral hemorrhage. Front Neurol. 2019;10:492.
25. Seidel G, Cangur H, Albers T, Burgemeister A, Meyer-Wiethe K. Sonographic evaluation of hemorrhagic transformation and arterial recanalization in acute hemispheric ischemic stroke. Stroke. 2009;40(1):119–23.
26. Niesen WD, Schlager A, Reinhard M, Fuhrer H. Transcranial sonography to differentiate primary intracerebral hemorrhage from cerebral infarction with hemorrhagic transformation. J Neuroimaging. 2018;28(4):370–3.
27. Ovesen C, Christensen AF, Krieger DW, Rosenbaum S, Havsteen I, Christensen H. Time course of early postadmission hematoma expansion in spontaneous intracerebral hemorrhage. Stroke. 2014;45(4):994–9.
28. Kaps M, Seidel G, Dorndorf W. Current status of transcranial color duplex ultrasound in the adult. Ultraschall Med. 1995;16(2):50–9.
29. Seidel G, Kaps M, Gerriets T, Hutzelmann A. Evaluation of the ventricular system in adults by transcranial duplex sonography. J Neuroimaging. 1995;5(2):105–8.
30. Gerriets T, Stolz E, Konig S, Babacan S, Fiss I, Jauss M, et al. Sonographic monitoring of midline shift in space-occupying stroke: an early outcome predictor. Stroke. 2001;32(2):442–7.
31. Motuel J, Biette I, Srairi M, Mrozek S, Kurrek MM, Chaynes P, et al. Assessment of brain midline shift using sonography in neurosurgical ICU patients. Crit Care. 2014;18(6):676.
32. Tang SC, Huang SJ, Jeng JS, Yip PK. Third ventricle midline shift due to spontaneous supratentorial intracerebral hemorrhage evaluated by transcranial color-coded sonography. J Ultrasound Med. 2006;25(2):203–9.
33. Horstmann S, Koziol JA, Martinez-Torres F, Nagel S, Gardner H, Wagner S. Sonographic monitoring of mass effect in stroke patients treated with hypothermia. Correlation with intracranial pressure and matrix metalloproteinase 2 and 9 expression. J Neurol Sci. 2009;276(1–2):75–8.
34. Bertram M, Khoja W, Ringleb P, Schwab S. Transcranial colour-coded sonography for the bedside evaluation of mass effect after stroke. Eur J Neurol. 2000;7(6):639–46.
35. Kiphuth IC, Huttner HB, Struffert T, Schwab S, Kohrmann M. Sonographic monitoring of ventricle enlargement in posthemorrhagic hydrocephalus. Neurology. 2011;76(10):858–62.
36. Gooding GA, Edwards MS. Hydrocephalus in adults. Ultrasound detection through surgically created cranial defects. Radiology. 1983;148(2):561–2.
37. Rainov NG, Weise JB, Burkert W. Transcranial Doppler sonography in adult hydrocephalic patients. Neurosurg Rev. 2000;23(1):34–8.
38. Newman WD, Hollman AS, Dutton GN, Carachi R. Measurement of optic nerve sheath diameter by ultrasound: a means of detecting acute raised intracranial pressure in hydrocephalus. Br J Ophthalmol. 2002;86(10):1109–13.
39. Niesen WD, Rosenkranz M, Weiller C. Bedside transcranial sonographic monitoring for expansion and progression of subdural hematoma compared to computed tomography. Front Neurol. 2018; 9:374.
40. Cattalani A, Grasso VM, Vitali M, Gallesio I, Magrassi L, Barbanera A. Transcranial color-coded duplex

sonography for evaluation of midline-shift after chronic-subdural hematoma evacuation (TEMASE): a prospective study. Clin Neurol Neurosurg. 2017;162:101–7.

41. Schoser BG, Riemenschneider N, Hansen HC. The impact of raised intracranial pressure on cerebral venous hemodynamics: a prospective venous transcranial Doppler ultrasonography study. J Neurosurg. 1999;91(5):744–9.

42. Robba C, Cardim D, Tajsic T, Pietersen J, Bulman M, Donnelly J, et al. Ultrasound non-invasive measurement of intracranial pressure in neurointensive care: a prospective observational study. PLoS Med. 2017;14(7):e1002356.

16 Vasospasm After Subarachnoid Hemorrhage

Mypinder Sekhon, Oliver Ayling, and Peter Gooderham

Contents

16.1 Introduction

While the incidence of ischemic stroke has declined in recent decades the incidence of aneurysmal subarachnoid hemorrhage (aSAH) has remained stable at 9 per 100,000 in the USA [1]. Furthermore, SAH accounts for ~5% of all strokes but is associated with very high morbidity and mortality [1–3]. The high rate of morbidity can be attributed to two overarching factors: early brain injury and what has been classically referred to as vasospasm [4]. Early brain injury is caused by the initial aneurysm rupture under high arterial pressure in the fixed-volume cranial vault, leading to damage of the brain parenchyma and raised intracranial pressure [2, 5]. Together this leads to neuronal ischemia and generation of a possible cascade of inflammation, microvasculature thrombi, cortical spreading depression, and neuronal apoptosis [6, 7]. Cerebral vasospasm is due to an abnormal narrowing of the cerebral arteries, after aneurysm rupture, that is associated

M. Sekhon (✉)
Division of Critical Medicine, Department of Medicine, Faculty of Medicine, University of British Columbia, Vancouver, BC, Canada

O. Ayling · P. Gooderham
Division of Neurosurgery, Department of Surgery, Faculty of Medicine, University of British Columbia, Vancouver, BC, Canada
e-mail: oliver.ayling@alumni.ubc.ca; peter.gooderham@vch.ca

C. Robba, G. Citerio (eds.), *Echography and Doppler of the Brain*, https://doi.org/10.1007/978-3-030-48202-2_16

with poor outcome [8]. Additional medical factors that lead to poor outcomes after aSAH include cardiac disturbances, lung injury, systemic inflammation, electrolyte abnormalities, and infection [9]. Broadly, the approach for treating patients after aSAH involves early aneurysm securing, with either microsurgical clipping or endovascular coiling, and the critical care management of these patients, much of which is dedicated to preventing, detecting, and treating cerebral vasospasm. The primary focus of this chapter is to discuss the diagnosis and management of cerebral vasospasm.

16.2 Pathophysiology of Cerebral Vasospasm and Delayed Cerebral Ischemia

Traditionally, cerebral vasospasm has been suggested to emanate from isolated vasoconstriction of the major intracranial cerebral vasculature but the underlying mechanisms which are responsible for this pathophysiologic phenomenon have remained elusive. Typically, the onset of cerebral vasospasm, accompanied by a reduction in the caliber of major cerebral vessels, occurs approximately 72 h after the initial sentinel subarachnoid hemorrhage [9–11]. The risk of cerebral vasospasms peaks at approximately 8–10 days after the initial hemorrhage and usually dissipates by 3–4 weeks after presentation [12]. This timeline suggests that pathophysiologic changes are occurring in the cerebral vasculature that require days to culminate in a reduction in the caliber of the major cerebral vessels. This increased cerebrovascular resistance is followed by a reduction in overall cerebral blood [13]. If the degree of cerebral oligemia and reduced cerebral oxygen delivery exceeds the metabolic demands of the cerebral parenchyma, then cerebral ischemia and anerobic metabolism ensue [14, 15]. These biochemical sequelae eventually result in malfunctioning of the associated neuronal tissue and clinical neurologic deficits arise which characterize the phenomenon of delayed cerebral ischemia [13, 16, 17]. If left untreated, this pathophysiology will lead to irreversible neuron cell loss and infarction of cerebral tissue [1, 18].

The precise mechanisms of the cerebral vasoconstriction which is seen in subarachnoid hemorrhage patients likely are the result of numerous pathophysiological sequelae. Specifically, underlying mechanisms involving calcium channel receptor signalling in the smooth muscle of the major cerebral vasculature likely play a role in the pathophysiology [1, 19]. This theory is supported by well-established literature demonstrating that the administration of nimodipine and use of intra-arterial calcium channel receptor antagonists have a clinical role in the management of cerebral vasospasm [20]. However, the clinical finding of cases of cerebral vasospasm which appear to be refractory to the administration of calcium channel receptor antagonists or the absence of a near-complete prevention of cerebral vasospasm with prophylactic nimodipine suggests that other mechanisms also play a role [1, 21].

Other mechanisms that appear to be involved in the onset of cerebral vasospasm include reduced nitric oxide signalling in the cerebral vasculature after subarachnoid hemorrhage. Nitric oxide signalling, emanating from an intricate interplay between the surrounding neurons and smooth muscle of the cerebral vasculature, is responsible for a significant portion of the control of cerebral blood flow in the cerebral parenchyma [21]. Depletion of circulating nitric oxide and its derivatives from hemosiderin deposits following subarachnoid hemorrhage has been proposed as a mechanism underpinning cerebral vasospasm [1]. Thus far, the literature does not strongly support the administration of nitric oxide analogues in the treatment of vasospasm or as prophylactic agents.

Finally, a key function of the cerebral vasculature is the maintaining of an auto-anticoagulant function within the vascular lumen to promote continual flow of cerebral blood flow in the major vessels but also in the microvasculature [1]. Tissue studies of patients with subarachnoid hemorrhage have revealed the finding of microvascular thrombosis in the cerebral microvasculature [1, 22]. This finding suggests that cerebral endothelial dysfunction may occur after subarachnoid hemorrhage and then downstream microvascular thrombosis results. The reduction of the intravascular lumen with microvascular thromboses limits cerebral blood flow and may cause reduced oxygen delivery with eventual delayed cerebral ischemia.

16.3 Diagnosis of Cerebral Vasospasm and Delayed Cerebral Ischemia

Due to recent advances in our understanding of the pathophysiology of cerebral vasospasm, largely demonstrating that pharmacological prevention of large-artery vasospasm did not lead to clinical improvements, there has been a shift to use the term delayed cerebral ischemia (DCI), rather than "vasospasm" [1]. Technically, vasospasm is a radiographic descriptor. DCI is a broad term that may include vasospasm. DCI is a diagnosis of exclusion and is defined as persistent neurological deterioration, that is presumably related to ischemia, when other causes of possible neurological deterioration have been excluded [1, 6]. In the setting of delayed neurological deterioration a plain CT and CT angiogram are completed [1, 5, 23]. DCI and arterial vasospasm are highly correlated but cerebral edema, aneurysmal rebleeding, hydrocephalus, seizure, infection, and electrolyte abnormalities (particularly hyponatremia) must be excluded. In a practical sense DCI and vasospasm are synonymous because when other causes are ruled out arterial vasospasm is attributed to the cause of DCI, although they can occur independently. Radiographic evidence of arterial vasospasm after aSAH occurs in ~70% of patients [2]. However, only half of the patients with radiographic vasospasm will become symptomatic and only half of those symptomatic patients will go on to have cerebral infarction [1, 2]. This may be explained by the fact that reduced cerebral blood flow and perfusion are only associated with severe angiographic vasospasm. Therefore, accurate diagnosis of arterial vasospasm is critical for two reasons: contemporary therapeutic measures after aSAH are targeted at vasospasm and it is necessary to exclude those patients with vasospasm detected radiographically but are asymptomatic and would therefore not benefit from treatment. Radiographic vasospasm is the term used for patients with radiographic evidence of vasospasm and without clinical sequalae attributed to the arterial narrowing [24]. Vasospasm may begin to develop 3 days after aSAH ictus, with the average maximal stenosis on the seventh day, and can persist for up to 14 days. It is rare to occur after 10 days [1].

Vasospasm is diagnosed clinically and radiographically. At the time of hospital admission, the risk of vasospasm can be predicted with the modified Fisher scale which indicates that larger volumes of subarachnoid blood are associated with higher rates of symptomatic vasospasm. Clinical assessment with serial neurological examinations to detect the presence of a new focal neurological deficit is fundamental for diagnosing DCI. A new-onset neurological deficit, which is usually gradual in onset, should be referable to a vascular territory that has evidence of vasospasm detected in concurrent radiographic studies (e.g., a new left pronator drift and radiographic evidence of right middle cerebral artery vasospasm) [1, 11, 21] (Fig. 16.1).

16.4 Transcranial Doppler Principles

Transcranial Doppler (TCD) has long maintained a central role in the detection of cerebral vasospasm as a supportive modality used to confirm the presence of clinical vasospasm [23]. TCD utilizes the principle of the Doppler effect, which encompasses the use of emitting and receiving sound waves from a receiver to detect the velocity of flow of a fluid within a compressible vessel [25]. The emission of sound waves from a source results in the bouncing off of structures within the vessel, principally red blood cells [26]. The return of the sound waves to a receiver is then interpreted as the velocity of flow of blood within a vessel and provides a directional component of the cerebral blood flow [27].

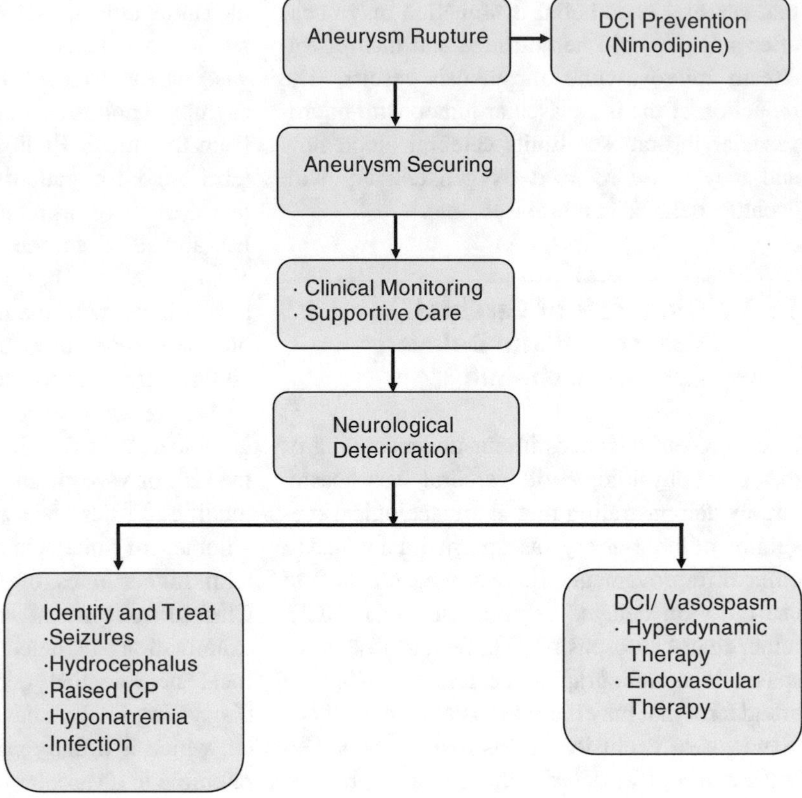

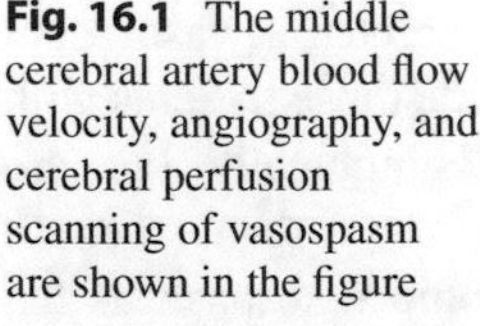
Fig. 16.1 The middle cerebral artery blood flow velocity, angiography, and cerebral perfusion scanning of vasospasm are shown in the figure

Utilizing specific windows of TCD insonation of the cerebral vessels and with knowledge of the cerebrovascular anatomy, an operator can then determine which specific blood vessel has been located and analyze its corresponding velocity of flow within it. The conventional windows that are used as part of clinical practice with TCD include the temporal, occipital, ophthalmic, and submandibular windows [28, 29]. The most often used temporal window is used to insonate the middle, anterior, and posterior cerebral arteries. Adequate insonation of these arteries is feasible in over 80% of patients after subarachnoid hemorrhage [30]. The proximal anterior cerebral and posterior cerebral arteries are also readily accessible from the temporal window [31, 32]. Less commonly, the occipital and ophthalmic windows are used to evaluate the distal posterior cerebral artery and anterior cerebral artery, respectively. The submandibular window provides access to the internal carotid artery, which provides a velocity reference point for the interpretation of the intracranial velocity dynamics of the major cerebral arteries [30].

TCD is noninvasive and can be performed at the bedside, allowing for frequent assessment of blood flow velocity of intracranial vessels. TCD provides an indirect measure of progressive cerebral arterial narrowing base on the velocities of blood flow. In general, blood flow velocities between 120 and 200 cm/s indicate vasospasm, with higher velocities associated with higher degrees of arterial stenosis [28, 32, 33]. Despite the simplicity of TCD it is susceptible to fluctuating measurements with blood pressure variations, is poor at assessing distal intracranial vasculature leading to false positives or negatives, and requires a skilled user to administer the test.

Accelerated velocities of the major cerebral vessels suggest cerebral vasospasm after subarachnoid hemorrhage; however, cerebral hyperemia may also account for this finding [26]. Therefore, analyzing the velocity of the flow in the internal carotid artery with reference to the

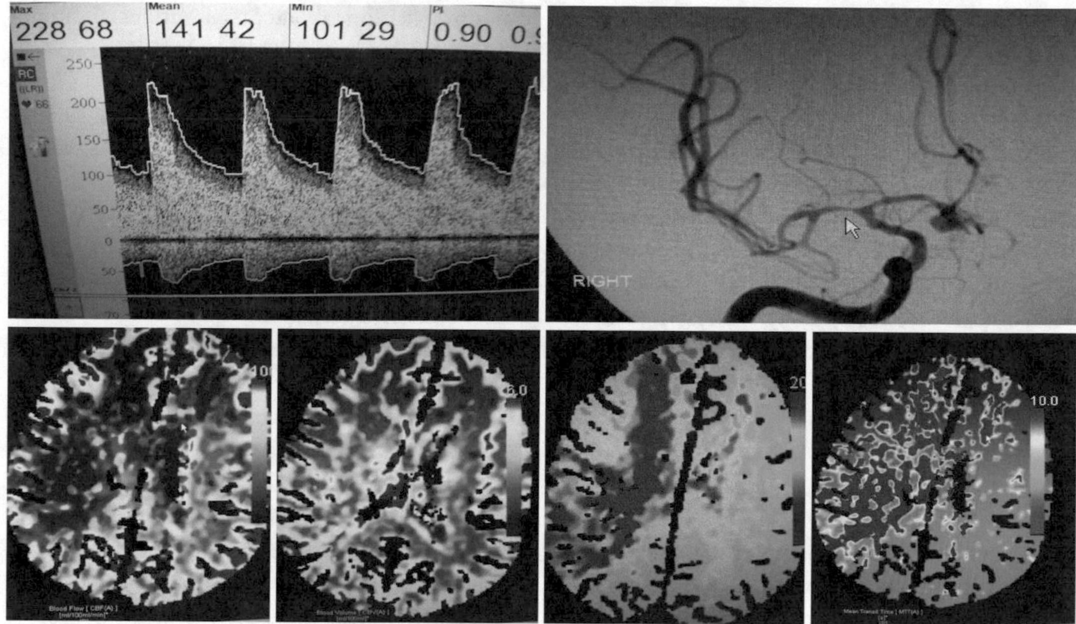

Fig. 16.2 Transcranial Doppler showing increased flow velocities on the middle cerebral artery compatible with vasospasm which can also be detected on angiography. CT perfusion demonstrates prolonged MTT and TTD with reduction of cerebral blood flow and maintenance of volume

simultaneous velocities of the major cerebral vessels can provide invaluable insights into the presence of cerebral vasospasm. Specifically, the Lindegaard ratio can be used to detect and grade the severity of vasospasm within the middle and anterior cerebral arteries. The Lindegaard ratio is calculated by using the middle or anterior cerebral artery velocity as the numerator and the extracranial carotid artery velocity as the denominator [34]. A ratio of 3–4 indicates mild vasospasm, 4–6 indicates moderate vasospasm, and greater than 6 suggests severe vasospasm [35]. The posterior cerebral artery is not used in the Lindegaard ratio due to its anatomical variance (Fig. 16.2).

16.5 Other Diagnostics of Cerebral Vasospasm

In the intensive care unit neurological examinations are often unable to be performed as patients may be sedated and ventilated; therefore imaging modalities to detect vasospasm are paramount. Transcranial Doppler (TCD), CT and digital subtraction angiography, and CT perfusion are useful tools to assess for the presence and impact of DCI [5, 23].

Catheter-based digital subtraction angiography is the gold standard for detection of cerebral vasospasm; however, CT angiography is largely replacing it as there is a strong correlation between the two modalities for detection of vascular narrowing and both exhibit high negative predictive value [20, 36]. Additionally, the lower risk profile and ease of use associated with CT angiography make it the most practical method for assessment of vasospasm in critically ill patients. Routine use of CT angiogram 3–5 days after aSAH is recommended to assess for vasospasm, particularly in the unexaminable patient. On angiography, vasospasm is classified, when compared to baseline imaging, as mild: <25%; moderate: 25–50%; and severe: >50% [2]. CT perfusion scanning is becoming increasingly employed to assess the functional status of cerebral blood flow as it detects cortical regions with reduced flow (indicative of ischemia) and blood volumes that are substantially reduced (completed infarction) [23]. CT perfusion scanning is associated with higher doses of radiation and longer scanning times than CT angiography which may limit its serial use. Recent meta-analysis data has demonstrated that CT perfusion, as compared to catheter angiogram, has high specificity (93%) and sensitivity (74%) for detecting vasospasm [23]. Other modalities have been utilized in this patient population to detect for vasospasm but their use is beyond the scope of this review (near-infrared spectroscopy, thermal diffuse flowmetry, microdialysis, oximetry).

16.6 Prevention of Vasospasm/Delayed Cerebral Ischemia

Fundamental to treating patients with aSAH is to maintain physiological parameters within a normal range in a neurointensive setting. Specifically, patients should be well hydrated with particular attention paid to normal sodium, hemoglobin, glucose, and temperature [4, 8, 11]. Additionally, after aneurysm securing, blood pressure may be maintained in a slightly hypertensive state [13, 14]. In combination, these factors are likely to promote a supportive environment for the injured brain by reducing edema, allowing adequate oxygen delivery, and decreasing a hypermetabolic state. However, there is no high-quality evidence that these measures will prevent DCI or vasospasm should they occur, but they may mitigate its impact.

To date, the highest quality of evidence for prevention of DCI is from a randomized controlled trial that demonstrated that administration of nimodipine significantly reduced the rates of cerebral infarction and poor outcome. Nimodipine is administered prophylactically at the time of admission and continued for 21 days, although cessation of the drug may be necessary if hypotension occurs and adequate cerebral perfusion cannot be maintained in the setting of vasospasm [1, 21, 37]. Interestingly, nimodipine, an L-type calcium channel antagonist, does not decrease angiographic vasospasm but does improve outcomes. However drugs such as clazosentan, an endothelin receptor antagonist, reduce rates of angiographic vasospasm but do not improve clinical outcomes, further highlighting that mechanisms other than large vessel vasospasm underline the mechanism of DCI [17, 21, 22]. Other medications to prevent DCI, such as magnesium and statins, have been studied in large trials but there is no evidence to support their use.

16.7 Management of Symptomatic Vasospasm

DCI attributed to arterial vasospasm is associated with high rates of morbidity and expeditious management is vital. A stepwise approach to the patient with symptomatic vasospasm is applied. The first-line management includes volume expansion with crystalloids and induced hypertension to increased cerebral perfusion and oxygenation [6, 19, 24]. Classically this has been referred to as triple-H therapy (hypervolemia, hypertension, hemodilution) but the term hyperdynamic therapy is preferred as hemodilution is likely associated with decreased cerebral oxygenation [17, 24, 38]. As such, crystalloid fluids are used to maintain euvolemia, with a central venous pressure of 8–10 mmHg and hematocrit greater than 30 [14]. Induced hypertension should lead to a rapid elevation in blood pressure and should be titrated to achieve a resolution in the neurological deficit. It is not uncommon to require a systolic blood pressure over 200 mmHg and as such patients are at risk of myocardial ischemia and pulmonary edema [19]. Induced hypertension should only be done after aneurysm securing and is performed with vasopressors (norepinephrine or phenylephrine) or inotropes (dobutamine or milrinone). Recent data, although limited, has suggested that the use of intravenous milrinone may be a useful medical therapy to treat vasospasm. Known as the “Montreal Protocol,” high doses of milrinone, often in conjunction with vasopressors, are administered to achieve a mean arterial pressure over 90 mmHg [39–48]. A clinical response from hyperdynamic therapy should be seen within several hours. If there is no clinical response or the patient is unable to tolerate sustained hypertension then the next step is endovascular management with intra-arterial calcium channel blockers or angioplasty. A catheter-based angiogram is performed to assess the sites of vasospasm and balloon angioplasty is deployed on stenotic proximal intracranial vessels, often with concomitant intra-arterial vasodilators such as verapamil [20, 36, 49, 50]. While there are no data from randomized trials for the use of endovascular therapies there are data from case series suggesting that it is efficacious as a rescue therapy in patients that do not respond to hyperdynamic therapy.

16.8 Conclusions

After aneurysm securing, following aSAH, the majority of efforts are focused on supportive care for patients in a neurointensive unit to maintain normal physiological parameters and optimize cerebral perfusion, as well as to closely monitor for signs of DCI. Nimodipine is used to prevent DCI while therapies to treat symptomatic vasospasm include hyperdynamic measures and endovascular methods.

References

1. Macdonald RL. Delayed neurological deterioration after subarachnoid haemorrhage. Nat Rev Neurol. 2014;10(1):44–58.
2. Li K, Barras CD, Chandra RV, et al. A review of the management of cerebral vasospasm after aneurysmal subarachnoid hemorrhage. World Neurosurg. 2019;126:513–27.
3. Lerch C, Yonekawa Y, Muroi C, Bjeljac M, Keller E. Specialized neurocritical care, severity grade, and outcome of patients with aneurysmal subarachnoid hemorrhage. Neurocrit Care. 2006;5(2):85–92. [Internet] [cited 2016 Jul 6] http://www.ncbi.nlm.nih.gov/pubmed/17099253
4. Bederson JB, Connolly ES, Batjer HH, et al. Guidelines for the management of aneurysmal subarachnoid hemorrhage: a statement for healthcare professionals from a special writing group of the Stroke Council, American Heart Association. Stroke. 2009;40(3):994–1025. [Internet] [cited 2015 Mar 2] http://www.ncbi.nlm.nih.gov/pubmed/19164800
5. Van Gijn J, Rinkel GJE. Subarachnoid haemorrhage: diagnosis, causes and management. Brain. 2001;124:249–78.
6. Francoeur CL, Mayer SA. Management of delayed cerebral ischemia after subarachnoid hemorrhage. Crit Care. 2016;20(1):277.
7. Kumar G, Shahripour RB, Harrigan MR. Vasospasm on transcranial Doppler is predictive of delayed cerebral ischemia in aneurysmal subarachnoid hemorrhage: a systematic review and meta-analysis. J Neurosurg. 2016;124(5):1257–64.
8. Rabinstein AA. Critical care of aneurysmal subarachnoid hemorrhage: state of the art. Acta Neurochir Suppl. 2015;120:239–42. [Internet] [cited 2015 Mar 20] http://www.ncbi.nlm.nih.gov/pubmed/25366630
9. Green DM, Burns JD, DeFusco CM. ICU management of aneurysmal subarachnoid hemorrhage. J Intensive Care Med. 2013;28(6):341–54.
10. Treggiari MM, Walder B, Suter PM, Romand J-A. Systematic review of the prevention of delayed ischemic neurological deficits with hypertension, hypervolemia, and hemodilution therapy following subarachnoid hemorrhage. J Neurosurg. 2003;98(5):978–84. [Internet] [cited 2015 Mar 20] http://www.ncbi.nlm.nih.gov/pubmed/12744357
11. Wolf S. Routine management of volume status after aneurysmal subarachnoid hemorrhage. Neurocrit Care. 2011;15(2):275–80. [Internet] [cited 2015 Mar 2] http://www.ncbi.nlm.nih.gov/pubmed/21748500
12. Muroi C, Seule M, Mishima K, Keller E. Novel treatments for vasospasm after subarachnoid hemorrhage. Curr Opin Crit Care. 2012;18:119–26.
13. Treggiari MM. Hemodynamic management of subarachnoid hemorrhage. Neurocrit Care. 2011;15(2):329–35. [Internet] [cited 2015 Mar 20] http://www.ncbi.nlm.nih.gov/pubmed/21786046
14. Treggiari MM, Deem S. Which H is the most important in triple-H therapy for cerebral vasospasm? Curr Opin Crit Care. 2009;15(2):83–6. [Internet] [cited 2015 Mar 20] http://www.ncbi.nlm.nih.gov/pubmed/19276798
15. Treggiari MM, Schutz N, Yanez ND, Romand J-A. Role of intracranial pressure values and patterns in predicting outcome in traumatic brain injury: a systematic review. Neurocrit Care. 2007;6(2):104–12. [Internet] [cited 2014 May 11] http://www.ncbi.nlm.nih.gov/pubmed/17522793
16. Durrant JC, Hinson HE. Rescue therapy for refractory vasospasm after subarachnoid hemorrhage. Curr Neurol Neurosci Rep. 2015;15(2):1–8.
17. Lee KH, Lukovits T, Friedman JA. "Triple-H" therapy for cerebral vasospasm following subarachnoid hemorrhage. Neurocrit Care. 2006;4(1):68–76. [Internet] [cited 2015 Mar 20] http://www.ncbi.nlm.nih.gov/pubmed/16498198
18. Nakae R, Yokota H, Yoshida D, Teramoto A. Transcranial doppler ultrasonography for diagnosis of cerebral vasospasm after aneurysmal subarach-

noid hemorrhage: mean blood flow velocity ratio of the ipsilateral and contralateral middle cerebral arteries. Neurosurgery. 2011;69(4):876–83.
19. Al-Mufti F, Amuluru K, Damodara N, et al. Novel management strategies for medically-refractory vasospasm following aneurysmal subarachnoid hemorrhage. J Neurol Sci. 2018;390:44–51.
20. Dabus G, Nogueira RG. Current options for the management of aneurysmal subarachnoid hemorrhage-induced cerebral vasospasm: a comprehensive review of the literature. Interv Neurol. 2013;2(1):30–51. [Internet] [cited 2015 Mar 18] http://www.pubmedcentral.nih.gov/articlerender.fcgi?artid=4031782&tool=pmcentrez&rendertype=abstract
21. Keyrouz SG, Diringer MN. Clinical review: prevention and therapy of vasospasm in subarachnoid hemorrhage. Crit Care. 2007;11(4):220.
22. Rowland MJ, Hadjipavlou G, Kelly M, Westbrook J, Pattinson KTS. Delayed cerebral ischaemia after subarachnoid haemorrhage: looking beyond vasospasm. Br J Anaesth. 2012;109(3):315–29.
23. Westermaier T, Pham M, Stetter C, et al. Value of transcranial Doppler, perfusion-CT and neurological evaluation to forecast secondary ischemia after aneurysmal SAH. Neurocrit Care. 2013; [Internet] [cited 2014 Apr 29];(Dci). http://www.ncbi.nlm.nih.gov/pubmed/23982597
24. Meyer R, Deem S, Yanez ND, Souter M, Lam A, Treggiari MM. Current practices of triple-H prophylaxis and therapy in patients with subarachnoid hemorrhage. Neurocrit Care. 2011;14(1):24–36. [Internet] [cited 2015 Mar 20]; http://www.ncbi.nlm.nih.gov/pubmed/20838932
25. Carrera E, Schmidt JM, Oddo M, et al. Transcranial Doppler for predicting delayed cerebral ischemia after subarachnoid hemorrhage. Neurosurgery. 2009;65(2):316–23. discussion 323-4 [Internet] [cited 2014 May 1] http://www.ncbi.nlm.nih.gov/pubmed/19625911
26. Purkayastha S, Sorond F. Transcranial Doppler ultrasound: technique and application. Semin Neurol. 2012;32(4):411–20.
27. White H, Venkatesh B. Applications of transcranial Doppler in the ICU: a review. Intensive Care Med. 2006;32(7):981–94.
28. Rigamonti A, Ackery A, Baker AJ. Transcranial Doppler monitoring in subarachnoid hemorrhage: a critical tool in critical care. Can J Anesth. 2008;55(2):112–23.
29. Bertuetti R, Gritti P, Pelosi P, Robba C. How to use cerebral ultrasound in the ICU. Minerva Anestesiol. 2020; [Internet] [cited 2020 Jan 16] http://www.ncbi.nlm.nih.gov/pubmed/31922373
30. Robba C, Cardim D, Sekhon M, Budohoski K, Czosnyka M. Transcranial Doppler: a stethoscope for the brain-neurocritical care use. J Neurosci Res. 2018;96(4):720.
31. Sadahiro H, Shirao S, Yoneda H, et al. Decreased flow velocity with transcranial color-coded duplex sonography correlates with delayed cerebral ischemia due to peripheral vasospasm of the middle cerebral artery. J Stroke Cerebrovasc Dis. 2016;25(10):2352–9.
32. Malhotra K, Conners JJ, Lee VH, Prabhakaran S. Relative changes in transcranial Doppler velocities are inferior to absolute thresholds in prediction of symptomatic vasospasm after subarachnoid hemorrhage. J Stroke Cerebrovasc Dis. 2014;23(1):31–6. [Internet] [cited 2014 Apr 29] http://www.ncbi.nlm.nih.gov/pubmed/22959107
33. Gonzalez NR, Boscardin WJ, Glenn T, Vinuela F, Martin NA. Vasospasm probability index: a combination of transcranial doppler velocities, cerebral blood flow, and clinical risk factors to predict cerebral vasospasm after aneurysmal subarachnoid hemorrhage. J Neurosurg. 2007;107(6):1101–12. [Internet] [cited 2014 May 1]; Available from http://www.ncbi.nlm.nih.gov/pubmed/18077946
34. Marshall SA, Nyquist P, Ziai WC. The role of transcranial Doppler ultrasonography in the diagnosis and management of vasospasm after aneurysmal subarachnoid hemorrhage. Neurosurg Clin N Am. 2010;21(2):291–303.
35. Rasulo FA, De Peri E, Lavinio A. Transcranial Doppler ultrasonography in intensive care. Eur J Anaesthesiol. 2008;25(SUPPL. 42):167–73.
36. Eddleman CS, Hurley MC, Naidech AM, Batjer HH, Bendok BR. Endovascular options in the treatment of delayed ischemic neurological deficits due to cerebral vasospasm. Neurosurg Focus. 2009;26(3):E6. [Internet] [cited 2015 Mar 20] http://www.ncbi.nlm.nih.gov/pubmed/19249962
37. Dorsch NW. A review of cerebral vasospasm in aneurysmal subarachnoid haemorrhage part II: management. J Clin Neurosci. 1994;1(2):78–92. [Internet] [cited 2015 Mar 20] http://www.ncbi.nlm.nih.gov/pubmed/18638735
38. Muench E, Horn P, Bauhuf C, et al. Effects of hypervolemia and hypertension on regional cerebral blood flow, intracranial pressure, and brain tissue oxygenation after subarachnoid hemorrhage. Crit Care Med. 2007;35(8):1844–51. [Internet] [cited 2015 Mar 20]; quiz 1852; http://www.ncbi.nlm.nih.gov/pubmed/17581487
39. Lannes M, Teitelbaum J, Corte P, Angle M. Milrinone and homeostasis to treat cerebral vasospasm associated with subarachnoid hemorrhage: the Montreal Neurological Hospital Protocol. Neurocrit Care. 2012;16:354–62.
40. Arakawa Y, Kikuta K, Hojo M, Goto Y, Ishii A, Yamagata S. Milrinone for the treatment of cerebral vasospasm after subarachnoid hemorrhage: report of seven cases. Neurosurgery. 2001;48(4):723–8. [Internet] [cited 2015 Mar 20]; http://www.ncbi.nlm.nih.gov/pubmed/11322432 discussion 728-30
41. Nishiguchi M, Ono S, Iseda K, Manabe H, Hishikawa T, Date I. Effect of vasodilation by milrinone, a phosphodiesterase III inhibitor, on vasospastic arteries after a subarachnoid hemorrhage in vitro and in vivo: effectiveness of cisternal injection of milrinone. Neurosurgery. 2010;66(1):158–64. [Internet]

[cited 2015 Mar 20] http://www.ncbi.nlm.nih.gov/pubmed/20023546; discussion 164

42. Romero CM, Morales D, Reccius A, et al. Milrinone as a rescue therapy for symptomatic refractory cerebral vasospasm in aneurysmal subarachnoid hemorrhage. Neurocrit Care. 2009;11(2):165–71. [cited 2015 Mar 20]; [Internet] Available from http://www.ncbi.nlm.nih.gov/pubmed/18202923
43. Schmidt U, Bittner E, Pivi S, Marota JJA. Hemodynamic management and outcome of patients treated for cerebral vasospasm with intra-arterial nicardipine and/or milrinone. Anesth Analg. 2010;110(3):895–902. [Internet] [cited 2015 Mar 20] http://www.ncbi.nlm.nih.gov/pubmed/20185665
44. Fraticelli AT, Cholley BP, Losser M, Saint MJ. Milrinone for the treatment of cerebral vasospasm after aneurysmal subarachnoid hemorrhage. Stroke. 2008;39:893–8.
45. Khajavi K, Ayzman I, Shearer D, et al. Prevention of chronic cerebral vasospasm in dogs with milrinone. Neurosurgery. 1997;40(2):354–62. [Internet] [cited 2015 Mar 20] ; discussion 362-3 http://www.ncbi.nlm.nih.gov/pubmed/9007870
46. Castro PB, Morales D, Reccius A, et al. Milrinone as a rescue therapy for symptomatic refractory cerebral vasospasm in aneurysmal subarachnoid hemorrhage. Neurocrit Care. 2009;11(2):165–71.
47. Fraticelli AT, Cholley BP, Losser M-R, Saint Maurice J-P, Payen D. Milrinone for the treatment of cerebral vasospasm after aneurysmal subarachnoid hemorrhage. Stroke. 2008;39(3):893–8. [Internet] [cited 2015 Mar 20] http://www.ncbi.nlm.nih.gov/pubmed/18239182
48. Sadamasa N, Yoshida K, Narumi O, Chin M, Yamagata S. Milrinone via lumbar subarachnoid catheter for vasospasm after aneurysmal subarachnoid hemorrhage. Neurocrit Care. 2014;21(3):470–5. [Internet] [cited 2015 Feb 20] http://www.ncbi.nlm.nih.gov/pubmed/24899113
49. Hänggi D, Beseoglu K, Turowski B, Steiger HJ. Feasibility and safety of intrathecal nimodipine on posthaemorrhagic cerebral vasospasm refractory to medical and endovascular therapy. Clin Neurol Neurosurg. 2008;110(8):784–90.
50. Kimball MM, Velat GJ, Hoh BL. Critical care guidelines on the endovascular management of cerebral vasospasm. Neurocrit Care. 2011;15(2):336–41. [Internet] [cited 2015 Mar 20] http://www.ncbi.nlm.nih.gov/pubmed/21761272

Brain US in the Neurological Settings

17

Piergiorgio Lochner and Andrea Naldi

Contents

Electronic Supplementary Material The online version of this chapter (https://doi.org/10.1007/978-3-030-48202-2_17) contains supplementary material, which is available to authorized users.

P. Lochner (✉)
Department of Neurology, Saarland University Medical Center, Homburg, Germany
e-mail: piergiorgio.lochner@uks.eu

A. Naldi
Department of Neuroscience "Rita Levi Montalcini", University of Turin, Turin, Italy

C. Robba, G. Citerio (eds.), *Echography and Doppler of the Brain*,
https://doi.org/10.1007/978-3-030-48202-2_17

17.1 Introduction

Brain ultrasonography (US) is a useful tool for the evaluation of cerebral structures both in the intensive care and neurological setting. The advantages of this approach include the high availability, inexpensiveness, and repeatability. Taken together, the different modalities for brain assessment may be broadly divided into those that allow the vascular flow examination and those used for the parenchyma visualization.

Combining different methods, transcranial color-coded duplex (TCCD) can depict the major cerebral arteries and veins, evaluating flow abnormalities and indirectly estimating intracranial pressure (ICP). In an acute stroke setting, TCCD allows the monitoring of patients who undergo intravenous thrombolysis and/or mechanical thrombectomy [1]. It can detect intracranial large-artery stenosis or occlusion and establish the collateral blood flow, as well as the hemodynamic effects of extra-intracranial occlusions in the case of cerebral ischemia [2]. In cases of symptomatic stenosis of the internal carotid artery, TCCD may identify patients at higher risk of developing hemodynamic infarctions, due to an exhausted cerebrovascular autoregulation [3].

In an outpatient setting, transcranial sonography can integrate the neurological clinical examination, facilitating the diagnosis of Parkinson's disease (PD) or other movement disorders [4]. Brain US may suggest and monitor atrophy in cases of suspected dementia by measuring the width of third ventricle and could be used as a screening tool in the large population of individuals with cognitive decline by detecting atrophy of the medial temporal lobe (MTL) [5].

Clinical applications with their relative main findings are summarized in Table 17.1.

Table 17.1 Clinical application of brain ultrasonography (morphological findings and basic/advanced transcranial color-coded duplex) derived in general ward and neurological intensive settings

Clinical application	Methods of brain ultrasonography	Role	Pathologic diagnostic criteria
Conditions with increased ICP AMS ICH SAH PRES Hydrocephalus CNS infections	ONSD, TCCD, PI, RI	Noninvasive ICP and CPP estimation Compliance and cerebrovascular dynamics	Significant ONSD ↑and correlation with LLS for AMS Significant ONSD ↑, ODE, ↑ PI and RI, ↑ of velocities of main cerebral arteries
IIH	ONSD, TCCD of venous system and jugular vein		Significant ONSD ↑, ODE, venous sinus stenosis Jugular vein anatomy alteration
Brain death	TCD, TCCD, ONSD	Noninvasive diagnosis of brain death	Reverberating flow, systolic spikes, or disappearance of previously registered Doppler flow signals
CSF hypotension	ONSD		Significant ONSD ↓; monitoring dynamic measurement
Acute ONs ON-MS	ONSD, OND	Supporting diagnosis	Significant ↑ ONSD, ODE in acute ONs OND ↓ in MS Atrophy of OND
Monitoring after mechanical thrombectomy Intracranial stenosis	TCCD	Monitoring	TIBI Doppler flow grade: 0, absent; 1, minimal; 2, blunted; 3, dampened; 4, stenotic; 5, normal MCA >220 cm/sec >50% (sensitivity 100%, specificity 100%)

Table 17.1 (continued)

Clinical application	Methods of brain ultrasonography	Role	Pathologic diagnostic criteria
Cerebral autoregulation and testing of metabolic coupling	BHI, apnea test CO2 inhalation test (5% CO2, 95% O2) Acetazolamide test	Metabolic coupling	Normal values = 1.2 + −0.6% %/sec A relative difference > as 15% argues against a relative impairment of CVR Exhausted CO2 reactivity: Flow increases below 10% = impaired CVR Mean increase approximately 10%
Movement disorder diseases	Brain US	Assessment of small deep brain structures	0.25 cm^2 moderately hyperechogenic (PD) Other anomalies: Hyperechogenicity of the thalamus, lenticular nucleus or caudate nucleus compared with the surrounding white matter is classified as abnormal echogenicity of the midbrain raphe Third ventricle enlargement
Dementia	Brain US	Assessment of small deep brain structures and medial temporal lobe evaluation	Third ventricle enlargement (6.0 and 7.5 mm for subjects < and ≥70 years of age, respectively) (M/F) ratio decrease

AMS acute mountain sickness, *BHI* breath holding index, *CNS* – central nervous system, *CCP* cerebral perfusion pressure, *CVR* cerebrovascular reactivity, *ICH* intracerebral hemorrhage, *LLS* Lake Louise score, *MCA* middle cerebral artery, *MTL* ratio of the height of the medial temporal lobe (MTL)/height of the choroidal fissure (M/F), *ODE* optic disc elevation, *OND* optic nerve diameter, *ONSD* optic nerve sheath diameter, *ONs* optic neuritis, *ON-MS* optic nerve/multiple sclerosis, *PD* Parkinson's disease, *PI* pulsatility index, *RI* resistivity index, *SAH* subarachnoid hemorrhage, *TIBI* thrombolysis in brain ischemia

$$\mathrm{BHI} = \frac{v_{\mathrm{apnea}} - v_{\mathrm{baseline}}}{v_{\mathrm{baseline}} \times t_{\mathrm{apnea}}} \times 100$$

Breath holding index (BHI), flow velocity (v), time (t in sec)

17.2 Pseudotumor Cerebri Syndrome

Idiopathic intracranial hypertension (IIH, also known as primary pseudotumor cerebri syndrome, PTCS) refers to disorders for which the mechanism of elevated ICP remains unknown. It is defined by an increase of ICP without neuroradiological abnormalities [6–8]. Increased ICP typically develops over a period of weeks or months. Typical signs and symptoms of IIH include headache, pulsatile tinnitus, transient visual obscurations, blurred vision, diplopia, and papilledema. Ultrasonography may be useful in several points of IIH. Firstly, it allows a real-time evaluation of the venous drainage that is postulated to be altered at the level of the internal jugular veins and/or cerebral venous sinuses. Nedelmann et al. found an internal jugular vein valvular insufficiency and an irregular leaflet structure on B-mode imaging in 70% of patients with PTCS, significantly higher than controls (30%, $p < 0.05$) [9]. However, these results were not confirmed by Lochner and colleagues who did not find differences in frequency of valvular competence among pathological and healthy subjects, so that no definitive conclusions can be made [10].

Transverse sinus stenosis has been reported in over than 90% of patients with IIH, but it is not clear if it represents the primary cause of raised ICP or, conversely, its consequence [11]. Independently of the mechanism, hemodynamic alterations of transverse sinus flow (turbulences and reverberation) have been detected by Naldi et al. who used venous TCCD for supporting the diagnosis of IIH in bilateral transverse sinus stenosis and for monitoring the efficacy of treatments by repeated measurements [12].

In addition to the vascular evaluation, the increased ICP in PTCS may be investigated by transorbital sonography (TOS) that may detect bulging of the optic nerve disc in the vitreal space and thickening of ONSD. Some studies addressed the role of TOS in supporting the diagnosis of primary IIH [10, 13, 14] and in a recent meta-analysis Lochner and colleagues demonstrated significantly higher values of ONSD in patients compared to controls (6.2–6.76 mm vs. 4.3–5.7 mm) [15]. This technique not only has proved to be useful in the diagnostic stage, but also appears to be particularly valuable in monitoring the effect of therapies. A bilateral decrease in ONSD has been demonstrated immediately after lumbar puncture (right 5.8 ± 0.7 mm, $p < 0.004$; left 5.9 ± 0.7 mm, $p < 0.043$) [13, 16]. Furthermore, a correlation between ONSD reduction and headache improvement has been observed by Lochner et al. after 6 months of treatment ($r = -0.477$, $p = 0.02$) [17].

17.3 Low-Pressure Syndromes, Cerebrospinal Fluid (CSF) Leaks, and Therapeutical Approaches: Intracranial Hypotension, Patch Test

Spontaneous or post-traumatic leak syndromes are recognized as important causes of headache. They are characterized by orthostatic headache, mostly occipital, varying in intensity and associated with neck pain or stiffness, nausea, or vomiting [18]. However, only a minority of spontaneous intracranial hypotension (SIH) cases present with classical symptoms, so it may be difficult to correctly diagnose this condition. The diagnosis of low-CSF syndromes is made combining clinical symptoms and diagnostic procedures such as cerebral and spinal magnetic resonance imaging (MRI) or CT myelography. It has been reported that TOS can be useful to support the diagnosis of low-CSF syndromes, showing a decrease in ONSD compared to normal ONSD. Moreover, some authors demonstrated a thickening of ONSD after the placement of epidural patching and in nine out of ten patients an increase of ONSD with successful lumbar epidural blood patching was shown [19]. In a case-control study, Fichtner et al. evaluated the ONSD modification measured in supine and upright positions in three groups of patients (symptomatic and asymptomatic SIH patients versus controls), observing a significant decrease in ONSD in the orthostatic compared to the supine position only in symptomatic patients [20].

17.4 Posterior Reversible Encephalopathy Syndrome (PRES)

Posterior reversible encephalopathy syndrome (PRES) is a clinical and radiological syndrome consisting of headache, visual changes, seizures, and imaging findings, including cerebral edema affecting the cerebral cortex and underlying white matter [21]. Typical MR findings include areas of hyperintensity in T2 and FLAIR imaging, most often involving the occipital and posterior parietal lobes [22]. It is argued that an impairment of cerebral autoregulation—resulting in arterial hypertension above the limit of cerebral autoregulation, breakdown of the blood-brain barrier (BBB), and subsequent brain edema—is the main underlying mechanism. In this context, brain US may be useful in demonstrating papilledema and can show an increase in ONSD, related to the severity of cerebral vasogenic edema (Fig. 17.1). These structural changes could therefore occur as a result of increased ICP or secondary to an inflammatory cause due to alteration of optic nerve pathways. So far there are only a few case series reporting ONSD abnormalities and papilledema in PRES [23, 24]. Monitoring of PRES using TOS can reveal a normalization of ONSD values following blood pressure control and resolution of symptoms [25].

17.5 Acute Mountain Sickness (AMS)

An increase in ICP is postulated in the pathophysiology of AMS. Ross et al. proposed the “tight-fit” hypothesis to explain the random nature of AMS. This theory postulates that some

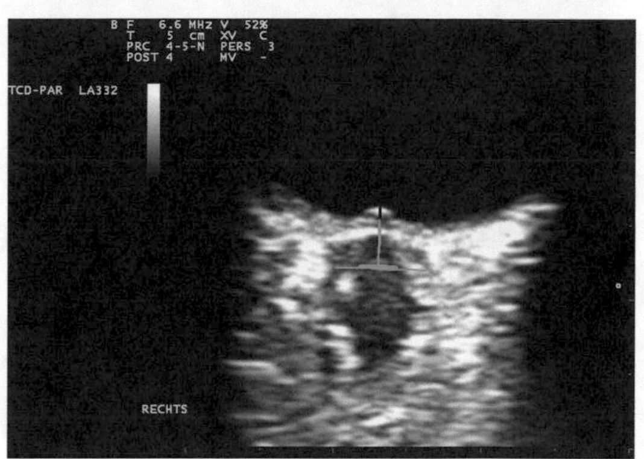

Fig. 17.1 Transorbital sonography in posterior reversible encephalopathy syndrome (PRES). Optic nerve sheath diameter (ONSD) and optic nerve diameter (OND) were measured 3 mm behind the papilla (vertical blue line) in an axial plane showing the optic nerve in its longitudinal course. The horizontal blue line indicates the OND (inner borders) and ONSD (external borders). The dark line denotes the optic disc elevation (ODE). The measurement was gauged between the fundus and the dome of the papilla

subjects have a low compliance to compensate for an increase in brain volume, and neuroimaging techniques support the hypothesis that hypoxia may increase cerebral arterial blood flow and venous volume, leading to increased ICP [26, 27]. The development of portable ultrasound equipment has made the evaluation of the cerebral compartment possible even at high altitude, including assessment of venous drainage, noninvasive estimation of ICP (through ONSD assessment), and semiquantitative measurement of cerebral blood flow.

It has been observed that ONSD rapidly enlarges after exposure to progressively increasing altitude [28–31]. In 69 out of 284 subjects who traveled at high altitude (4240 m) through Pheriche, Nepal, and with clinical symptoms of AMS, Fagenholz et al. observed a significant increase in ONSD to 5.34 mm [95% CI 5.18–5.51 mm] vs. 4.46 mm (95% CI 4.39–4.54 mm) in the 218 other subjects without evidence of altitude illness ($p < 0.0001$) [32].

Given that measurement of middle cerebral artery blood flow velocity (MCAv) using transcranial Doppler/duplex ultrasound (TCD/TCCD) is relatively easy to perform, some studies demonstrated reductions in dynamic cerebral autoregulation in hypoxia [33, 34]. In particular, Horiuchi et al. showed a dynamic decrease of cerebral autoregulation at a progressive reduction of fractional inspired O2 [35]. Feddersen showed that early physiological and pathophysiological changes occur at high altitudes, reflecting mechanisms of adaptation such as brain activity measured by cerebral blood flow velocity (CBFV) with transcranial Doppler sonography (TCD) [36]. The venous system also appears to be modified at high altitudes. Wilson demonstrated in five out of seven subjects a marked venous distension after 3 h of hypoxia (FiO2 = 12%), more prominent than the arterial dilation [37].

17.6 Optic Neuritis and Non-arteritic Ischemic Optic Neuropathy

Transorbital sonography (TOS) represents a promising imaging tool for supporting the diagnosis and monitoring the follow-up of acute optic neuritis. Some case-control studies have shown a significant thickening of the optic nerve (ON). This swelling can be caused by an abnormal increase in permeability of the blood-brain barrier (BBB) and subsequently by inflammation due to increased perineural subarachnoid fluid [38]. TOS is particularly sensitive for detecting the thickening of ON and its sheaths at an early stage of inflammation. In a longitudinal study, the authors found an increase of markers of inflammation and neurodegeneration, correlating with abnormalities of ONSD and OND, persisting in patients with constant visual deficits [39]. Moreover, some studies demonstrated papillitis with a swollen disc in 6–43% of patients, depending on when the diagnostic study was performed [40–46]. Furthermore, other studies revealed ON atrophy in patients affected by a more severe and chronic form of MS, suggesting that the sequential measurement of ON can reveal atrophy [47, 48]. In contrast to acute optic neuritis, in non-arteritic ischemic optic neuropathy (nAION), two authors did not report any change in ONSD [40, 42].

17.7 Hydrocephalus

Hydrocephalus is a common condition characterized by an imbalance between production and absorption of CSF related to primary or secondary cerebral pathologies, determining CSF accumulation within the ventricular system [49]. Ventricles can be assessed with ultrasound through the temporal window, appearing as anechoic structures (corresponding to CSF) surrounded by the hyperechogenic borders of the cerebral ventricles. While almost the entire ventricular system can be evaluated in the fetus and newborn because of the absence of cranial bones, in adults the temporal acoustic window may only allow the partial assessment of the third and lateral ventricles.

In adults, echographic measurements of the width of the third ventricle and the frontal horns of both lateral ventricles show a good correlation to those obtained by cerebral CT scan ($r = 0.83$–0.96 and $r = 0.86$–0.92, respectively) and a good rate of interobserver ($r = 0.9$ for third ventricle and $r = 0.87$ for lateral ventricle) and intraobserver reproducibility correlation coefficient ($r = 0.93$ for lateral ventricle) [50, 51]. In clinical contexts, a direct visualization of the lateral ventricles may be useful to establish indications to surgical revision, especially after external ventricular drainage, as demonstrated in posthemorrhagic hydrocephalus where a cutoff value of 5.5 mm increase of the lateral ventricle width was associated to the necessity to reposition the drainage (sensitivity 100% and specificity 83%) [52]. In a recent report, TCCD allowed to detect a hydrocephalus secondary to traumatic brain injury with endoventricular vegetation and to monitor its reduction after insertion of an external ventricular drainage and administration of intrathecal antibiotic therapy [53]. Ertl and colleagues evaluated the predictive role of ONSD measurements in patients with idiopathic normal pressure hydrocephalus in response to CSF removal (Fisher test). They found that the variability of ONSD values between supine and upright position (ONSD-V) had a good correlation with the clinical response to Fisher test (AUC = 0.93, sensibility 83%, and specificity 100% with a ONSD-V cutoff value of −0.23 mm), providing information to support the selection of patients eligible for shunt placement [54].

In addition to ventricular evaluation, TCCD has been used to study changes in vascular Doppler parameters (resistive and pulsatility index, RI-PI) in intracranial arteries in the setting of hypertensive hydrocephalus. In this setting, increased RI and PI have been documented, reflecting elevated ICP; furthermore, the rapid ICP reduction secondary to ventriculoperitoneal shunting determined marked changes of TCD parameters [55].

In conclusion, ultrasonography of the ventricular system appears to be a reliable tool for monitoring patients after surgery and for selecting those who require shunting, potentially representing a noninvasive alternative to repeated CT scans. In addition, TCCD may allow a direct visualization of ventricular drain and may help to establish displacement or obstructions, leading to surgical repositioning.

17.8 Infections of Central Nervous System

Transcranial sonography in the setting of CNS infections has found a wider application in infants and newborns because of the favorable acoustic window. In these patients, the role of brain sonography ranges from the preliminary assessment of suspected bacterial meningitis to the monitoring of therapies and disease complications.

In the newborn with bacterial meningitis, the main sonographic findings include ventriculitis, ventriculomegaly/hydrocephalus, echogenic and widened sulci, subdural effusions, empyema, and parenchymal changes (cerebritis, brain abscess) [56]. A further description of these findings is outside the scope of this chapter and comprehensive explanations are available elsewhere [57].

In adults, the attention has been mainly focused on vascular changes that may occur during cerebral infections. In acute bacterial meningitis, the mean cerebral blood flow in the arteries of the Willis circle showed a significant increase compared to healthy controls, reflecting arteriopathy, vasospasm, and possible stenosis; however, these findings were not predictive of outcome. In addition, raised arterial flow velocities detected by TCCS did not necessarily reflect the arterial stenosis documented by MR angiography, probably because several factors influence cerebral blood flow, including inflammatory hyperemia, elevated intracranial pressure, body temperature, use of mechanical ventilation, sedation of patients, systemic conditions, and arterial CO_2 [58]. Among bacterial infections, Haring and colleagues documented a transient increased flow in the middle cerebral artery (up to 100% of the baseline values) that was mainly related to pneumococcal meningitis; conversely, no flow changes in the basal cerebral artery were observed in viral infections [59]. Similar findings have been demonstrated in cryptococcal meningitis in HIV-negative patients [60]. Altogether, although increased blood velocity in the cerebral basal arteries has been detected, the significance of vascular changes in acute bacterial meningitis has to be confirmed in larger populations.

While cerebral arterial flow does not appear to be compromised in CNS viral infections, alterations of the venous drainage have been demonstrated in herpes simplex virus encephalitis (HSVE). By using TCCS, Doepp and colleagues recorded a significant increase of blood flow velocity in the basal vein of Rosenthal at the affected side in five patients with temporal HSVE. Interestingly, these flow changes were more homogeneous than those observed in the basal cerebral artery. They concluded that drainage flow study of the basal vein of Rosenthal could be an additional diagnostic tool in these patients, both in the acute phase and in monitoring the activity of the disease [61].

The possible role of ONSD evaluation in brain infections has also been studied in CNS tuberculosis. The rationale resides in the increased intracranial pressure that can emerge after the hypersensitivity reaction following cerebral invasion (meningitis, inflammation, secondary hydrocephalus). ONSD was significantly increased compared to controls (5.81 mm vs. 4.37, $p < 0.001$), providing useful information about the development of raised intracranial pressure in these patients [62].

17.9 Intracranial Stenosis and Systemic Vasculitis

Intracranial stenosis accounts for 8–10% of ischemic strokes and is more common in the Asiatic population [63]. In a large cohort of patients Baumgartner et al. confirmed the reliability of TCCD in detecting intracranial stenosis comparing TCCD data with the gold standard method, arterial digital subtraction angiography. These authors established velocimetric TCCD criteria for ≥50% and <50% basal cerebral artery narrowing of intracranial stenosis (Fig. 17.2) [64]. Intracranial

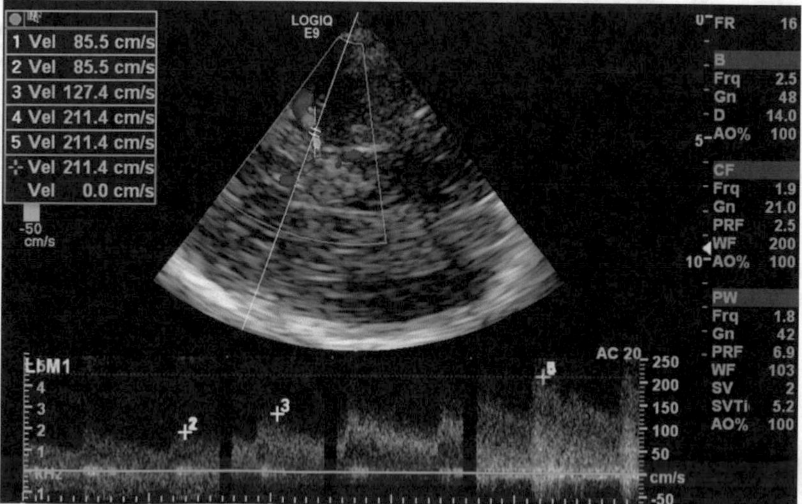

Fig. 17.2 Transcranial color-coded duplex (TCCD) shows raised flow velocities in the proximal segment of the middle cerebral artery (211.4 cm/s, corresponding to a stenosis >50%)

stenosis may be caused due to progressive atheromatic disease in the presence of vascular risk factors or, rarely, may be related to systemic vasculitis. In the latter case, the integrative evaluation of extracranial large arteries may provide further information showing typical structural changes secondary to vessel inflammation. These alterations consist of a characteristic homogeneous, midechoic, circumferential wall or intimal thickening and may determine progressive lumen stenosis, occlusion, or aneurysmatic dilation [65]. Among systemic vasculitis, the mostly known ultrasonographic sign can be seen in giant cell arteritis, the so-called halo sign consisting of a perivascular and hypoechoic circumferential area around the superficial temporal artery denoting edema and vessel inflammation [66]. A similar sign may be present in Takayasu arteritis (Macaroni sign) [67]. In both vasculitis, TCCD and extracranial color-coded duplex may allow an easy and fast evaluation of the efficacy of treatments.

17.10 Parenchymal B Sonography in Neurodegenerative Diseases

Bone window patency is the essential premise for brain parenchymal sonography, ranging from excellent to missing visibility of intracranial structures. Through the temporal window, bones, parenchyma, and CSF may be visualized and the last one is usually used as a marker of conventional B-mode for intracranial orientation. The examination should be started in the axial planes. In Fig. 17.3, the midbrain is visible as a butterfly-shaped hypoechogenic structure surrounded by the basal cisterns. By tilting the probe 10° above, the diencephalic plane is depicted (Fig. 17.4).

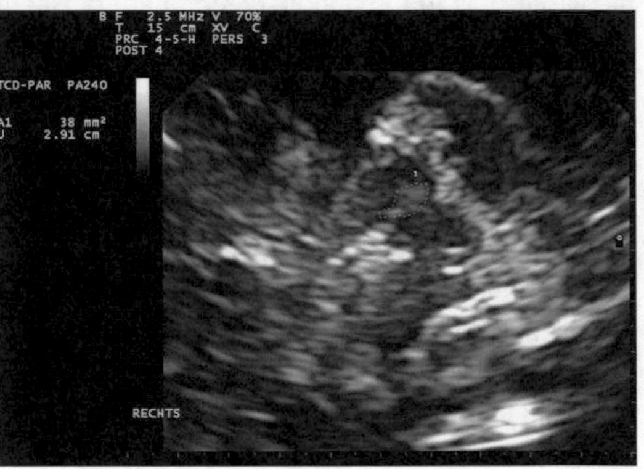

Fig. 17.3 Transcranial brain sonography: assessment of the echogenic area of substantia nigra, using the transtemporal approach, where the butterfly shape of the midbrain is visualized. Increased area (38 mm^2) bounded in green indicates the substantia nigra (SN). The visualization and measurement of SN can be facilitated by zooming the image. Note that the cutoff values for the discrimination between normoechogenic and hyperechogenic substantia nigra can slightly differ with different ultrasound systems

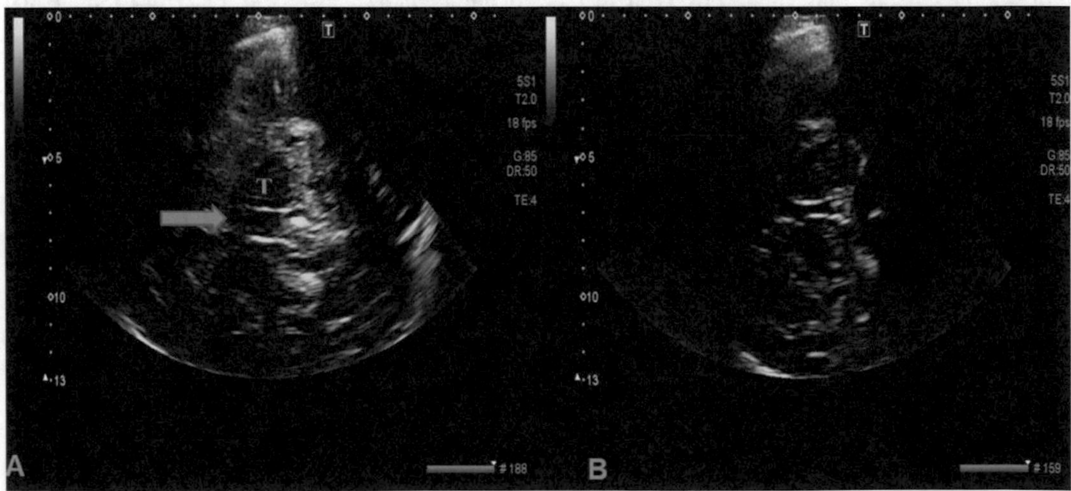

Fig. 17.4 (**a**) Magnification of the diencephalic plane. The third ventricle (blue arrow) is represented by the hyperechogenic lines between both hypogenic thalami (T); the hyperechogenic rounded epiphysis is identified at the end of the double-track structure of the third ventricle. Clear enlargement of third ventricle. (**b**) Typical normal appearance of the basal ganglia and third ventricle plane without zooming the image

In this plane, the third ventricle, the thalami, and the epiphysis may be recognized. The determination of the width of the third ventricle is easy for the identification of the double-track image of the ependyma [51].

It has been shown that in patients with cognitive decline the mean diameter of the third ventricle was significantly wider (6 mm ± 2) than in subjects with normal cognitive testing results (4.6 mm ± 1.8) [68]. Yilmaz R. et al. identified the presence of medial temporal lobe (MTL) atrophy by measuring in coronal or transcoronal plane the ratio between MTL and choroidal fissure height (M/F). The M/F ratio was significantly smaller in the Alzheimergroup on both sides [5]. Thus, brain sonography of the MTL could represent a potential and noninvasive screening technique for suspected dementias.

Increased echogenicity of the substantia nigra is a characteristic finding in idiopathic Parkinson's disease (PD), occurring in more than 90% of the patients (Fig. 17.3) [69].

From a pathological point of view, hyperechogenicity is probably due to increased tissue iron content. Various independent groups demonstrated a high intraobserver reliability of substantia nigra (SN) determination using planimetric measurements of the echogenic area or semi-quantitative visual grading [70, 71]. Notably the finding of a hyperechoic substantia nigra and other parenchymal abnormalities may support the discrimination of Parkinson's disease from atypical parkinsonian syndromes and essential tremor [4, 72–74].

17.11 Conclusion

The noninvasive nature, portability, accuracy, and progressively higher resolution of sonography for vascular and parenchymal cerebral evaluation as well as the technological advances in the available ultrasound systems have improved the applications of brain sonography in patients with chronic disorders and acute neurocritical diseases.

Novel technologies, such as the in-time fusion of TCCD with MRI image automated detection, promise an even wider application in the coming years [75].

References

1. Saqqur M, Khan K, Derksen C, Alexandrov A, Shuaib A. Transcranial Doppler and transcranial color duplex in defining collateral cerebral blood flow. J Neuroimaging. 2018;28(5):455–76. https://doi.org/10.1111/jon.12535.
2. Sacco RL, Kargman DE, Gu Q, Zamanillo MC. Race-ethnicity and determinants of intracranial atherosclerotic cerebral infarction. The Northern Manhattan Stroke Study. Stroke. 1995;26(1):14–20.
3. Reinhard M, Müller T, Roth M, Guschlbauer B, Timmer J, Hetzel A. Bilateral severe carotid artery stenosis or occlusion - cerebral autoregulation dynamics and collateral flow patterns. Acta Neurochir. 2003;145(12):1053–9. discussion 1059-60
4. Walter U, Dressler D, Probst T, Wolters A, Abu-Mugheisib M, Wittstock M, et al. Transcranial brain sonography findings in discriminating between parkinsonism and idiopathic Parkinson disease. Arch Neurol. 2007;64:1635–40.
5. Yilmaz R, Pilotto A, Roeben B, Preische O, Suenkel U, Heinzel S, et al. Structural ultrasound of the medial temporal lobe in Alzheimer's disease. Ultraschall Med. 2017;38(3):294–300. https://doi.org/10.1055/s-0042-107150.
6. Amico DD, Curone M, Ciasca P, Cammarata G, Melzi L, Bussone G, et al. Headache prevalence and clinical features in patients with idiopathic intracranial hypertension (IIH). Neurol Sci. 2013;34(Suppl 1):S147–9. https://doi.org/10.1007/s10072-013-1388-7.
7. Friedman DI, Liu GT, Digre KB. Revised diagnostic criteria for the pseudotumor cerebri syndrome in adults and children. Neurology. 2013;81:1159–65. https://doi.org/10.1212/WNL.0b013e3182a55f17.
8. Raoof N, Sharrack B, Pepper IM, Hickman SJ. The incidence and prevalence of idiopathic intracranial hypertension in Sheffield, UK. Eur J Neurol. 2011;18:1266–8. https://doi.org/10.1111/j.1468-1331.2011.03372.
9. Nedelmann M, Kaps M, Mueller-Forell W. Venous obstruction and jugular valve insufficiency in idiopathic intracranial hypertension. J Neurol. 2009;256(6):964–9.
10. Lochner P, Brigo F, Zedde ML, Sanguigni S, Coppo L, Nardone R, et al. Feasibility and usefulness of ultrasonography in idiopathic intracranial hypertension or secondary intracranial hypertension. BMC Neurol. 2016;16:85. https://doi.org/10.1186/s12883-016-0594-3.
11. Farb RI, Vanek I, Scott JN, Mikulis DJ, Willinsky RA, Tomlinson G, et al. Idiopathic intracranial hypertension: the prevalence and morphology of sinovenous stenosis. Neurology. 2003;60(9):1418–24.

12. Naldi A, Lochner P, Canu P, Settembre R, Alessi S, Sanguigni S. Transcranial color-coded sonography for monitoring idiopathic intracranial hypertension. Ultraschall Med. 2018; https://doi.org/10.1055/a-0783-2541.
13. Bäuerle J, Nedelmann M. Sonographic assessment of the optic nerve sheath in idiopathic intracranial hypertension. J Neurol. 2011;258(11):2014–9. https://doi.org/10.1007/s00415-011-6059-0.
14. Lochner P, Nardone R, Tezzon F, Coppo L, Brigo F. Optic nerve sonography to monitor treatment efficacy in idiopathic intracranial hypertension: a case report. J Neuroimaging. 2013;23:533–4. https://doi.org/10.1111/jon.12005.
15. Lochner P, Fassbender K, Knodel S, Andrejewski A, Lesmeister M, Wagenpfeil G, et al. B-mode transorbital ultrasonography for the diagnosis of idiopathic intracranial hypertension: a systematic review and meta-analysis. Ultraschall Med. 2019;40(2):247–52. https://doi.org/10.1055/a-0719-4903.
16. Chen LM, Wang LJ, Hu Y, Jiang XH, Wang YZ, Xing YQ. Ultrasonic measurement of optic nerve sheath diameter: a non-invasive surrogate approach for dynamic, real-time evaluation of intracranial pressure. Br J Ophthalmol. 2019;103:437–41.https://doi.org/10.1136/bjophthalmol-2018-312934.
17. Lochner P, Fassbender K, Lesmeister M, Nardone R, Orioli A, Brigo F, et al. Ocular ultrasound for monitoring pseudotumor cerebri syndrome. J Neurol. 2018;265:356–61. https://doi.org/10.1007/s00415-017-8699-1.
18. Headache Classification Committee of the International Headache Society (IHS). The international classification of headache disorders, 3rd edition. Cephalalgia. 2018;38:1–211. https://doi.org/10.1177/0333102417738202.
19. Dubost C, Le Gouez A, Zetlaoui PJ, Benhamou D, Mercier FJ, Geeraerts T. Increase in optic nerve sheath diameter induced by epidural blood patch: a preliminary report. Br J Anaesth. 2011;107:627–30. https://doi.org/10.1093/bja/aer186.
20. Fichtner J, Ulrich CT, Fung C, Knüppel C, Veitweber M, Jilch A, et al. Management of spontaneous intracranial hypotension—Transorbital ultrasound as discriminator. J Neurol Neurosurg Psychiatry. 2016;87(6):650–5. https://doi.org/10.1136/jnnp-2015-310853.
21. Fugate JE, Claassen DO, Cloft HJ, Kallmes DF, Kozak OS, Rabinstein AA. Posterior reversible encephalopathy syndrome: associated clinical and radiologic findings. Mayo Clin Proc. 2010;85:427–32. https://doi.org/10.4065/mcp.2009.0590.
22. Ollivier M, Bertrand A, Clarençon F, Gerber S, Deltour S, Domont F, et al. Neuroimaging features in posterior reversible encephalopathy syndrome: a pictorial review. J Neurol Sci. 2017;15(373):188–200. https://doi.org/10.1016/j.jns.2016.12.007.
23. Caputo ND, Fraser RM, Abdulkarim J. Posterior reversible encephalopathy syndrome presenting as papilledema. Am J Emerg Med. 2012;30:835. e835-837. https://doi.org/10.1016/j.ajem.2011.03.016.
24. Lochner P, Mader C, Nardone R, Cantello R, Orioli A, Brigo F. Usefulness of ultrasonography in posterior reversible encephalopathy syndrome. Neurol Sci. 2014;35:475–7. https://doi.org/10.1007/s10072-013-1562-y.
25. Lochner P, Nardone R, Brigo F, Tamber MS, Zuccoli G. The diagnosis of posterior reversible encephalopathy syndrome. Lancet Neurol. 2015;14:1074–5. https://doi.org/10.1016/S1474-4422(15)00256-2.
26. Ross RT. The random nature of cerebral mountain sickness. Lancet. 1985;1:990–1.
27. Lawley JS, Alperin N, Bagci AM, Lee SH, Mullins PG, Oliver SJ, et al. Normobaric hypoxia and symptoms of acute mountain sickness: elevated brain volume and intracranial hypertension. Ann Neurol. 2014;75:890–8. https://doi.org/10.1002/ana.24171.
28. Lawley JS, Oliver SJ, Mullins P, Morris D, Junglee NA, Jelleyman C, et al. Optic nerve sheath diameter is not related to high altitude headache: a randomized controlled trial. High Alt Med Biol. 2012;13:193–9. https://doi.org/10.1089/ham.2012.1019.
29. Strapazzon G, Brugger H, Dal Cappello T, Procter E, Hofer G, Lochner P. Factors associated with optic nerve sheath diameter during exposure to hypobaric hypoxia. Neurology. 2014;82:1914–8. https://doi.org/10.1212/WNL.0000000000000457.
30. Sutherland AI, Morris DS, Owen CG, Bron AJ, Roach RC. Optic nerve sheath diameter, intracranial pressure and acute mountain sickness on Mount Everest: a longitudinal cohort study. Br J Sports Med. 2008;42:183–8. https://doi.org/10.1136/bjsm.2007.045286.
31. Lochner P, Falla M, Brigo F, Pohl M, Strapazzon G. Ultrasonography of the optic nerve sheath diameter for diagnosis and monitoring of acute mountain sickness: a systematic review. High Alt Med Biol. 2015;16:195–203. https://doi.org/10.1089/ham.2014.1127.
32. Fagenholz PJ, Gutman JA, Murray AF, Noble VE, Camargo CA Jr, Harris NS. Optic nerve sheath diameter correlates with the presence and severity of acute mountain sickness: evidence for increased intracranial pressure. J Appl Physiol. 2009;106:1207–11. https://doi.org/10.1152/japplphysiol.01188.2007.
33. Iwasaki K, Ogawa Y, Shibata S, Aoki K. Acute exposure to normobaric mild hypoxia alters dynamic relationships between blood pressure and cerebral blood flow at very low frequency. J Cereb Blood Flow Metab. 2007;27:776–84.
34. Subudhi AW, Grajzel K, Langolf RJ, Roach RC, Panerai RB, Davis JE. Cerebral autoregulation index at high altitude assessed by thigh-cuff and transfer function analysis techniques. Exp Physiol. 2015;100:173–81. https://doi.org/10.1113/expphysiol.2014.082479.
35. Horiuchi M, Endo J, Dobashi S, Kiuchi M, Koyama K, Subudhi AW. Effect of progressive normobaric hypoxia on dynamic cerebral autoregulation. Exp Physiol. 2016;101(10):1276–84. https://doi.org/10.1113/EP085789.

36. Feddersen B, Neupane P, Thanbichler F, Hadolt I, Sattelmeyer V, Pfefferkorn T, et al. Regional differences in the cerebral blood flow velocity response to hypobaric hypoxia at high altitudes. J Cereb Blood Flow Metab. 2015;35(11):1846–51. https://doi.org/10.1038/jcbfm.2015.142.
37. Wilson MH, Imray CH, Hargens AR. The headache of high altitude and microgravity--similarities with clinical syndromes of cerebral venous hypertension. High Alt Med Biol. 2011;12(4):379–86. https://doi.org/10.1089/ham.2011.1026.
38. Youl BD, Turano G, Miller DH, Towell AD, MacManus DG, Moore SG, et al. The pathophysiology of acute optic neuritis. An association of gadolinium leakage with clinical and electrophysiological deficits. Brain. 1991;114(Pt 6):2437–50.
39. Lochner P, Cantello R, Fassbender K, Lesmeister M, Nardone R, Siniscalchi A, et al. Longitudinal assessment of transorbital sonography, visual acuity, and biomarkers for inflammation and axonal injury in optic neuritis. Dis Markers. 2017;2017:5434310. https://doi.org/10.1155/2017/5434310.
40. Dehghani A, Giti M, Akhlaghi MR, Karami M, Salehi F. Ultrasonography in distinguishing optic neuritis from nonarteritic anterior ischemic optic neuropathy. Adv Biomed Res. 1:3. https://doi.org/10.4103/2277-9175.94425.
41. Elvin A, Andersson T, Soderstrom M. Optic neuritis. Doppler ultrasonography compared with MR and correlated with visual evoked potential assessments. Acta Radiol. 1998;39:243–8.
42. Gerling J, Janknecht P, Hansen LL, Kommerell G. Diameter of the optic nerve in idiopathic optic neuritis and in anterior ischemic optic neuropathy. Int Ophthalmol. 1997;21:131–5.
43. Karami M, Janghorbani M, Dehghani A, Riahinejad M. Orbital Doppler evaluation of blood flow velocities in optic neuritis. Korean J Ophthalmol. 2012;26:116–22. https://doi.org/10.3341/kjo.2012.26.2.116.
44. Lochner P, Cantello R, Brigo F, Coppo L, Nardone R, Tezzon F, et al. Transorbital sonography in acute optic neuritis: a case-control study. AJNR Am J Neuroradiol. 2014;35:2371–5. https://doi.org/10.3174/ajnr.A4051.
45. Neroev VV, Karlova IZ, Zaitseva OV, Kruzhkova GV, Boiko AN. Role of ultrasonic B-scanning in differential diagnosis and prognosis of the course of optic neuritis. Vestn oftalmol. 2001;117:25–9.
46. Stefanovic IB, Jovanovic M, Krnjaja BD, Veselinovic D, Jovanovic P. Influence of retrobulbar neuritis and papillitis on echographically measured optic nerve diameter. Vojnosanit Pregl. 2010;67:32–5.
47. Carraro N, Servillo G, Sarra VM, Bignamini A, Pizzolato G, Zorzon M. Optic nerve and its arterial-venous vascularization: an ultrasonologic study in multiple sclerosis patients and healthy controls. J Neuroimaging. 2014;24:273–7. https://doi.org/10.1111/j.1552-6569.2012.00758.x.
48. Candeliere Merlicco A, Gabaldón Torres L, Villaverde González R, Fernández Romero I, Aparicio Castro E, Lastres Arias MC. Transorbital ultrasonography for measuring optic nerve atrophy in multiple sclerosis. Acta Neurol Scand. 2018;138(5):388–93. https://doi.org/10.1111/ane.12976.
49. Venkataramana NK. Hydrocephalus Indian scenario—a review. J Pediatr Neurosci. 2011;6(Suppl 1):S11–22. https://doi.org/10.4103/1817-1745.85704.
50. Becker G, Bogdahn U, Strassburg HM, Lindner A, Hassel W, Meixensberger J, et al. Identification of ventricular enlargement and estimation of intracranial pressure by transcranial color-coded real-time sonography. J Neuroimaging. 1994;4(1):17–22.
51. Seidel G, Kaps M, Gerriets T, Hutzelmann A. Evaluation of the ventricular system in adults by transcranial duplex sonography. J Neuroimaging. 1995;5(2):105–8.
52. Kiphuth C, Huttner HB, Struffert T, Schwab S, Köhrmann M. Sonographic monitoring of ventricle enlargement in posthemorrhagic hydrocephalus. Neurology. 2011;76(10):858–62. https://doi.org/10.1212/WNL.0b013e31820f2e0f.
53. Robba C, Simonassi F, Ball L, Pelosi P. Transcranial color-coded duplex sonography for bedside monitoring of central nervous system infection as a consequence of decompressive craniectomy after traumatic brain injury. Intensive Care Med. 2019;45(8):1143–4. https://doi.org/10.1007/s00134-018-5405-4.
54. Ertl M, Aigner R, Krost M, Karnasová Z, Müller K, Naumann M, et al. Measuring changes in the optic nerve sheath diameter in patients with idiopathic normal-pressure hydrocephalus: a useful diagnostic supplement to spinal tap tests. Eur J Neurol. 2017;24(3):461–7. https://doi.org/10.1111/ene.13225.
55. Rainov NJ, Weise JB, Burkert W. Transcranial Doppler sonography in adult hydrocephalic patients. Neurosurg Rev. 2000;23:34–8.
56. Gupta N, Grover H, Bansal I, Hooda K, Sapire JM, Anand R, et al. Neonatal cranial sonography: ultrasound findings in neonatal meningitis - a pictorial review. Quant Imaging Med Surg. 2017;7(1):123–31. https://doi.org/10.21037/qims.2017.02.01.
57. Yikilmaz A, Taylor GA. Sonographic findings in bacterial meningitis in neonates and young infants. Pediatr Radiol. 2008;38(2):129–37.
58. Lu CH, Chang HW, Lui CC, Huang CR, Chang WN. Cerebral haemodynamics in acute bacterial meningitis in adults. QJM. 2006;99(12):863–9.
59. Haring HP, Rötzer HK, Reindl H, Berek K, Kampfl A, Pfausler B, et al. Time course of cerebral blood flow velocity in central nervous system infections. A transcranial Doppler sonography study. Arch Neurol. 1993;50(1):98–101.
60. Chang WN, Lu CH, Chang HW, Lui CC, Tsai NW, Huang CR, et al. Time course of cerebral hemodynamics in cryptococcal meningitis in HIV-negative adults. Eur J Neurol. 2007;14(7):770–6.
61. Doepp F, Valdueza JM, Schreiber SJ. Serial ultrasound assessment of the basal vein of Rosenthal in HSV encephalitis. Ultrasound Med Biol. 2006;32(4):473–7.

62. Sangani SV, Parikh S. Can sonographic measurement of optic nerve sheath diameter be used to detect raised intracranial pressure in patients with tuberculous meningitis? A prospective observational study. Indian J Radiol Imaging. 2015;25(2):173–6. https://doi.org/10.4103/0971-3026.15586.
63. Wong LKS. Global burden of intracranial atherosclerosis. Int J Stroke. 2006;1:158–9. https://doi.org/10.1111/j.1747-4949.2006.00045.x.
64. Baumgartner RW, Mattle HP, Schroth G. Assessment of >/=50% and <50% intracranial stenoses by transcranial color-coded duplex sonography. Stroke. 1999;30(1):87–92.
65. Muratore F, Pipitone N, Salvarani C, Schmidt WA. Imaging of vasculitis: state of the art. Best Pract Res Clin Rheumatol. 2016;30(4):688–706. https://doi.org/10.1016/j.berh.2016.09.010.
66. Habib HM, Essa AA, Hassan AA. Color duplex ultrasonography of temporal arteries: role in diagnosis and follow-up of suspected cases of temporal arteritis. Clin Rheumatol. 2012;31(2):231–7. https://doi.org/10.1007/s10067-011-1808-0.
67. Maeda H, Handa N, Matsumoto M, Hougaku H, Ogawa S, Oku N, et al. Carotid lesions detected by B-mode ultrasonography in Takayasu's arteritis: "macaroni sign" as an indicator of the disease. Ultrasound Med Biol. 1991;17(7):695–701.ù
68. Wollenweber FA, Schomburg R, Probst M, Schneider V, Hiry T, Ochsenfeld A, et al. Width of the third ventricle assessed by transcranial sonography can monitor brain atrophy in a time- and cost-effective manner—results from a longitudinal study on 500 subjects. Psychiatry Res. 2011;191(3):212–6. https://doi.org/10.1016/j.pscychresns.2010.09.010.
69. Berg D, Behnke S, Seppi K, Godau J, Lerche S, Mahlknecht P, et al. Enlarged hyperechogenic substantia nigra as a risk marker for Parkinson's disease. Mov Disord. 2013;28(2):216–9. https://doi.org/10.1002/mds.25192.
70. Berg D, Roggendorf W, Schröder U, Klein R, Tatschner T, Benz P, et al. Echogenicity of the substantia nigra: association with increased iron content and marker for susceptibility to nigrostriatal injury. Arch Neurol. 2002;59:999–1005.
71. van de Loo S, Walter U, Behnke S, Hagenah J, Lorenz M, Sitzer M, et al. Reproducibility and diagnostic accuracy of substantia nigra sonography for the diagnosis of Parkinson's disease. J Neurol Neurosurg Psychiatry. 2010 Oct;81(10):1087–92. https://doi.org/10.1136/jnnp.2009.196352.
72. Gaenslen A, Unmuth B, Godau J, Liepelt I, Di Santo A, Schweitzer KJ, et al. The specificity and sensitivity of transcranial ultrasound in the differential diagnosis of Parkinson's disease: a prospective blinded study. Lancet Neurol. 2008;7:417–24. https://doi.org/10.1016/S1474-4422(08)70067-X.
73. Stockner H, Sojer M, Seppi K, Mueller J, Wenning GK, Schmidauer C, et al. Midbrain sonography in patients with essential tremor. Mov Disord. 2007;22:414–7.
74. Walter U. How to measure substantia nigra hyperechogenicity in Parkinson disease: detailed guide with video. J Ultrasound Med. 2013;32(10):1837–43. https://doi.org/10.7863/ultra.32.10.1837.
75. Ewertsen C. Image fusion between ultrasonography and CT, MRI or PET/CT for image guidance and intervention—a theoretical and clinical study. Dan Med Bull. 2010;57:B4172.

Brain Death

18

Charu Mahajan, Indu Kapoor,
and Hemanshu Prabhakar

Contents

Brain death is an irreversible cessation of all functions of brain, including brainstem. The three cardinal features include coma, absence of brainstem reflexes and apnoea. It is reasonable that the time between the diagnosis and declaration of brain death should be short, so that organ harvesting for the purpose of transplantation can be carried out before their function gets compromised.

C. Mahajan · I. Kapoor · H. Prabhakar (✉)
Department of Neuroanaesthesiology
and Critical Care, Neurosciences Center,
All India Institute of Medical Sciences,
New Delhi, India

18.1 Pathophysiology of Brain Death

The main inciting event which leads to brain damage is the rise in intracranial pressure. Any severe head injury, cerebrovascular accident or cerebral anoxia due to any reason causes neuronal damage. The ensuing inflammatory cascade of events leads to activation of various neurotransmitters, dysregulation of ion channels and damage to blood-brain barrier, resulting in progressively increasing cerebral oedema. As a result, the intracranial pressure becomes high, and the low-pressure bridging veins get compressed resulting in increase in cerebral venous pressure [1]. As the intracranial pressure further increases, the cerebral blood flow decreases inside the intracranial cavity. With loss of autoregulation, the cerebral perfusion becomes

C. Robba, G. Citerio (eds.), *Echography and Doppler of the Brain*,
https://doi.org/10.1007/978-3-030-48202-2_18

pressure dependent and there is risk of global hypoperfusion with any decrease in blood pressure. This further perpetuates the damage and ultimately a state of irreparable and irreversible damage follows. The blood flow inside the intracranial cavity completely ceases and swollen brain may herniate through foramen magnum or dural folds. Herniation may lead to permanent brainstem damage affecting major vital centres and cranial nerves leading to the clinical state of brain death. The pressure gradients generated inside the cranial cavity can also cause early brainstem herniation and focal ischemia of the vital control centres resulting in death.

18.2 Diagnosis

It is primarily a clinical diagnosis and ancillary tests are not mandatory to perform and are categorised as optional only. However, in situations when examination cannot be completed or results obtained are uncertain, the role of ancillary tests becomes important (Table 18.1). The confirmatory tests establish either loss of electrical activity or cessation of blood flow. These are

- Four-vessel cerebral angiography
- EEG
- Evoked potentials
- Transcranial Doppler (TCD)
- Radionuclide imaging
- CTA/CT perfusion/MRA
- Cervical colour Doppler sonography

Table 18.1 Conditions where clinical examination cannot be performed or is uncertain

Hypotension
Hypoxemia
Hypothermia
Metabolic disturbances
Maxillofacial trauma
Pupillary abnormalities
Toxic levels of certain drugs like TCA, anticholinergic, aminoglycosides, anti-epileptics, chemotherapeutic drugs, neuromuscular blocking agents
High cervical cord injury
Sleep apnoea
Chronic pulmonary disease leading to CO_2 retention
Spinal reflexes

The criteria of their use in the diagnosis of brain death vary worldwide. The demonstration of absent cerebral flow is included as a mandatory test in France and in children below 1 year of age in Italy. It is also essential to carry out these tests in the presence of confounding factors or in situations where brainstem reflexes cannot be carried out. Similarly, EEG is required as a mandatory test in Italy, Japan and France and is one of the most commonly used tests though country-specific variations exist. However, it is rendered unreliable under the effect of sedatives and hypothermia. Cerebral angiography is considered the gold standard for diagnosis of cerebral circulatory arrest (CCA). However, it is invasive, needs transportation of patient and is time consuming. The other tests like radionuclide imaging and perfusion scans are expensive and time consuming. The possibility of false results, susceptibility to confounding factors and non-standardisation affect the other diagnostic modalities [2].

One of these ancillary tests is transcranial Doppler (TCD) which has been considered as an optional confirmatory test for the diagnosis of BD in several guidelines across the world [3, 4]. It uses ultrasonography for assessing blood flow in basal cerebral arteries and helps in the confirmation of cerebral circulatory arrest. The reported sensitivity and specificity range from 70 to 100% and 97 to 100%, respectively [5, 6]. The agreement between TCD and angiography for confirmation of BD has been found to be 100% [7]. In Europe, cerebral angiography is the most common first-line test followed by TCD for confirmation of BD [8]. However at many places angiography is less preferred over TCD because of its invasiveness. In another retrospective study, TCD was seen to be useful as a first-line confirmatory test or as a specific prognosticator in such cases. The early and repetitive examinations depicting CCA pattern are particularly useful in such cases [9]. Both TCD and transcranial colour-coded sonography can be used as confirmatory tests. The colour duplex scanning has an additional advantage that it allows direct visualisation of the vessel lumen. The waveform patterns obtained are similar in both. The advantages and disadvantages of TCD are listed in Table 18.2.

Table 18.2 Advantages and disadvantages of TCD

Advantages	Disadvantages
1. Bedside tool 2. Non-invasive 3. Repeatable 4. Relatively inexpensive 5. Portable 6. Quick	1. Needs trained personnel 2. Inability to differentiate cerebral blood flow cessation from absent acoustic window 3. False negative in patients with open or expansible skulls

The results of a meta-analysis by Chang and colleagues suggest that transcranial Doppler is a highly accurate ancillary test for brain death confirmation. However, as transcranial Doppler evaluates cerebral circulatory arrest and not the brainstem function, this limitation needs to be taken into account when interpreting the results of the meta-analysis [10].

18.3 TCD Procedure

It involves use of a low-frequency ultrasonography transducer (2 MHz) placed at relatively thin bone windows to insonate the basal intracranial arteries and estimate cerebral blood flow velocity. The major vessels studied by TCD are internal carotid artery (ICA), middle cerebral artery (MCA), anterior cerebral artery (ACA), posterior cerebral artery (PCA), basilar artery and vertebral artery. The different bone windows used for TCD are transtemporal, suboccipital, transorbital and submandibular. The ultrasonic waves emitted from transducer are reflected back from moving erythrocytes with a change in frequency that is directly proportional to the velocity of moving cells. The blood flow towards and away from the probe is displayed as positive waveform and negative waveform with respect to baseline. The different arteries are identified based on the window used, depth of insonation and direction of waveform. Cerebral blood flow velocity (CBFV) is derived from a standard equation which uses speed of incident wave, wave pulse frequency and change in angle of incident and reflector beam. It is also dependent on several other physiologic factors. Other than the calculation of CBFV, waveform analysis provides information about parameters like cerebrovascular resistance, autoregulatory status, estimation of cerebral perfusion pressure (CPP) and intracranial pressure (ICP) also. The CBFV gives an indirect estimation of intracranial vessel diameter. Increase in CBFV can be seen in conditions of hyperdynamic flow, stenosis or vasospasm. Similarly, decrease in CBFV points towards hypotension, increased ICP or decrease in intracranial blood flow as seen in brain death.

Before carrying out TCD, few prerequisites have been defined for diagnosing CCA. These include established cause of coma consistent with irreversible loss of brain function, exclusion of hypotension, hypothermia, metabolic derangements and clinical evaluation by two experts showing no evidence of cerebral and brainstem function [11]. The patient should be normocapnic, tachycardia should not be >120/min and systolic blood pressure should be >90 mm Hg. An experienced trained physician should be available for carrying out TCD examination. The cerebral circulatory arrest precedes brain death by approximately 24 h. This is the period when TCD is especially useful for early confirmation of brain death and organ retrieval [12].

The technical prerequisites of TCD [13] for diagnosing CCA are:

- A high-pass filter ≤50 Hz should be used.
- Gain should be increased.
- Sample volume should be set at ≥15 mm.
- Envelope should be switched off.

During TCD examination, bilateral insonation should be performed by placing probes either at temporal bone for MCA or at suboccipital transcranial window for vertebrobasilar vessels.

Calculation of CPP can be done non-invasively by TCD and it correlates well with the CPP measured by invasive ICP monitor. The positive predictive value for diagnosing CPP <60 mm Hg is 94% [14]. It is more useful as a trend monitor rather than considering an absolute value.

A diagnosis of CCA on TCD is confirmed if following waveforms are obtained on two examinations performed at least 30 min apart. The appearance of following waveforms is due to the different stages of progressively increasing ICP (Figs. 18.1 and 18.2).

- An oscillating waveform (systolic forward flow and diastolic reverse flow)
- Short systolic spikes
- Disappearance of intracranial flow

With increase in ICP, higher pulsatility is evident in cerebral arteries (high pulsatility index). At the point when ICP is equal to the diastolic blood pressure, the brain is perfused only in systolic cycle and when end-diastolic velocity is zero. Gradually, as ICP equals to the mean blood pressure, the blood flow ceases during both

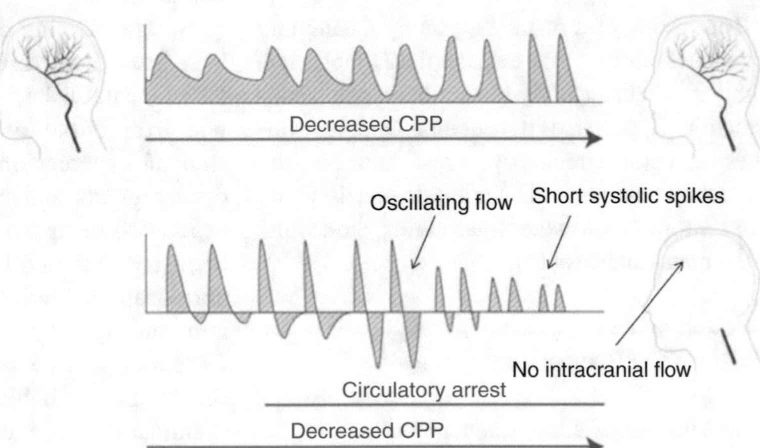

Fig. 18.1 Changes in intracranial arterial waveform with progressively increasing intracranial pressure and reducing cerebral perfusion pressure; oscillating flow, short systolic spikes and finally no flow, all corresponding to circulatory arrest (lower graph)

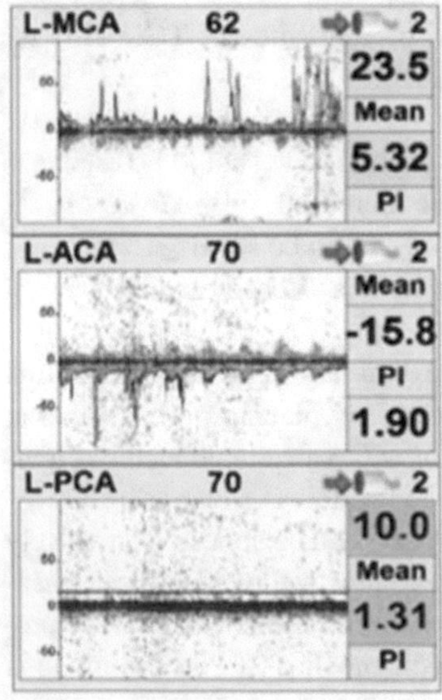

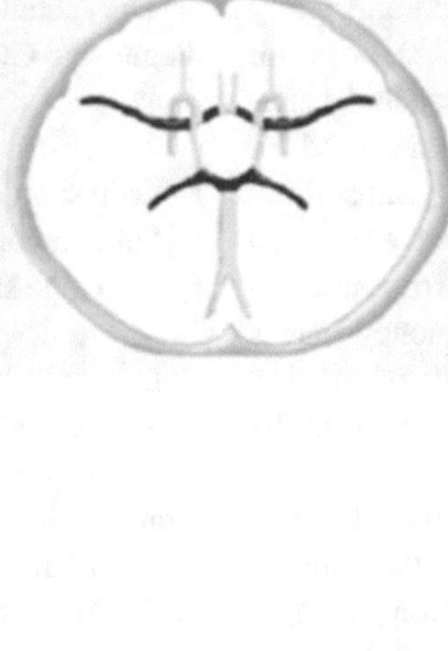

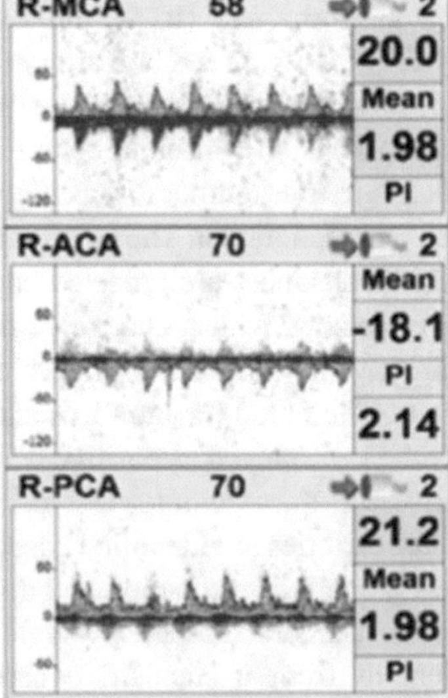

Fig. 18.2 Transcranial Doppler in brain death. Transcranial Doppler shows reverberating or oscillating pattern of flow in all but the left posterior cerebral artery (L-PCA, right inferior corner rectangle) where there is complete absence of flow. Findings confirm brain death. Reverberating or absent flow is diagnostic of brain death. "Reprinted from Seminars in Ultrasound, CT and MRI, 39 (5), Tanvir Rizvi, Prem Batchala, Sugoto Mukherjee. Brain Death: Diagnosis and Imaging Techniques, 515–529, Copyright (2019) with permission from Elsevier"

cycles. The point at which ICP increases to such an extent that no blood can flow into intracranial cavity is evident as oscillatory waveform with equal area under positive and negative waves. This may be explained by the elasticity and compliance of arterial musculature. The systolic forward flow in large basal arteries and diastolic reverse flow produced by microcirculatory obstruction result in zero net flow. This to and fro movement can be appreciated in patent arteries. This usually corresponds to the angiographic picture of CCA [15]. Gradually, with ICP reaching systolic blood pressure, low-amplitude short systolic spikes are seen ending up in total disappearance of waveforms. The systolic peak is less than 50 cm/s and lasts for less than 200 ms in early systole, with absent flow signal during rest of the cycle. Disappearance of intracranial blood flow indicates cerebral circulatory arrest. A mean CBFV in MCA <10 cm/s for more than 30 min is not compatible with survival. It is better to insonate both MCA and BA for demonstration of CCA with a repeat test performed at an interval of 30 min to ensure irreversibility of finding. Corroborating these findings with extracranial demonstration of similar blood flow changes bilaterally in common carotid artery, ICA, VA is also important. On the other hand, flow in external carotid arteries will be normal as the arrest of blood flow usually occurs at the level of carotid bifurcation. Absent cerebral blood flow has to be differentiated from ultrasonic transmission problems. A previous successful examination through the same window and waveforms depictive of brain death seen on the opposite site usually rules out ultrasonic transmission problem.

Dominguez-Roldan studied the difference in waveforms in patients who were brain dead having a supratentorial or infratentorial lesion. In patients with supratentorial lesions, the oscillatory flow pattern was more common. However in patients with infratentorial lesions, systolic spikes were more commonly seen [16].

Use of TCD for central retinal vessel waveform analysis and blood flow variables may have a potential to be developed as an ancillary test in paediatric population to determine brain death [17].

18.3.1 False-Positive and False-Negative Results

The typical waveforms indicative of brain death are produced as a result of changes between ICP and cerebral blood flow. There are certain situations when typical TCD waveforms indicative of CCA are not identified. In such cases, persistent blood flow pattern may be seen in patients with decompressive craniectomies, skull fractures and intraventricular drains; in small children with open fontanelle; or in patients with brainstem injuries [18]. The loss of ICP generation fails to elicit changes in intracranial CBF. Such conditions require other confirmatory studies for diagnosis of brain death. TCD is highly accurate as an ancillary test but it should be remembered that it evaluates CCA rather than brainstem death.

False-positive TCD findings may also be seen in aneurysm rupture at the time when there is a sudden surge in ICP. Also, in the early stage after cardiac arrest, there will be CCA before the patient's circulation returns. In both these situations, CCA is transient and the patient cannot be labelled as brain dead. A repeat examination performed 30 min later will show normal waveforms. Other conditions in which false-positive findings are obtained are ICA distal occlusion and aortic insufficiency. Thus, this makes clinical examination and fulfilment of prerequisites for performing the TCD ultrasonography important.

An inexperienced operator may be unable to insonate the vessel or misinterpret the waveforms. Thus, it is operator dependent and extremely essential to have a trained physician. The transorbital window can be used in such cases to visualise carotid siphon [19].

Thus, TCD is an ancillary test used for confirmation of clinical diagnosis of brain death. It should be considered in conjunction with the clinical condition. If performed by a trained operator, it is a quite sensitive and specific test.

18.3.2 Other Tests

Few other tests are also useful for diagnosis of brain death though these are not validated as confirmatory tests.

18.3.2.1 Cervical Colour Doppler

In cases where insonation window is absent or definitive flow patterns cannot be ascertained, the cervical colour Doppler may be used to confirm CCA. The procedure is performed bilaterally in a technique similar to TCD using 5 or 7.5 MHz Doppler probe but through a cervical approach. This helps to visualise the flow patterns in extracranial ICA and VA. The submandibular and suboccipital window are used for insonation of extracranial ICA and VA, respectively. The waveform patterns indicative of CCA are same as discussed before. ICA occlusion and anatomical conditions may preclude successful examination. The sensitivity for confirming CCA has been found to be 78–80% and has been suggested to be considered as a complementary test [20].

Still, CCD has not been included in the list of standard ancillary tests. However, it is especially of help in patients having absent bone window or when TCD-trained physician is not available.

18.3.2.2 Optic Nerve Sheath Diameter

The optic nerve is covered by a dural sheath containing cerebrospinal fluid inside it which is in direct continuation with intracranial subarachnoid space. This optic nerve is loosely attached to dural sheath in the retrobulbar part. At the time of increase in ICP, there is shift of CSF into this distensible part (3 mm behind the globe) giving rise to increase in optic nerve sheath diameter which is thus taken as a surrogate of raised ICP. This diameter can be measured by CT, MRI or ultrasound.

Ultrasonography for optic nerve sheath diameter is a simple, non-invasive, rapid bedside test for diagnosis of raised ICP. High-frequency linear probes (7.5–10 MHz) are placed gently on closed upper eyelid of a patient in an axial plane to visualise the retrobulbar area. The globe appears as a round dark structure with optic nerve seen as black strip-like structure at the back of the globe. The probe is adjusted to display the entry of optic nerve into the globe at the centre of the image. After freezing this picture, callipers are used to measure the ONSD at 3 mm behind the papilla. A mean of three readings of ONSD is calculated to obtain the final value. ONSD measurement as a surrogate for ICP can be especially useful to screen patients when invasive monitoring is not possible or not indicated.

A value ranging from 4.8 to 6 mm correlates with increased ICP [21]. Brain death is a state of tremendous increase in ICP and this should be evident on ONSD also. Studies have shown that mean ONSD is much greater in patients who were brain dead (0.72 ± 0.05 versus 0.53 ± 0.06) [22]. Moreover, a range of ONSD values from 0.68 to 0.75 cm with ICP values from 28 to 54 mm Hg have been noted in brain-dead patients [23]. The ONSD is significantly higher in patients with BD but it cannot differentiate BD patients from comatose patients who have raised ICP but are not clinically brain dead [24]. The patients with decompressive craniectomies will not have an ICP rise to an extent of inducing cessation of intracerebral blood flow. As a result, ONSD values fail to provide reliable information in such patients [23].

Thus, ONSD is a non-invasive test which can be quickly performed and sustained trend of high values points towards cerebral deterioration and possibly brain death if corrective measures fail.

To conclude, ultrasound when used for detection of CCA has advantages of being a non-invasive, inexpensive, complication free and a quick technique. TCD is the most reliable and sensitive ultrasonographic technique for confirmation of CCA. For this reason, it is now coming up as a first-line ancillary test more often in country-specific guidelines.

References

1. Nakagawa Y, Tsuru M, Yada K. Site and mechanism for compression of the venous system during experimental intracranial hypertension. J Neurosurg. 1974;41:427–34.

2. Wijdicks EFM. Brain death worldwide: accepted fact but no global consensus in diagnostic criteria. Neurology. 2002;58:20.
3. Wijdicks EFM, Varelas PN, Gronseth GS, Greer DM. Evidence-based guideline update: determining brain death in adults: Report of the Quality Standards Subcommittee of the American Academy of Neurology. Neurology. 2010;74:1911–8. 181e242a8
4. Walter U, Schreiber J, Kaps M. Doppler and duplex sonography for the diagnosis of the irreversible cessation of brain function ('brain death'): current guidelines in Germany and neighbouring countries. Ultraschall Med. 2016;37:558–78.
5. De Freitas GR, Andre C. Sensitivity of transcranial Doppler for confirming brain death: a prospective study of 270 cases. Acta Neurol Scand. 2006;113:426–32.
6. Kuo JR, Chen CF, Chio CC, et al. Time dependent validity in the diagnosis of brain death using transcranial Doppler sonography. J Neurol Neurosurg Psychiatry. 2006;77:646–9.
7. Poularas J, Karakitsos D, Kouraklis A, Kostakis A, De Groot E, et al. Comparison between transcranial color Doppler ultrasonography and angiography in the confirmation of brain death. Transplant Proc. 2006;38:1213–7.
8. Citerio G, Murphy PG. Brain death: the European perspective. Semin Neurol. 2015;35:139–44.
9. Sharma D, Souter MJ, Moore AE, Lam AM. Clinical experience with transcranial Doppler ultrasonography as a confirmatory test for brain death: a retrospective analysis. Neurocrit Care. 2011;14:370–6.
10. Chang JJ, Tsivgoulis G, Katsanos AH, Malkoff MD, Alexandrov AV. Diagnostic accuracy of transcranial Doppler for brain death confirmation: systematic review and meta-analysis. AJNR Am J Neuroradiol. 2016;37:408–14.
11. Hassler W, Steinmetz H, Gawlowski J. Transcranial Doppler ultrasonography in raised intracranial pressure and in intracranial circulatory arrest. J Neurosurg. 1988;68:745–51.
12. Dosemeci L, Dora B, Yilmaz M, Cengiz M, Balkan S, Ramazanoglu A. Utility of transcranial Doppler ultrasonography for confirmatory diagnosis of brain death: two sides of the coin. Transplantation. 2004;77:71–5.
13. Widder B, Görtler M, Widder G. Doppler- und Duplexsonographie der hirnversorgenden. Arterien. 6th ed. Berlin: Springer; 2004.
14. Czosnyka M, Matta BF, Smielewski P, Kirkpatrick PJ, Pickard JD. Cerebral perfusion pressure in head injured patients: a noninvasive assessment using transcranial Doppler ultrasonography. J Neurosurg. 1998;88:802–8.
15. Hassler W, Steinmetz H, Pirschel J. Transcranial Doppler study of intracranial circulatory arrest. J Neurosurg. 1989;71:195–201.
16. Dominguez-Roldan JM, Garcia-Alfaro C, Jimenez-Gonzalez PI, Rivera-Fernandez V, Hemandez-Hazanas F, Perez-Bemal J. Brain death due to supratentorial masses: diagnosis using transcranial Doppler ultrasonography. Transplant Proc. 2004;36:2898–900.
17. Riggs BJ, Choen JS, Shivakumar B, et al. Doppler ultrasonography of the central retinal vessels in children with brain death. Pediatr Crit Care Med. 2017;18:258–64.
18. Cabrer C, Dominguez-Roldan MM, Trias E, Paredas D, et al. Persistence of intracranial diastolic flow in transcranial Doppler sonography exploration of patients in brain death. Transplant Proc. 2003;35:1642–3.
19. Dominguez-Roldan JM, Jimenez Gonzalez PI, Garcia-Alfaro V, Rivera-Fernandez V, Hernandez HF. Diagnosis of brain death by transcranial Doppler ultrasonography: solutions for cases of difficult sonic windows. Transplant Proc. 2004;36: 2896–7.
20. Pedicelli A, Bartocci M, Lozupone E, D'Argento F, Alexandre A, Garignano G, et al. The role of cervical color Doppler ultrasound in the diagnosis of brain death. Neuroradiology. 2019;61:137–45.
21. Kristiansson H, Nissborg E, Bartek J Jr, Andresen M, Reinstrup P, Romner B. Measuring elevated intracranial pressure through noninvasive methods: a review of the literature. J Neurosurg Anesthesiol. 2013;25:372–85.
22. Arijana L-H, Simicevic DJ, Popovic IM, Puretic MB, Cvetkovic VV, Gopcevic A, et al. New trends in neurosonology and cerebral hemodynamics - an update. Pers Med. 2012;1:414–6.
23. Toscano M, Spadetta G, Pulitano P, Rocco M, Di Piero V, Mecarelli O, Vicenzini E. Optic nerve sheath diameter ultrasound evaluation in intensive care unit: possible role and clinical aspects in neurological critical patients daily monitoring. Biomed Res Int. 2017;2017:7.
24. Topcuoglu MA, Arsava EM, Bas DF, Kozak HH. Transorbital ultrasonographic measurement of optic nerve sheath diameter in brain death. J Neuroimaging. 2015;25:906–9.

Part VI

Pathology and Clinical Applications: Applications in Neurosurgery

19 Intraoperative Echo in TBI

Carlo Giussani, Erik Pietro Sganzerla, Francesco Prada, and Andrea Di Cristofori

Contents

C. Giussani (✉) · E. P. Sganzerla
Department of Medicine and Surgery, Neurosurgery Unit, Università degli Studi Milano Bicocca, Milan, Italy

Neurosurgery Unit, Azienda Socio-Sanitaria Territoriale, Ospedale San Gerardo, Monza, Italy
e-mail: carlo.giussani@unimib.it

F. Prada
Ultrasound NeuroImaging and Therapy Lab, Fondazione IRCCS Istituto Neurologico C. Besta, Milan, Italy

Department of Neurological Surgery, University of Virginia, Charlottesville, VA, USA

A. Di Cristofori
Neurosurgery Unit, Azienda Socio-Sanitaria Territoriale, Ospedale San Gerardo, Monza, Italy

19.1 Introduction

Traumatic brain injuries (TBIs) are common neurosurgical emergencies that, in many cases, require fast decision-making and management [1–5]. In particular, surgery in these cases may inopportunely lack appropriate planning and traumatic brain lesions may change over time from the first radiological picture to the time of surgery [6, 7]. For example, traumatic brain lesions such as epidural hematoma, subdural hematomas, or cerebral contusions can increase or develop in the first few hours or minutes after a TBI and this can occur in the gap between imaging and surgery [8, 9].

In the typical scenario of a tertiary care hospital, a patient arrives to a trauma center, undergoes brain CT scan and a whole-body CT scan, and then a surgical decision is made [4].

C. Robba, G. Citerio (eds.), *Echography and Doppler of the Brain*,
https://doi.org/10.1007/978-3-030-48202-2_19

During the time lapse between the radiology department and the operating room post-traumatic intracranial hematomas and brain contusions might develop or increase in size. Such evolution might obviously affect patients' prognosis and outcome but it also affects the management of the patient during surgery that may be performed blindly, especially in case of development of contralateral hematomas or in case of growing hematomas [9]. Furthermore this same scenario can occur intraoperatively, when the opening of a close system such as the skull is modified, leading to changes in blood inflow and outflow and CSF dynamics, ultimately changing brain perfusion and intracranial pressure.

In such an emergency setting, a real-time intraoperative imaging modality can be of help in evaluating a lesion under development, allowing a real-time scanning of the surgical field.

Intraoperative imaging techniques available in neurosurgery are computed tomography (CT) scan, magnetic resonance imaging (MRI), and ultrasound (US). The first two techniques are very accurate but they are cost and time consuming and they could not be useful in an emergency setting especially for the amount of time needed to achieve a full brain scan [10]. Intraoperative US (ioUS) is less expensive than the first two techniques and it does not require radiology technicians or dedicated personnel, nor involve the use of ionizing radiations. Such characteristics make ioUS available in many neurosurgical centers and 24/7 [10, 11].

In current neurosurgical settings, ioUS is mainly used in B-mode to perform a morphological evaluation of the surgical field, in order to localize superficial and deep-seated lesions after bone flap removal; fusion imaging with preoperative imaging allows orientation and comparison with other imaging modalities [12, 13]. Ultrasound is nowadays a multiparametric imaging modality with advanced functions [14]:

- Color Doppler scans in order to locate vessels and understand their integrity after surgery [15, 16]
- Sonoelastograms that are able to assess mechanical properties of brain tissues [17–19]
- Contrast-enhanced scans that are able to describe pathological brain tissue and to perform perfusion studies able to understand the areas of secondary damage [20–22]

For its versatility, the use of ioUS is becoming more widespread and it is now a fundamental tool in the neurosurgical equipment [11]. In fact, intraoperative real-time imaging has demonstrated to have several advantages over preoperative imaging since anatomy can change during surgery due to brain shifting and physiopathological and surgically induced tissue deformation [23]. Despite the extensive literature reporting the cost-effective benefits of ioUS and the increased quality of imaging through the years, neurosurgeons do not generally consider ioUS as a user-friendly technique [24]. This is mainly related with the fact that ioUS is not used a standard diagnostic tool, the topographic anatomy is not clear, and it employs scans that differ from the three standard preoperative orthogonal planes since pictures are mainly acquired in 2D along several variable planes different from the three standard ones. These problems can be overcome by an appropriate training which requires daily elective practice to better understand probe and image orientations, to increase the ability to interpret anatomy and to reduce the time spent to understand the pictures acquired [24].

Nowadays, ioUS is mainly used for neuro-oncological, epilepsy, and vascular neurosurgery. In the neuro-oncological and epilepsy setting, ioUS is used to localize the lesion, to check for complete resection at the end of surgery, and to correct the neuro-navigation according to the brain shift during the surgical removal of the tumor [12, 13, 15, 20, 21, 25, 26]. Contrast-enhanced US (CEUS) is used for better definition of a lesion and to better define the perilesional tissue, while color Doppler technique might be useful in some cases with major vessel encasement. Moreover, some advanced reports deal with the utility of sonoelastogram in understanding the mechanical properties of the brain and differentiating between low-grade and high-grade gliomas [17, 19, 20]. For what concerns vascular neurosurgical cases, ioUS is mainly used for arteriovascular malformation (AVM) localization and color Doppler or angiosonographic studies of AVMs or dural arteriovenous fistulas in order to define the intraoperative occlusion of the malformation after surgery [15, 16, 27, 28].

Moreover, in some cases, ioUS is used for external ventricular drain (EVD) placement [29], especially when free-hand technique is at high risk of malpositioning, and drainage of cystic lesions like brain abscesses [30].

In case of TBIs, ioUS is not routinely used in neurosurgical procedure and, despite its real-time capacities, has not been employed to understand during surgery the evolution of the dramatically dynamic phenomena that occurs in trauma patients. Also ioUS does not have nowadays a definitive role in defining the prognosis and outcome of patients undergoing surgery for major brain injuries. As a consequence only few series of patients or case reports have been reported in the literature regarding the utility of ioUS; most of them deal with decompressive craniectomy (DC) for ICP control after failure of medical management [31, 32]. Besides these, some experimental models have been described in order to understand the potential utility of ioUS [33].

In this chapter we are going to describe the multiple options that ioUS can offer in the surgery of major TBIs in an emergency setting.

19.2 Utility of ioUS in TBI

Performing surgery in patients with traumatic brain lesions is like interfering on the natural history of a major TBI without having control on it. As a consequence, during the time lapse between the diagnostic CT scan and the postoperative CT scan, each patient can develop post-traumatic lesions other than the one for which surgery is being done.

Routine use of ioUS may be of help in order to control during surgery if a patient is developing other post-traumatic lesions such as posterior fossa hematomas or homolateral and contralateral hematomas since ioUS allows to explore contralateral hemisphere and posterior fossa structures.

Moreover, an intraoperative picture of brain parenchyma may be of help in order to understand the persistence of brain shift or uncus herniation after a decompressive craniectomy (DC). Finally, evaluating the dimensions of ventricles in some cases may lead to a direct placement of an EVD under US guidance which can reduce the risk of malpositioning.

Furthermore, advanced ioUS modalities such as CEUS and SEG might be helpful in understanding vessel integrity and tissue perfusion, highlighting contusions, and showing parenchymal edema/elasticity.

19.2.1 Intraoperative Use of US

In an emergency setting it is difficult to routinely use ioUS since surgery needs quick decision-making and a fast performance. As a matter of facts, reports about ioUS use in TBIs mainly regard case reports or small case series of patients undergoing DC after failure of medical management.

In this small burden of papers, of some note is the study by Hepner and colleagues that report the use of CEUS in patients undergoing DC for ICP control [31]. In their work, they report the results of cerebral perfusion measured with CEUS in a series of six patients undergoing DC. In particular, it has been shown that cerebral perfusion can increase after DC and that CEUS during ioUS can be used as a reference for post-craniectomy check of the brain perfusion at the bedside of the patient during the stay in ICU. Patients without the bone flap can be explored with US with or without CEUS and in some cases secondary damage can be seen like areas of hypoperfusion due to uncontrolled ICP [31, 34].

Another interesting study is the one by He and colleagues [32]. In their study they showed the potential utility of CEUS in patients undergoing resection of contused brain showing how CEUS was able to identify more hypo-perfused brain tissue than the standard US.

Other few experiences are available in literature but they deal with experiences of small groups of patients or of case reports [7]. This is mainly related with the fact that there is still not a routine use of ioUS in TBIs during surgical procedures and this might be due to:

- Difficult management of a new imaging technique in an emergency setting
- No known benefits about the usefulness of routinary use of ioUS in patients with TBIs

19.2.2 Possible Scenarios

As reported above, surgery for TBI can present some obstacles that requires some changes from what was briefly planned preoperatively. In particular, patients can present unexpected bleedings due to a damage of major vessels, hematomas in the contralateral hemisphere, and further evolution of hidden contusions after release of the intracranial pressure.

Contralateral hematomas can be considered a common complication of major TBIs but they do not generally require surgical intervention. In fact, bilateral small contusions can be considered a common finding such as evolution of small subdural hematomas without significant mass effect. In fact, surgical management of contralateral site hemorrhages is considered a rare event and about 50 case series are reported in literature [6–9]. Such hematomas especially occur after evacuation of acute subdural hematomas (ASDH). In quite all cases such event occurs immediately during surgery and it requires a quick planning of a new surgical procedure. Only a couple of case reports dealt with the fast management of such complications using ioUS. The most interesting and well described is the one from Pil Soo Kim et al. [7]: in their experience, the use of ioUS determined a fast shifting from a unilateral surgery to a bilateral surgery that allowed to minimize the secondary damage due to a fast-growing contralateral hematoma. According to their experience, ioUS can allow to check for complications after surgery in TBIs while the patient is still in the operating room. This is in line with our experience as reported in the explanatory cases of this chapter.

Another clinical scenario can involve patients with post-traumatic hematomas managed conservatively. In fact, sometimes post-traumatic hematomas can be managed conservatively in the first instance but some of them require a delayed surgical evacuation due to increase of perilesional edema. In these cases, colliquation of blood allows endoscopic evacuation of the clot that can be guided by ioUS. In fact ioUS can be used for localizing the clot and for checking the volume of hematoma after evacuation. In other cases, hematomas can be liquid enough in order to be drained under US guidance [35].

Finally, in case of brain swelling due to TBIs it might be necessary at the end of a DC to place an EVD. In these cases, EVD placement can be considered challenging even for experienced neurosurgeons since usually ventricles are collapsed due to the brain edema. In such a scenario, the presence of a large bone defect is of help in order to use the US probe and place an EVD under US guidance [29].

19.2.3 Explanatory Cases

19.2.3.1 Case n. 1

Seventy-six-year-old lady presenting to the A&E department intubated on the scene after a brain injury with left-sided anisocoria and GCS 3 due to sedation. The CT scan at presentation (see Fig. 19.1) documented the presence of a left-sided ASDH with a rounded isodense lesion in the right frontal lobe without any mass effect. Due to the clinical presentation and the radiological focal hematoma, it was decided to perform a left-sided craniotomy for evacuation of the ASDH. During surgery, a sudden brain swelling was experienced after clot evacuation. For this reason, a B-mode ioUS scan was performed that documented a right-sided post-traumatic frontal hematoma with mass effect and a midline shift (see Fig. 19.1). Due to the documented formation of the hematoma, it was decided to perform a right-sided frontal craniotomy. At the opening of

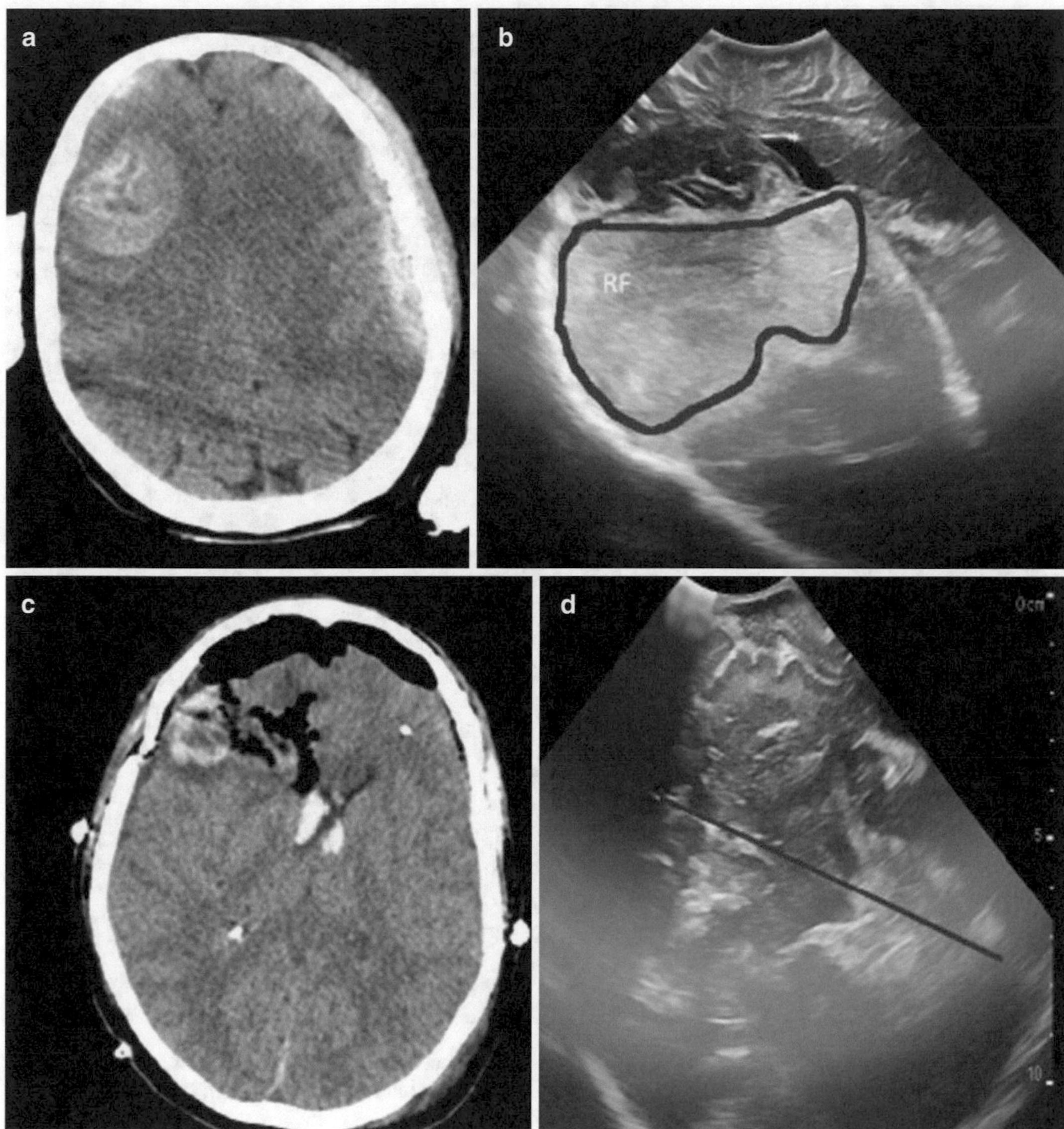

Fig. 19.1 Explanatory case n. 1. (**a**) Preoperative brain CT scan showing a right-sided frontal rounded contusion and a left-sided extradural hematoma. (**b**) Intraoperative US after left-sided craniotomy showing a big right frontal contusion with midline shift and intraventricular clot (*RF* right frontal lobe; *left ventricle). (**c**) Postoperative CT scan. (**d**) Intraoperative US after removal of the right frontal hematoma

the dura, a large right frontal hematoma was found. Postoperative CT scan of the brain documented the surgical cavity and clot removal.

19.2.3.2 Case n. 2

A 10-month-old baby boy fell from the changing table having a traumatic head injury from a 1.3 m height. He was transported to the A&E department where he started having intractable seizure. He was intubated by the emergency team and he underwent an antiepileptic treatment and a subsequent fast brain MRI that showed a large frontal contusion without significant mass effect (see Fig. 19.2a). The EEG showed a persistent seizure after suspension of sedation despite anticonvulsive therapy. Given this finding we decided to

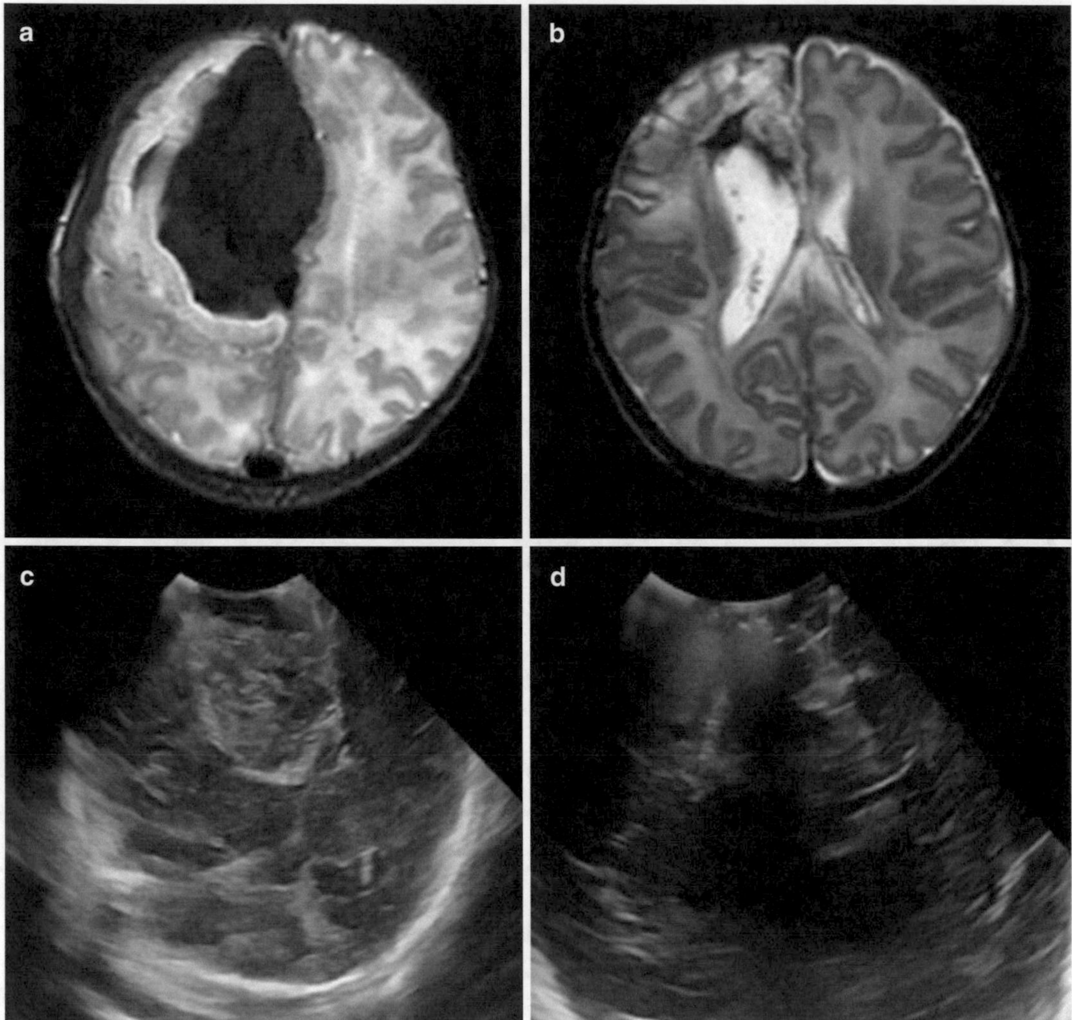

Fig. 19.2 Explanatory case n. 2. (**a**) Preoperative brain MRI showing a right frontal hematoma. (**b**) Postoperative brain MRI showing the surgical cavity in the frontal lobe. (**c**) Intraoperative US showing the right frontal lobe hematoma. (**d**) Intraoperative US showing the surgical cavity

evacuate the hematoma with a small frontal craniotomy and a minimally invasive procedure through a small corticectomy. IoUS was performed and it was helpful to quantify the amount of blood before opening the dura mater (Fig. 19.2c) and after clot removal in order to understand if there were any blood remnants (see Fig. 19.2d). Postoperative scans showed removal of the clot without complications in the surgical cavity (see Fig. 19.2b).

After surgery the baby slowly resolved the grand mal seizures and recovered in a couple of weeks returning back to home.

This case is of interest because of its rarity and because it brings light on the potential use of US in the emergency setting in case of pediatric TBIs. In fact, in some cases involving newborns and infants with open anterior fontanel, US can be performed at the bedside and it is particularly important in case of unstable conditions that do not allow transfer to the radiology department. In these cases, US through the bregmatic fontanel can be used to briefly exclude significant lesions with mass effect or midline shift or it can be used to observe the evolution of TBIs. In case of minor injuries, it can also be used to avoid a brain CT scan and to reduce the exposure to ionizing radiations.

19.3 Future Perspectives

Routine use of ioUS allows to open further perspectives in prognosis stratification of patients with major TBIs. In fact, ioUS can be performed as a baseline evaluation of the brain at the moment of surgery that can be used for future comparisons during the ICU recovery [31]. Moreover, it can be used as a way to estimate the primary and secondary brain damage at the beginning of the clinical history of a patient [32]. As a matter of fact, the majority of the published studies deal with the role of US in patients who have undergone DC [31, 32, 34, 36]. The presence of a large bone defect determines the possibility to explore the brain with the US probe without the interference of the skull that, in many cases, makes the brain inaccessible to the US.

One of the issues in comparing the preoperative and postoperative findings is the region of interest to be used in order to appreciate US changes in terms of perfusion or brain elasticity. As proposed by Hepner et al. in 2006, comparison of brain perfusion with CEUS can be performed using the first burr hole performed for the DC as "the region of interest" (ROI) for further postoperative comparisons [31]. Moreover, they were able to perform the preoperative scans with a small burr hole probe. In their study acquisition of perfusion data was performed only on six patients but they assessed that DC was related with an improvement of brain perfusion at the postoperative US scans. With this perspective, future studies may be directed to distinguish between patients with low response to DC and patients with a good response to DC.

In a study by He and colleagues the utility of ioUS with CEUS in traumatic brain injuries was reported on a series of 32 patients [32]. In one group they performed standard ioUS while in the other group they performed ioUS with CEUS. They showed interesting results about the information that CEUS can add to the normal US. In fact, according to their study, CEUS can show the difference between vital brain and hypo-perfused dead-brain tissue that can appear normal at the standard US. Findings about vital or dead brain can change the surgical plan in case of resection of brain contusion or in case of surgery of intraparenchymal hematomas. As a matter of fact, in the study by He et al. it was found that CEUS demonstrated a larger hypo-perfused brain area around the contused brain tissue than was planned to be removed. In those cases of brain with low perfusion at CEUS, neurosurgeons planned a larger brain resection. Despite their interesting findings, their study had some limitations such as the lack of a longitudinal follow-up in order to understand if removal of perilesional damaged brain can increase patient's outcome reducing the secondary brain damage due to cytotoxic edema, or the simple resection of the contused area could lead to a recovery of the perilesional area.

Moreover, starting from this point, brain stiffness at the time of DC may be studied with the systematic performance of elastosonography with ioUS. In fact, one of the new frontiers in brain US is the study of brain elastance. Elastance can be measured applying the US probe on the brain surface and it can give information about pathological conditions of the brain, like it has been described in experimental models of ischemic strokes in mice or in case of patients with brain tumors [17, 37].

Moreover, changes of stiffness may reflect changes of brain perfusion. In a previous work by Xu and colleagues it was found that in a rodent model of ischemic stroke there were changes in brain elastograms due to reduction of brain perfusion and increase of brain edema [38]. The same research group studied a rodent model of TBI [33]. In their study, they found that US elastography is able to detect changes in the fluid content of the brain after a mild brain trauma. In a speculative way, given these reports and the raising knowledge about MR elastography, it will be possible to prognosticate the outcome of a patient with high ICP and with repeated measures of brain elastance with brain US. Moreover, comparison with intraoperative findings will possibly allow to distinguish patients with poor prognosis from patients with a good outcome.

References

1. Carney N, Totten AM, O'Reilly C, et al. Guidelines for the management of severe traumatic brain injury, fourth edition. Neurosurgery. 2016;80(1):6.
2. Management of Concussion/mTBI Working Group. VA/DoD clinical practice guideline for management of concussion/mild traumatic brain injury. J Rehabil Res Dev. 2009;46:CP1–68.
3. Vella MA, Crandall ML, Patel MB. Acute management of traumatic brain injury. Surg Clin North Am. 2017;97:1015–30.
4. Murray GD, Brennan PM, Teasdale GM. Simplifying the use of prognostic information in traumatic brain injury. Part 2: graphical presentation of probabilities. J Neurosurg. 2018;128:1621–34.
5. Brennan PM, Murray GD, Teasdale GM. Simplifying the use of prognostic information in traumatic brain injury. Part 1: the GCS-pupils score: an extended index of clinical severity. J Neurosurg. 2018;128:1612–20.
6. Shen J, Pan JW, Fan ZX, Zhou YQ, Chen Z, Zhan RY. Surgery for contralateral acute epidural hematoma following acute subdural hematoma evacuation: five new cases and a short literature review. Acta Neurochir. 2013;155:335–41.
7. Kim PS, Yu SH, Lee JH, Choi HJ, Kim BC. Intraoperative transcranial sonography for detection of contralateral hematoma volume change in patients with traumatic brain injury. Korean J Neurotrauma. 2017;13:137.
8. Su T-M, Lee T-H, Chen W-F, Lee T-C, Cheng C-H. Contralateral acute epidural hematoma after decompressive surgery of acute subdural hematoma: clinical features and outcome. J Trauma. 2008;65:1298–302.
9. Choi YH, Lim TK, Lee SG. Clinical features and outcomes of bilateral decompression surgery for immediate contralateral hematoma after craniectomy following acute subdural hematoma. Korean J Neurotrauma. 2017;13:108.
10. Moiyadi A, Shetty P. Objective assessment of utility of intraoperative ultrasound in resection of central nervous system tumors: a cost-effective tool for intraoperative navigation in neurosurgery. J Neurosci Rural Pract. 2011;02:004–11.
11. Pino M, Imperato A, Musca I, et al. New hope in brain glioma surgery: the role of intraoperative ultrasound. A Review. Brain Sci. 2018;8:202.
12. Velthoven V. Intraoperative ultrasound imaging: comparison of pathomorphological findings in US versus CT, MRI and intraoperative findings. In: Bernays RL, Imhof H-G, Yonekawa Y, editors. Intraoperative imaging neurosurgery. Vienna: Springer Vienna; 2003. p. 95–9.
13. Sun H, Zhao JZ. Application of intraoperative ultrasound in neurological surgery. Minim Invasive Neurosurg. 2007;50:155–9.
14. Mannaerts CK, Wildeboer RR, Postema AW, Hagemann J, Budäus L, Tilki D, Mischi M, Wijkstra H, Salomon G. Multiparametric ultrasound: evaluation of greyscale, shear wave elastography and contrast-enhanced ultrasound for prostate cancer detection and localization in correlation to radical prostatectomy specimens. BMC Urol. 2018;18:98.
15. Prada F, Del Bene M, Faragò G, DiMeco F. Spinal dural arteriovenous fistula: is there a role for intraoperative contrast-enhanced ultrasound? World Neurosurg. 2017;100:712.e15–8.
16. Bartels E. Evaluation of arteriovenous malformations (AVMs) with transcranial color-coded duplex sonography: does the location of an AVM influence its sonographic detection? J Ultrasound Med. 2005;24:1511–7.
17. Prada F, Del Bene M, Moiraghi A, et al. From grey scale B-mode to elastosonography: multimodal ultrasound imaging in meningioma surgery—pictorial essay and literature review. Biomed Res Int. 2015;2015:1–13.
18. Del Bene M, Perin A, Casali C, Legnani F, Saladino A, Mattei L, Vetrano IG, Saini M, DiMeco F, Prada F. Advanced ultrasound imaging in glioma surgery: beyond gray-scale B-mode. Front Oncol. 2018;8:576.
19. Chauvet D, Imbault M, Capelle L, Demene C, Mossad M, Karachi C, Boch A-L, Gennisson J-L, Tanter M. In vivo measurement of brain tumor elasticity using intraoperative shear wave elastography. Ultraschall Med. 2016;37:584–90.
20. Prada F, Bene MD, Fornaro R, et al. Identification of residual tumor with intraoperative contrast-enhanced ultrasound during glioblastoma resection. Neurosurg Focus. 2016;40:E7.
21. Mattei L, Prada F, Marchetti M, Gaviani P, DiMeco F. Differentiating brain radionecrosis from tumour recurrence: a role for contrast-enhanced ultrasound? Acta Neurochir. 2017;159:2405–8.
22. Sastry R, Bi WL, Pieper S, Frisken S, Kapur T, Wells W, Golby AJ. Applications of ultrasound in the resection of brain tumors: ultrasound in brain tumor resection. J Neuroimaging. 2017;27:5–15.
23. Reinertsen I, Lindseth F, Askeland C, Iversen DH, Unsgård G. Intra-operative correction of brain-shift. Acta Neurochir. 2014;156:1301–10.
24. Giussani C, Riva M, Djonov V, Beretta S, Prada F, Sganzerla E. Brain ultrasound rehearsal before surgery: a pilot cadaver study: cerebral ultrasound in cadaveric heads. Clin Anat. 2017;30:1017–23.
25. Coburger J, Scheuerle A, Pala A, Thal D, Wirtz CR, König R. Histopathological insights on imaging

results of intraoperative magnetic resonance imaging, 5-aminolevulinic acid, and intraoperative ultrasound in glioblastoma surgery. Neurosurgery. 2017;81:165–74.

26. Prada F, Gennari AG, Del Bene M, Bono BC, Quaia E, D'Incerti L, Villani F, Didato G, Tringali G, DiMeco F. Intraoperative ultrasonography (ioUS) characteristics of focal cortical dysplasia (FCD) type II b. Seizure. 2019;69:80–6.
27. Unsgård G, Rao V, Solheim O, Lindseth F. Clinical experience with navigated 3D ultrasound angiography (power Doppler) in microsurgical treatment of brain arteriovenous malformations. Acta Neurochir. 2016;158:875–83.
28. Prada F, Del Bene M, Saini M, Ferroli P, DiMeco F. Intraoperative cerebral angiosonography with ultrasound contrast agents: how I do it. Acta Neurochir. 2015;157:1025–9.
29. Manfield JH, Yu KKH. Real-time ultrasound-guided external ventricular drain placement: technical note. Neurosurg Focus. 2017;43:E5.
30. Park H, Lee Y, Oh S, Lee HJ. Successful treatment with ultrasound-guided aspiration of intractable methicillin-resistant *Staphylococcus aureus* brain abscess in an extremely low birth weight infant. Pediatr Neurosurg. 2015;50:210–5.
31. Heppner P, Ellegala DB, Durieux M, Jane JA, Lindner JR. Contrast ultrasonographic assessment of cerebral perfusion in patients undergoing decompressive craniectomy for traumatic brain injury. J Neurosurg. 2006;104:738–45.
32. He W, Wang L-S, Li H-Z, Cheng L-G, Zhang M, Wladyka CG. Intraoperative contrast-enhanced ultrasound in traumatic brain surgery. Clin Imaging. 2013;37:983–8.
33. Xu ZS, Yao A, Chu SS, Paun MK, McClintic AM, Murphy SP, Mourad PD. Detection of mild traumatic brain injury in rodent models using shear wave elastography: preliminary studies. J Ultrasound Med. 2014;33:1763–71.
34. Sarà M, Sorpresi F, Guadagni F, Pistoia F. Real-time ultrasonography in craniectomized severely brain injured patients. Ultrasound Med Biol. 2009;35:169–70.
35. Sadahiro H, Nomura S, Goto H, Sugimoto K, Inamura A, Fujiyama Y, Yamane A, Oku T, Shinoyama M, Suzuki M. Real-time ultrasound-guided endoscopic surgery for putaminal hemorrhage. J Neurosurg. 2015;123:1151–5.
36. Bobinger T, Huttner HB, Schwab S. Bedside ultrasound after decompressive craniectomy: a new standard? Neurocrit Care. 2017;26:319–20.
37. Prada F, Del Bene M, Rampini A, et al. Intraoperative strain elastosonography in brain tumor surgery. Oper Neurosurg. 2019;17:227–36.
38. Xu ZS, Lee RJ, Chu SS, Yao A, Paun MK, Murphy SP, Mourad PD. Evidence of changes in brain tissue stiffness after ischemic stroke derived from ultrasound-based elastography. J Ultrasound Med. 2013;32:485–94.

Neurosonology in Tropical Medicine

20

David Clark and Peter John Ashton Hutchinson

Contents

D. Clark (✉) · P. J. A. Hutchinson
National Institute of Health Research Global Health Research Group on Neurotrauma, Cambridge University Hospitals and University of Cambridge, Cambridge, UK

Division of Neurosurgery, Addenbrooke's Hospital, Cambridge, UK
e-mail: dj.clark@cantab.net; pjah2@cam.ac.uk

20.1 Introduction

'Tropical medicine' refers to the field of medicine that deals with pathologies, both infectious and non-infectious, that are prevalent in tropical and subtropical regions. Many of the diseases in this

C. Robba, G. Citerio (eds.), *Echography and Doppler of the Brain*,
https://doi.org/10.1007/978-3-030-48202-2_20

region result from poverty, poor sanitation, infrastructure and inadequate health sources [1]. Although infectious diseases have historically been the greatest challenge to healthcare providers in these regions, ageing populations and rapid urbanisation mean non-communicable diseases (such as trauma and cerebrovascular disease) are becoming increasingly prevalent in low- and middle-income countries (LMICs). Neurosonological techniques are a relatively inexpensive, non-invasive method of obtaining detailed information on intracranial pressure and haemodynamics. As such, neurosonology represents an exciting opportunity to better understand and improve the management of neurological conditions prevalent in the tropics where advanced diagnostic modalities such as neuroimaging or invasive multimodality neuromonitoring are not routinely available. In this chapter, we aim to review the literature on the role of neurosonology in a number of neurological diseases typically encountered by doctors and other healthcare professionals working in tropical medicine and propose that it remains an underutilised technique in this environment. In addition, recommendations are made to help ensure effective and responsible implementation of neurosonology for those wishing to adopt it into their own tropical medicine practice.

20.2 Neurosonology in Neurological Infections in the Tropics

Neurosonology in tropical neurological infections has two main applications—transcranial Doppler ultrasound (TCD) and ultrasound optic nerve sheath diameter (ONSD) as non-invasive methods to diagnose raised intracranial pressure (ICP) in low-resource settings where invasive methods are unavailable or impractical, and TCD to evaluate vasculopathy secondary to infection. In the sections that follow, we present a brief overview of the epidemiology, clinical features, diagnosis and treatment of each condition followed by a review of perturbations in intracranial haemodynamics associated with each pathology and, finally, the role of neurosonology in their clinical management. We have decided to focus on five neurological infections that are prevalent in many tropical and subtropical countries—HIV, tuberculous meningitis, cryptococcal meningitis, neurocysticercosis and cerebral malaria. The role of neurosonology in central nervous system infections that are also prevalent in temperate regions (such as meningoencephalitides, brain abscesses and subdural empyema due to various aetiologies) is not covered here as this is discussed in greater detail elsewhere.

20.3 Human Immunodeficiency Virus

The incidence of stroke in LMICs is increasing, especially in young populations [2]. HIV infection is an important risk factor for stroke in endemic regions [3]. HIV-associated vasculopathy is an important cause of HIV-related ischaemic stroke [4, 5] and can be defined as intimal hyperplasia more than expected for age in an HIV patient, which includes several pathological findings including accelerated atherosclerosis, non-atherosclerotic vasculopathy, vasculitis and small-vessel disease [6].

Two authors have published their experience of the use of TCD examination to assess vasculopathy in HIV infection [7, 8]. Brilla et al. found that both mean blood flow velocities of the MCAs were reduced and cerebral vasoreactivity (assessed using increase in mean blood flow velocity after administration of intravenous acetazolamide) was impaired in HIV-infected individuals (n = 31) relative to healthy controls (n = 10) [7]. Similarly, Chow et al. found that cerebral vasoreactivity (assessed using the response of cerebral blood flow to inhaled carbon dioxide) was impaired in 65 antiretroviral therapy-treated, virally suppressed HIV-infected individuals relative to 28 healthy controls [8]. The exact significance of these findings remains unclear but points to the possibility of intracranial endothelial dysfunction in response to chronic HIV infection.

In addition to HIV-associated vasculopathy, coagulopathy, cardiothromboembolism and, importantly, opportunistic infections are postulated to be important causes of HIV-related ischaemic stroke [4, 5]. A review of important opportunistic infections (specifically tuberculous and cryptococcal meningitis) common in HIV, their cerebrovascular complications and the role of neurosonology in their diagnosis and monitoring is presented below.

20.4 Tuberculous Meningitis

Over ten million cases of tuberculosis were estimated to occur in 2015 [9]. Tuberculous meningitis (TBM) is the most common manifestation of neurological involvement in TB and at least 100,000 cases are thought to occur worldwide annually [10]. Mortality in TBM admitted to intensive care units is 40–53% with over 60% having a poor functional outcome [11, 12].

20.4.1 Intracranial Hypertension in TBM

TBM is associated with intracranial hypertension [13]. The pathophysiology of intracranial hypertension in TBM is postulated to be due to hydrocephalus (mostly communicating hydrocephalus), cerebral oedema and mass effect due to tuberculomas [14]. The gold standard of measurement of intracranial pressure is invasive monitoring with an intraparenchymal probe or ventriculostomy—however, these devices are expensive and, as such, are not readily available in the low-resource settings where TBM is most prevalent. Opening pressure (OP) on lumbar puncture (LP) is an alternative and an LP would also help to confirm the diagnosis of TBM microbiologically—however, such one-off OP measurements are not particularly accurate at reflecting ICP. Moreover, performing an LP in a patient with obstructive hydrocephalus or a tuberculoma may precipitate tonsillar herniation and death—this is a particularly pertinent issue in low-resource settings with unreliable access to neuroimaging where a pre-procedure CT scan is not guaranteed. In addition, unreliable supply chains in low-resource settings mean sterile manometers are not always available. Finally, many patients in regions where TBM is endemic refuse lumbar puncture due to complex, deeply entrenched negative cultural perceptions [15].

ONSD measured by ultrasound is able to determine the presence of intracranial hypertension with reasonable accuracy in TBM [16]. However, its potential role in the management of TBM has yet to be established. Ultrasound ONSD could be of great utility in the diagnosis of neurological deterioration in TBM—a raised ONSD in a patient deteriorating neurologically could signify the development of hydrocephalus which would warrant an urgent CT scan and possibly neurosurgical intervention, whereas a normal ONSD in the same patient may indicate other complications of TBM such as hyponatraemia, seizures or stroke.

20.4.2 Tuberculous Meningitis-Related Vasculopathy

Stroke is a recognised complication of tuberculous meningitis—rates reported in the literature vary from 15% to 60% depending on the method of diagnosis [17–19]. The pathophysiology of stroke in TBM remains poorly defined, but vasculopathy associated with TBM is now a recognised phenomenon and histopathological studies have demonstrated infiltrative, proliferative and necrotising changes in those intracranial vessels passing through the basal meningeal exudate typical of this pathology [20]. Vasospasm has also been suggested as being implicated, particularly due to, histologically, the presence of fibrinoid necrosis in the absence of infiltrative changes and the observation that angiographic findings correlate poorly with the presence of infarction [20, 21]. On CT and MRI, infarcts in the 'TB zone' in the anterior basal ganglia (caudate head, anteromedial thalamus and anterior limb of the internal capsule) [21, 22] are most commonly observed although other areas can also be affected. Angiographically, narrowing of the supraclinoid internal carotid artery and proximal anterior cerebral and middle cerebral arteries are most commonly observed [23–25].

Transcranial Doppler ultrasound has been used for the diagnosis and monitoring of TBM vasculopathy. To our knowledge, five authors have published their experience of using TCD to diagnose and monitor TBM-related vasculopathy (Table 20.1) [26–30]. Kilic et al. identified three phases of TBM vasculopathy based on clinical and sonographic findings (Table 20.2) [30]. Interestingly, the authors likened the findings on TCD examination in phase 1 to those seen in the early stages of acute vasospasm following aneurysmal subarachnoid haemorrhage (SAH) [30]. If vasospasm is involved in the pathophysiology of stroke in TBM and TCD is able to identify it reliably, TCD could be used to guide the treatment of TBM-induced vasospasm with management options that have already proven successful in vasospasm associated with SAH (for example, through pharmacologically induced hypertension). A single-centre, open-label, randomised controlled trial demonstrated that 'triple H' therapy (hypervolaemia-hypertension-haemodilution—used extensively in vasospasm in SAH) is safe and feasible in TBM and a trend towards improvement in focal neurological deficits and mentation was found [28]—however, the conclusions that can be drawn from this study are limited given its small sample size ($n = 12$).

20.5 Cryptococcal Meningitis

Cryptococcal meningitis (CrM) is an infection of the central nervous system with fungi in the species *Cryptococcus*—specifically, *C. neoformans* and *C. gattii* [31]. It almost always occurs in the setting of HIV infection. It has been esti-

Table 20.1 Studies using TCD to evaluate TBM vasculopathy

Author	Year	Country	Subjects	Comparison	Major findings
Tai [26]	2016	Malaysia	Adults (16–75 years) with TBM ($n = 36$)	None	Mean blood flow velocity was elevated (>120 cm/s) in the MCA in 11 patients, bilaterally in 6 LR was elevated (>3) in ten patients 80% of patients with TBM vasculopathy based on TCD criteria also had narrowing on CTA or MRA
Van Toorn [27]	2014	South Africa	Children (<13 years) with TBM ($n = 20$)	None	Bilateral peak systolic velocity was high (>140 cm/s) in both MCAs in 70% Side-to-side differences in MCA flow velocities in 4/8 children with radiologically proven infarcts
Arunodaya [28]	2009	India	Adults (15–49 years) with TBM receiving triple H (hypervolaemia-hypertension-haemodilution) therapy ($n = 7$)	Adults (23–35 years) with TBM receiving standard management ($n = 5$)	Randomised controlled trial No significant difference in mortality Trend towards improvement in motor deficit and mental state in triple H group TCD evidence of 'focal high velocities' in MCA in five patients—three patients showed resolution of these changes after HHH therapy on serial TCD exams
Lu [29]	2007	Taiwan	TBM and cryptococcal meningitis ($n = 15$)	None	27% of patients had stenosis in at least one major intracranial artery Risk of poor outcome at 6 months was greater in patients with one or more intracranial stenoses (odds ratio 5.3)
Kilic [30]	2002	Turkey	Children (age 2–24 years) with TBM (n = 20)	None	Three phases of TBM-related vasculopathy identified

Table 20.2 Phases of TBM vasculopathy on TCD described by Kilic et al. [30]

Phase	Clinical features	TCD findings
1	Temporary focal neurological deficits that resemble transient ischaemic attacks clinically, GCS is 15	Increased mean blood flow velocity Normal to moderately reduced PI
2	Focal neurological deficit(s) with no loss of consciousness, GCS is 12–14	Reduced mean blood flow velocity Reduced PI
3	Impaired consciousness, GCS is <12	Mean blood flow velocity < 40 cm/s PI is very low and can approach 0 Near-complete absence of blood flow in at least one basal artery

mated that almost one million new cases of CrM occur per year in HIV-infected individuals, causing over 600,000 deaths [32] of which the vast majority are in sub-Saharan Africa. CrM commonly presents with chronic fever, headache and malaise with minimal neck stiffness or photophobia. Diagnosis is confirmed by India ink staining of CSF, detection of cryptococcal polysaccharide antigen by latex agglutination test or lateral flow assay and/or culture of the organism. The mainstay of treatment is with amphotericin B and flucytosine for induction, followed by fluconazole for maintenance. Antiretroviral therapy in HIV-positive patients should also be instituted in a timely fashion. Finally, symptomatic and supportive management should be provided, including for raised intracranial pressure.

20.5.1 Intracranial Hypertension in CrM

Approximately half of HIV-infected patients with CrM will have an opening pressure (OP) of >25 cmH_2O on lumbar puncture (LP), with almost 40% having an OP of >35 cmH_2O [33, 34]. Moreover, raised CSF pressure has been associated with increased acute mortality [34] and the measurement and management of CSF pressure are recommended in practice guidelines [35]—serial therapeutic lumbar puncture with volumes of 30 mL being removed is reasonable, although temporary external lumbar drainage [36, 37] and ventriculoperitoneal shunting are occasionally necessary and warranted if available. However, as discussed above with regard to TBM, CrM is endemic in regions where performing a LP with manometry may not always be feasible. Nabeta el al. found that sonographic optic nerve sheath diameter was able to predict OP with manometry with reasonable accuracy in a cohort of 98 HIV-positive Ugandan adults with CrM [38], although the authors proposed no specific recommendations for its use in guiding the management of raised ICP in CrM. Future studies are warranted to investigate the potential utility of sonographic optic nerve sheath diameter in guiding the management of raised ICP in CrM.

20.5.2 Vasculopathy in CrM

Reported prevalence of stroke in CrM is between 4% and 32% [39–41], less than TBM. The pathophysiology of stroke in CrM is thought to be similar to TBM, where a basal meningeal exudate surrounding the arteries of the circle of Willis results in a vasculopathy [40]. Two authors have reported on the use of TCD in the evaluation of CrM-related vasculopathy [29, 42].

20.6 Neurocysticercosis

Neurocysticercosis (NCC), an infection of the central nervous system (CNS) and the meninges with the larval stage of *Taenia solium*, is the most common helminthic infection of the CNS worldwide and is endemic in most Latin American countries, sub-Saharan Africa and large regions of Asia [43]. Cysticerci develop in (intraparenchymal NCC) and around (extraparenchymal NCC) the CNS—the most common reasons for presentation are epilepsy and intracranial hypertension [44]. Diagnosis of NCC is often difficult in low-resource settings and criteria constitute a mix of findings on history and examination, lumbar puncture, serology neuroimaging and response to cysticercal drugs. Treatment is with anthelmintic therapy.

20.6.1 Intracranial Hypertension in Neurocysticercosis

Intracranial hypertension can be caused by arachnoiditis, granular ependymitis, mass effect of cysts located in basal subarachnoidal cisterns or obstruction of CSF pathway by ventricular cysts [15]. To our knowledge, no studies using neurosonology to diagnose and/or monitor intracranial hypertension in NCC patients have been published to date and this is a potential avenue for research in regions where the disease is endemic.

20.6.2 Vasculopathy in NCC

NCC-related stroke causes considerable morbidity and mortality—in areas where it is endemic, up to 10% of strokes in the population may be due to NCC [45]. Cysticerci release immunomodulators to dampen the host's local inflammatory response to their presence [46]. When the parasites die, the host's response is no longer restricted and the inflammatory cascade that ensues results in arachnoiditis. Histopathology demonstrates an inflammatory arteriopathy in vessels adjacent to the degenerating parasite, known in the literature as 'cysticercal arteritis' [46]. Approximately 6% of all patients with symptomatic NCC have angiographic evidence of cysticercal arteritis [47], although this increases to 21–53% in the presence of subarachnoid cysticercosis [47, 48]. The middle cerebral artery and posterior cerebral artery are most commonly affected. NCC-related stroke can be classified into four main groups: focal NCC with small vessel involvement, focal NCC with large vessel involvement, diffuse NCC with small vessel involvement and diffuse NCC with large vessel involvement [46]. Small vessel involvement is defined as normal angiographic findings; large vessel involvement is defined as angiographic or TCD evidence of narrowing or occlusion of intracranial arteries.

Cantu et al. published a case series on the use of TCD in the evaluation of nine patients with subarachnoid cysticercosis and stroke [49]. Four patients had a stenotic pattern in a major intracranial vessel on TCD examination and two had an occlusive pattern. Of these, three patients with stenotic patterns had resolved at follow-up TCD following discharge but both patients with occlusive patterns had persistent occlusion. Of note, of the three cases with a lacunar infarct on MRI, both cerebral angiography and TCD examination were normal. On the basis of these existing findings in the literature, Marquez and Arauz have proposed diagnostic criteria for NCC-related stroke, which require evidence of cysticercal arteritis [46] for which suggestive findings on TCD examination (increased peak systolic velocity in a vessel supplying an ischaemic region or, when diffuse NCC is present, in any vessel) are considered an acceptable indicator.

Early diagnosis and subsequent monitoring of cysticercotic arteritis are important, as commencement of steroids can reverse clinical deterioration [50] by reducing the local inflammatory response affecting the meninges and blood vessels elicited by the degenerating parasite [51].

20.7 Cerebral Malaria

Over 200 million cases of malaria occur per year and greater than 400,000 of these cases are fatal [52]. The vast majority of these cases occur in sub-Saharan Africa in children under the age of 5. Severe malaria can be defined as a confirmed malarial infection in the presence of one or more of a series of conditions, including impaired consciousness, acidosis, hyperlactaemia, hypoglycaemia, severe anaemia, acute kidney injury, jaundice, pulmonary oedema, significant bleeding, hyperparasitaemia or shock. Cerebral malaria (CM) is the most devastating manifestation of severe malaria and is one of the most common non-traumatic encephalopathies in the world [53]. Evidence from autopsy studies suggests that adhesion of parasitised erythrocytes (PEs) to the microvascular endothelium leading to their sequestration in microvessels is the pathological hallmark of adult and paediatric CM [54, 55]. CM can be defined clinically as coma in the presence of a peripheral *Plasmodium falciparum* parasitaemia in the absence of another identifiable cause of coma [56]. However, approximately one-quarter of patients meeting this clinical definition do not have evidence of sequestration of parasitised RBCs at autopsy [55]. Impaired consciousness in the context of severe malaria may be due to other causes such as a prolonged postictal state following febrile seizure or metabolic derangements such as acidosis or hypoglycaemia [57]. More recently, the presence of malarial retinopathy has been suggested as an important diagnostic sign for paediatric CM [58]. Malarial retinopathy accurately predicts the degree of sequestration of parasitised red blood cells (PRBCs) in the cerebral microvasculature [55, 59], presence of brain haemorrhages [60] and prognosis [61]. As such, it has been proposed that retinopathy-positive (RN-positive) paediatric CM is a distinct entity in which neurovascular disturbance is a characteristic component of the pathophysiology of the disease. Mortality from retinopathy-positive (RN-positive) paediatric CM remains high at approximately 14% [62] despite appropriate treatment with artesunate. Moreover, approximately one-third of survivors of RN-positive paediatric CM will develop long-term neurological sequelae, including epilepsy, motor, sensory or language deficits [63]. Despite this, the pathophysiology of paediatric CM remains poorly understood and few adjunctive therapies to antimalarials have been developed that are successful in improving the outcome [64].

20.7.1 Raised Intracranial Pressure in Paediatric CM

All children with paediatric CM develop intracranial hypertension and intracranial hypertension has been associated with a less favourable outcome in paediatric CM [65]. Intracranial hypertension (ICH) has been demonstrated in African children by raised cerebrospinal fluid (CSF) opening pressure on lumbar puncture (LP) [66–68] and intraparenchymal intracranial pressure (ICP) monitoring [65]. The pathophysiology of ICH in paediatric CM remains unclear. Increased brain volume has previously been demonstrated in African children using CT (defined as loss of CSF spaces) [69] and MRI [70]. Various mechanisms have been proposed for this increased brain volume, including vasogenic oedema due to blood-brain barrier (BBB) breakdown [71, 72], cytotoxic oedema from impaired perfusion leading to cell death [73], sequestration of PRBCs in postcapillary venules leading to obstruction and vascular congestion [54], diffuse cerebral microhaemorrhages [72] and hyperaemia due to seizures, anaemia and/or fever leading to autoregulatory dysfunction.

Like TBM and CrM, ICP monitoring and LP are often unavailable in the regions where paediatric CM is most prevalent and optic nerve sheath diameter (ONSD) on ultrasound has been investigated as a possible alternative. Beare et al. scanned 112 Malawian children, 101 with retinopathy-positive cerebral malaria and 11 with malaria and impaired consciousness [74]. An ONSD of 4.3 mm or more was considered abnormal, based on normative values previously established in this population [75]. ONSD was found to predict morbidity but not mortality in paediatric CM and did not detect raised ICP as frequently as OP on LP. Murphy et al. performed scans on 30 Ugandan children with severe malaria (including cerebral malaria, based on the WHO definition) [76]. All children with CM had raised ONSD and raised ONSD was associated with a diagnosis of CM relative to other severe malarial syndromes. A relatively inexpensive, non-invasive method of detecting intracranial hypertension could be of great value in diagnosing raised ICP in paediatric CM in low-resource settings and thereby helping develop adjunct therapies. In addition, it may help distinguish patients with paediatric CM from those with severe malarial syndromes and impaired consciousness due to other pathologies (e.g., acidosis or electrolyte derangement).

20.7.2 Transcranial Doppler in Paediatric CM

Four authors have published their experience on the use of TCD in paediatric CM (see Table 20.3) [76–79]. The largest and most comprehensive study to date was published by O'Brien et al. in 2018—160 Congolese children with retinopathy-positive cerebral malaria and 155 comparison patients (severe malaria syndrome with no impaired consciousness) underwent TCD examination [77]. Based on findings on TCD examination, they stratified patients into five phenotypic groups—low flow, hyperaemia, microvascular obstruction, vasospasm and isolated posterior hyperaemia (Table 20.4). Low flow may be due to hypovolaemia (due to vomiting, reduced fluid input or insensible losses) or increased intracranial pressure (resulting in reduced cerebral perfusion pressure) and hyperaemia is found with

Table 20.3 Studies using TCD to evaluate vasculopathy related to paediatric CM

Author	Year	Country	Subjects	Comparison	Major findings
O'Brien [77]	2018	DRC	CM (WHO criteria) + malarial retinopathy No SCD, advanced HIV or severe malnutrition (n = 160)	Severe malaria with a BCS of 5 (*n* = 155)	Neurovascular changes in RN-positive CM can be categorised into five phenotypic groups: 1. Low flow (28%) 2. Hyperaemia (26%) 3. Microvascular obstruction (22%) 4. Vasospasm (13%) 5. Isolated posterior hyperaemia (4%) Impaired autoregulation (THRT) on day 1
Murphy [76]	2011	Uganda	Children hospitalised with malaria (*n* = 31) Subjects were then stratified into those with and without a severe malarial syndrome as defined by WHO criteria (SMA, CM, LA or respiratory distress syndrome with hypoxia)	None	6/31 subjects had mean blood flow velocity > 2 SD below published values for age (2 with CM, 1 with SMA and 3 with hospitalised malaria without severe malaria) 3/31 subjects had mean blood flow velocity > 2 SD above published values for age (all with SMA) Elevated PI in 2 patients with CM
Clavier [78]	1999	Benin	CM (WHO criteria)	1. SMA (WHO criteria) without impaired consciousness 2. Healthy outpatients	Peak systolic and diastolic flow velocity is statistically greater in CM and SMA patients relative to healthy controls
Newton [79]	1996	Kenya	CM (WHO criteria)	Healthy children, or those who had recently recovered from non-cerebral malaria or were anaemic	30% had documented evidence of increased cerebral blood flow velocity (CBFV) in the MCA 80% of the patients with paediatric CM surviving with a focal neurological deficit demonstrated evidence of abnormalities on TCD

Table 20.4 Phenotypic groups on TCD examination in paediatric CM as defined by O'Brien et al. [77]

Group	Findings on TCD examination
Microvascular obstruction	Normal systolic flow velocity Reduced diastolic flow velocity Increased PI
Hyperaemia	Increased systolic flow velocity Increased diastolic flow velocity Loss of dicrotic notch LR < 3
Vasospasm	Increased systolic flow velocity Increased diastolic flow velocity Presence of dicrotic notch LR > 3
Low flow	Decreased systolic flow velocity Decreased diastolic flow velocity Decreased mean flow velocity
Isolated posterior hyperaemia	Increased systolic flow velocity, increased diastolic flow velocity and increased mean flow velocity in the basilar artery All three measurements normal in both MCAs

seizures, fever or anaemia—all common physiological derangements in severe malarial syndromes. Microvascular obstruction is a histopathological hallmark of paediatric CM and the authors proposed that this pathological process is particularly prominent in this phenotypic group on TCD evaluation.

Thirteen percent of patients had TCD evidence of vasospasm. Autopsies of patients with cerebral malaria demonstrate morphological characteristics consistent with spastic constriction of arterioles in the cerebral microvasculature [80]. Moreover, in the murine model of CM, mice demonstrate evidence of widespread cerebral vasoconstriction [81, 82]. Interestingly, nimodipine (a calcium channel antagonist used to prevent subarachnoid haemorrhage-associated vasospasm) significantly improves survival in these mice. Akin to TBM, if vasospasm is implicated in the pathophysiology of paediatric CM and TCD can reliably identify it, this opens up the possibility of the investigation of TCD-guided adjunctive management for this pathological process.

Cerebrovascular autoregulation (CA) is the homeostatic process of regulation of cerebral blood flow (CBF) in response to changes in cerebral perfusion pressure (CPP). O'Brien et al. assessed CA using the transient hyperaemic response ratio (THRR)—autoregulation was impaired (THRR < 1.1) in the CM group and THRR was significantly lower than in the control group. Newton et al. found that in two Kenyan children with paediatric CM and severe intracranial hypertension (HTN—ICP >40 mmHg and cerebral perfusion pressure < 40 mmHg for >15 min), a linear relationship was observed between cerebral perfusion pressure (CPP) and flow velocity in the MCA, consistent with impaired autoregulation [79]. However, the same relationship was not observed in children with mild or moderate intracranial HTN leading the investigators to conclude that autoregulation was only impaired in a small proportion of paediatric CM patients with critically raised ICP. A recent MRI study in 16 Zambian retinopathy-positive paediatric CM patients who survived their illness without neurological deficit demonstrated symmetrical cortical swelling with underlying white matter changes [83], clinical and radiological findings consistent with posterior reversible encephalopathy syndrome (PRES). A similar study of 11 Indian survivors of CM (5 adults, 6 children) who also demonstrated a complete recovery without deficit showed evidence of vasogenic oedema in a predominantly posterior distribution, again consistent with PRES [84]. Interestingly, 4% of patients in O'Brien et al.'s cohort had TCD findings described as 'isolated posterior hyperaemia'—however, MRI scans were not performed in this study due to lack of facilities [77]. PRES is defined as a disorder of reversible subcortical vasogenic brain oedema in patients with acute neurological symptoms [85]. The pathophysiology of PRES (of any aetiology) remains unclear. Two prevailing theories have emerged [86], both of which suggest an impairment of cerebrovascular autoregulation. The first theory states that uncontrolled hypertension leads to cerebral hyperperfusion due to impaired cerebrovascular autoregulation. In the second, hypertension leads to an inappropriately excessive autoregulatory compensation in the form of cerebral vasoconstriction resulting in hypoperfusion, ischaemia and vasogenic oedema. The presence of clinical and radiological findings consistent with PRES in paediatric CM patients is further evidence for autoregulatory dysfunction in the pathophysiology of the disease.

20.8 Neurosonology in Non-infectious Diseases in Tropical Regions

20.8.1 Sickle Cell Anaemia

Stroke in SCD is associated with an occlusive vasculopathy involving the distal internal carotid artery and proximal anterior and middle cerebral arteries [87–89] and the risk of stroke is significantly higher in children with elevated time-averaged mean maximum blood flow velocity in major intracranial vessels on TCD examination [90, 91]. This led to the Stroke Prevention Trial in Sickle Cell Anemia (STOP), which demonstrated such a positive effect of chronic transfusion therapy (CTT) for the primary prevention of stroke in sickle cell disease patients with elevated cerebral blood flow velocities that the trial was stopped early by the study's data and safety monitoring board [92]. The use of TCD to guide the decision to institute transfusion therapy in SCD is now well established in high-income countries. In LMICs, chronic transfusion therapy is often not possible due to a lack of transfusion medicine services and prohibitive costs. Hydroxyurea is an alternative treatment and the TCD With Transfusions Changing to Hydroxyurea (TWiTCH) study demonstrated that hydroxyurea was not inferior to transfusions in the primary prevention of stroke in SCD in children with abnormal cerebral blood flow velocities who had been on CTT for at least 1 year [93]. Given the greater ease of access to hydroxyurea than CTT for patients in LMICs, a recent feasibility trial of hydroxyurea in Nigerian children with SCD and abnormal cerebral blood flow velocities was successfully conducted [94].

20.8.2 Hydrocephalus

There are estimated to be more than 383,000 cases of childhood hydrocephalus each year, with the majority of these cases occurring in Africa, Latin America and South East Asia [95] due to the high prevalence of meningitis and neural tube defects. The use of neurosonology for the diagnosis of hydrocephalus and shunt malfunction would potentially be of great value in these patients, where access to neuroimaging is unreliable. Furthermore, in the absence of expensive equipment intraoperative neuronavigation that is widespread in operating theatres in high-income countries, there is great potential for intraoperative ultrasound to assist surgeons in low-resource settings in ventricular catheterisation as well as other routine tasks such as tumour localisation in addition to the use of surface anatomy and craniometric measurements.

20.8.3 Traumatic Brain Injury

The Global Burden of Disease estimated that there were 27 million new cases of TBI worldwide in 2016, the majority of which occurred in LMICs [96]. The control of intracranial hypertension by invasive ICP monitoring remains the cornerstone of severe TBI management in high-income countries, based on the Brain Trauma Foundation guidelines [97]. As per the other pathologies discussed in this chapter, invasive ICP monitoring is not available in many low- and middle-income countries (LMICs) primarily due to its prohibitive cost. Moreover, the value of ICP monitoring in LMICs has been the subject of much discussion in the neurosurgical literature in recent years. The Benchmark Evidence from South American Trials: Treatment of Intracranial Pressure (BEST-TRIP) trial compared care guided by ICP monitoring to that guided by imaging and clinical examination (ICE) alone in six intensive care units in Bolivia and Ecuador [98]. They concluded that 'care focused on maintaining monitored intracranial pressure at 20 mm Hg or less was not shown to be superior to care based on imaging and clinical examination'.

However, the publication of the findings from BEST:TRIP and their interpretation prompted considerable debate in the literature and some have interpreted the trial as indicating that ICP monitoring has no role in low-resource settings. As such, a consensus-based interpretation was subsequently published by the authors [99]. Of note, one of the statements included was that the findings from the trial should be 'applied cautiously to regions with much different treatment milieu'. In consideration of this, it should be noted that there is considerable variability in the resources available for neurotrauma care between and even within LMICs. For example, many hospitals in sub-Saharan Africa and Asia do not have the capacity to perform serial CT scans on severe TBI patients or regularly administer neuroprotective treatments (such as mannitol, hypertonic saline or barbiturates) to them as was done in in the ICE arm of the study. Moreover, there is emerging evidence to suggest that ICP monitoring does add benefit in certain, specific settings in LMICs. A single-centre retrospective cohort study from Kerala in India found that ICP monitoring of severe TBI patients with diffuse brain injury was associated with a decreased need for neuroprotective management, radiation exposure and length of ICU stay [99]. In addition, improved functional outcome was observed at 1 month (although this was not observed at 3 and 6 months). As such, given the barriers to deploying ICP monitoring in many institutions in LMICs, an inexpensive, accurate method of estimating ICP may be of benefit in guiding treatment decisions in TBI in this population. To our knowledge, no studies have been published examining the utility of neurosonology in managing moderate and severe TBI in low-resource settings where ICP monitoring is unavailable but, at the time of publication, research projects are ongoing in Ethiopia and Zambia. This research area is one of the most promising potential applications of neurosonology in tropical medicine, especially as a means of augmenting existing clinical practise guidelines for moderate and severe TBI in LMICs which rely on imaging and clinical examination alone.

20.9 Implementation of Neurosonology in Health Systems in Low- and Middle-Income Countries

In this chapter, we have presented a number of possible applications of neurosonology in the diagnosis and monitoring of tropical diseases. As such, we propose that these techniques represent an exciting avenue for improving understanding of the pathobiological basis of these often neglected diseases and refining their management. However, prior to the implementation of a new technology in a hospital or clinic in a low-resource setting, a comprehensive needs assessment should be conducted and the impact on the health system considered in detail. Initial enthusiasm regarding the potential of new technology in low-resource settings can result in well-meaning clinicians and academics indirectly causing harm to already fragile health systems. For example, introduction of neurosonological methods as cheaper alternatives to invasive ICP monitoring in intensive care (which remains the gold standard) in an LMIC could have the unintended consequence of discouraging hospital administrators from acquiring intraparenchymal ICP probes in the future if and when funding does become available. Other practical considerations for implementation of medical equipment in low-resource environments, such as protecting delicate electronics from power surges and arrangements for repair when the equipment breaks down, are also extremely important. Finally, a plan for training of local staff (to such a level that they feel confident teaching others) is essential if the equipment is being donated by clinicians who are not permanently based in the country in which it will be used. The UK Tropical Health and Education Trust (THET) has produced a toolkit to help decide whether or not medical equipment donation is appropriate in these situations and how to do so effectively [100].

References

1. Rupali P. Introduction to tropical medicine. Infect Dis Clin N Am. 2019;33(1):1–15.
2. Feigin VL, Forouzanfar MH, Krishnamurthi R, Mensah GA, Connor M, Bennett DA, et al. Global and regional burden of stroke during 1990–2010: findings from the global burden of disease study 2010. Lancet. 2014;383(9913):245–54.
3. Benjamin LA, Corbett EL, Connor MD, Mzinganjira H, Kampondeni S, Choko A, et al. HIV, antiretroviral treatment, hypertension, and stroke in Malawian adults: a case-control study. Neurology. 2016;86(4):324–33.
4. Benjamin LA, Allain TJ, Mzinganjira H, Connor MD, Smith C, Lucas S, et al. The role of human immunodeficiency virus-associated vasculopathy in the etiology of stroke. J Infect Dis. 2017;216(5):545–53.
5. Connor M. Stroke in patients with human immunodeficiency virus infection. J Neurol Neurosurg Psychiatry. 2007;78(12):1291.
6. Benjamin LA, Bryer A, Lucas S, Stanley A, Allain TJ, Joekes E, et al. Arterial ischemic stroke in HIV: defining and classifying etiology for research studies. Neurol Neuroimmunol Neuroinflamm. 2016;3(4):e254.
7. Brilla R, Nabavi DG, Schulte-Altedorneburg G, Kemény V, Reichelt D, Evers S, et al. Cerebral vasculopathy in HIV infection revealed by transcranial Doppler: a pilot study. Stroke. 1999;30(4):811–3.
8. Chow FC, Boscardin WJ, Mills C, Ko N, Carroll C, Price RW, et al. Cerebral vasoreactivity is impaired in treated, virally suppressed HIV-infected individuals. AIDS. 2016;30(1):45–55.
9. WHO. Global tuberculosis report. 21st ed; 2016.
10. Wilkinson RJ, Rohlwink U, Misra UK, van Crevel R, Mai NTH, Dooley KE, et al. Tuberculous meningitis. Nat Rev Neurol. 2017;13(10):581–98.
11. Misra UK, Kalita J, Bhoi SK. Spectrum and outcome predictors of central nervous system infections in a neurological critical care unit in India: a retrospective review. Trans R Soc Trop Med Hyg. 2014;108(3):141–6.
12. Cantier M, Morisot A, Guérot E, Megarbane B, Razazi K, Contou D, et al. Functional outcomes in adults with tuberculous meningitis admitted to the ICU: a multicenter cohort study. Crit Care. 2018;22(1):210.
13. Visudhiphan P, Chiemchanya S. Hydrocephalus in tuberculous meningitis in children: treatment with acetazolamide and repeated lumbar puncture. J Pediatr. 1979;95(4):657–60.
14. Donovan J, Figaji A, Imran D, Phu NH, Rohlwink U, Thwaites GE. The neurocritical care of tuberculous meningitis. Lancet Neurol. 2019;18(8):771–83.
15. Thakur KT, Mateyo K, Hachaambwa L, Kayamba V, Mallewa M, Mallewa J, et al. Lumbar puncture refusal in sub-Saharan Africa: a call for further understanding and intervention. Neurology. 2015;84(19):1988–90.
16. Sangani SV, Parikh S. Can sonographic measurement of optic nerve sheath diameter be used to detect raised intracranial pressure in patients with tuberculous meningitis? A prospective observational study. Indian J Radiol Imaging. 2015;25(2):173–6.
17. Lammie GA, Hewlett RH, Schoeman JF, Donald PR. Tuberculous cerebrovascular disease: a review. J Infect. 2009;59(3):156–66.
18. Misra UK, Kalita J, Maurya PK. Stroke in tuberculous meningitis. J Neurol Sci. 2011;303(1–2):22–30.
19. Shukla R, Abbas A, Kumar P, Gupta RK, Jha S, Prasad KN. Evaluation of cerebral infarction in tuberculous meningitis by diffusion weighted imaging. J Infect. 2008;57(4):298–306.
20. Rojas-Echeverri LA, Soto-Hernández JL, Garza S, Martínez-Zubieta R, Miranda LI, García-Ramos G, et al. Predictive value of digital subtraction angiography in patients with tuberculous meningitis. Neuroradiology. 1996;38(1):20–4.
21. Nair PP, Kalita J, Kumar S, Misra UK. MRI pattern of infarcts in basal ganglia region in patients with tuberculous meningitis. Neuroradiology. 2009;51(4):221–5.
22. Hsieh FY, Chia LG, Shen WC. Locations of cerebral infarctions in tuberculous meningitis. Neuroradiology. 1992;34(3):197–9.
23. Dalal PM. Observations on the involvement of cerebral vessels in tuberculous meningitis in adults. Adv Neurol. 1979;25:149–59.
24. Lehrer H. The angiographic triad in tuberculous meningitis. A radiographic and clinicopathologic correlation. Radiology. 1966;87(5):829–35.
25. Mathew NT, Abraham J, Chandy J. Cerebral angiographic features in tuberculous meningitis. Neurology. 1970;20(10):1015–23.
26. Tai MS, Sharma VK. Role of transcranial Doppler in the evaluation of vasculopathy in tuberculous meningitis. PLoS One. 2016;11(10):e0164266.
27. van Toorn R, Schaaf HS, Solomons R, Laubscher JA, Schoeman JF. The value of transcranial Doppler imaging in children with tuberculous meningitis. Childs Nerv Syst. 2014;30(10):1711–6.
28. Gujjar AR, Srikanth SG, Umamaheshwara Rao GS. HHH regime for arteritis secondary to TB meningitis: a prospective randomized study. Neurocrit Care. 2009;10(3):313–7.
29. Lu CH, Chang WN, Chang HW, Chung KJ, Tsai NW, Lui CC, et al. Clinical relevance of intracranial arterial stenoses in tuberculous and cryptococcal meningitis. Infection. 2007;35(5):359–63.
30. Kiliç T, Elmaci I, Ozek MM, Pamir MN. Utility of transcranial Doppler ultrasonography in the diagnosis and follow-up of tuberculous meningitis-related vasculopathy. Childs Nerv Syst. 2002;18(3–4):142–6.
31. Williamson PR, Jarvis JN, Panackal AA, Fisher MC, Molloy SF, Loyse A, et al. Cryptococcal meningitis: epidemiology, immunology, diagnosis and therapy. Nat Rev Neurol. 2017;13(1):13–24.

32. Park BJ, Wannemuehler KA, Marston BJ, Govender N, Pappas PG, Chiller TM. Estimation of the current global burden of cryptococcal meningitis among persons living with HIV/AIDS. AIDS. 2009;23(4):525–30.
33. Jarvis JN, Bicanic T, Loyse A, Namarika D, Jackson A, Nussbaum JC, et al. Determinants of mortality in a combined cohort of 501 patients with HIV-associated cryptococcal meningitis: implications for improving outcomes. Clin Infect Dis. 2014;58(5):736–45.
34. Graybill JR, Sobel J, Saag M, van Der Horst C, Powderly W, Cloud G, et al. Diagnosis and management of increased intracranial pressure in patients with AIDS and cryptococcal meningitis. The NIAID Mycoses Study Group and AIDS Cooperative Treatment Groups. Clin Infect Dis. 2000;30(1):47–54.
35. Perfect JR, Dismukes WE, Dromer F, Goldman DL, Graybill JR, Hamill RJ, et al. Clinical practice guidelines for the management of cryptococcal disease: 2010 update by the Infectious Diseases Society of America. Clin Infect Dis. 2010;50(3):291–322.
36. Manosuthi W, Sungkanuparph S, Chottanapund S, Tansuphaswadikul S, Chimsuntorn S, Limpanadusadee P, et al. Temporary external lumbar drainage for reducing elevated intracranial pressure in HIV-infected patients with cryptococcal meningitis. Int J STD AIDS. 2008;19(4):268–71.
37. Macsween KF, Bicanic T, Brouwer AE, Marsh H, Macallan DC, Harrison TS. Lumbar drainage for control of raised cerebrospinal fluid pressure in cryptococcal meningitis: case report and review. J Infect. 2005;51(4):e221–4.
38. Nabeta HW, Bahr NC, Rhein J, Fossland N, Kiragga AN, Meya DB, et al. Accuracy of noninvasive intraocular pressure or optic nerve sheath diameter measurements for predicting elevated intracranial pressure in cryptococcal meningitis. Open Forum Infect Dis. 2014;1(3):ofu093.
39. Mishra AK, Arvind VH, Muliyil D, Kuriakose CK, George AA, Karuppusami R, et al. Cerebrovascular injury in cryptococcal meningitis. Int J Stroke. 2018;13(1):57–65.
40. Lan SH, Chang WN, Lu CH, Lui CC, Chang HW. Cerebral infarction in chronic meningitis: a comparison of tuberculous meningitis and cryptococcal meningitis. QJM. 2001;94(5):247–53.
41. Tjia TL, Yeow YK, Tan CB. Cryptococcal meningitis. J Neurol Neurosurg Psychiatry. 1985;48(9):853–8.
42. Chang WN, Lu CH, Chang HW, Lui CC, Tsai NW, Huang CR, et al. Time course of cerebral hemodynamics in cryptococcal meningitis in HIV-negative adults. Eur J Neurol. 2007;14(7):770–6.
43. Garcia HH, Nash TE, Del Brutto OH. Clinical symptoms, diagnosis, and treatment of neurocysticercosis. Lancet Neurol. 2014;13(12):1202–15.
44. Garcia HH, Del Brutto OH, Peru CWGi. Neurocysticercosis: updated concepts about an old disease. Lancet Neurol. 2005;4(10):653–61.
45. Alarcón F, Hidalgo F, Moncayo J, Viñán I, Dueñas G. Cerebral cysticercosis and stroke. Stroke. 1992;23(2):224–8.
46. Marquez JM, Arauz A. Cerebrovascular complications of neurocysticercosis. Neurologist. 2012;18(1):17–22.
47. Cantú C, Barinagarrementeria F. Cerebrovascular complications of neurocysticercosis. Clinical and neuroimaging spectrum. Arch Neurol. 1996;53(3):233–9.
48. Barinagarrementeria F, Cantú C. Frequency of cerebral arteritis in subarachnoid cysticercosis: an angiographic study. Stroke. 1998;29(1):123–5.
49. Cantú C, Villarreal J, Soto JL, Barinagarrementeria F. Cerebral cysticercotic arteritis: detection and follow-up by transcranial Doppler. Cerebrovasc Dis. 1998;8(1):2–7.
50. Bouldin A, Pinter JD. Resolution of arterial stenosis in a patient with periarterial neurocysticercosis treated with oral prednisone. J Child Neurol. 2006;21(12):1064–7.
51. Mahanty S, Garcia HH. Perú CWGi. Cysticercosis and neurocysticercosis as pathogens affecting the nervous system. Prog Neurobiol. 2010;91(2):172–84.
52. WHO. World malaria report. Geneva: WHO; 2015.
53. Mishra SK, Newton CR. Diagnosis and management of the neurological complications of falciparum malaria. Nat Rev Neurol. 2009;5(4):189–98.
54. Ponsford MJ, Medana IM, Prapansilp P, Hien TT, Lee SJ, Dondorp AM, et al. Sequestration and microvascular congestion are associated with coma in human cerebral malaria. J Infect Dis. 2012;205(4):663–71.
55. Taylor TE, Fu WJ, Carr RA, Whitten RO, Mueller JS, Fosiko NG, et al. Differentiating the pathologies of cerebral malaria by postmortem parasite counts. Nat Med. 2004;10(2):143–5.
56. Newton CR, Taylor TE, Whitten RO. Pathophysiology of fatal falciparum malaria in African children. Am J Trop Med Hyg. 1998;58(5):673–83.
57. Allen S, O'Donnell A, Alexander N. Causes of coma in children with malaria in Papua New Guinea. Lancet. 1996;348(9035):1168–9.
58. Beare NA, Taylor TE, Harding SP, Lewallen S, Molyneux ME. Malarial retinopathy: a newly established diagnostic sign in severe malaria. Am J Trop Med Hyg. 2006;75(5):790–7.
59. Barrera V, Hiscott PS, Craig AG, White VA, Milner DA, Beare NA, et al. Severity of retinopathy parallels the degree of parasite sequestration in the eyes and brains of Malawian children with fatal cerebral malaria. J Infect Dis. 2015;211(12):1977–86.
60. White VA, Lewallen S, Beare N, Kayira K, Carr RA, Taylor TE. Correlation of retinal haemorrhages with brain haemorrhages in children dying of cerebral malaria in Malawi. Trans R Soc Trop Med Hyg. 2001;95(6):618–21.
61. Beare NA, Southern C, Chalira C, Taylor TE, Molyneux ME, Harding SP. Prognostic significance

and course of retinopathy in children with severe malaria. Arch Ophthalmol. 2004;122(8):1141–7.
62. Villaverde C, Namazzi R, Shabani E, Opoka RO, John CC. Clinical comparison of retinopathy-positive and retinopathy-negative cerebral malaria. Am J Trop Med Hyg. 2017;96(5):1176–84.
63. Birbeck GL, Molyneux ME, Kaplan PW, Seydel KB, Chimalizeni YF, Kawaza K, et al. Blantyre Malaria Project Epilepsy Study (BMPES) of neurological outcomes in retinopathy-positive paediatric cerebral malaria survivors: a prospective cohort study. Lancet Neurol. 2010;9(12):1173–81.
64. Varo R, Crowley VM, Sitoe A, Madrid L, Serghides L, Kain KC, et al. Adjunctive therapy for severe malaria: a review and critical appraisal. Malar J. 2018;17(1):47.
65. Newton CR, Crawley J, Sowumni A, Waruiru C, Mwangi I, English M, et al. Intracranial hypertension in Africans with cerebral malaria. Arch Dis Child. 1997;76(3):219–26.
66. Newton CR, Kirkham FJ, Winstanley PA, Pasvol G, Peshu N, Warrell DA, et al. Intracranial pressure in African children with cerebral malaria. Lancet. 1991;337(8741):573–6.
67. Schmutzhard E, Gerstenbrand F. Cerebral malaria in Tanzania. Its epidemiology, clinical symptoms and neurological long term sequelae in the light of 66 cases. Trans R Soc Trop Med Hyg. 1984;78(3):351–3.
68. Thapa BR, Marwaha RK, Kumar L, Mehta S. Cerebral malaria in children: therapeutic considerations. Indian Pediatr. 1988;25(1):61–5.
69. Newton CR, Peshu N, Kendall B, Kirkham FJ, Sowunmi A, Waruiru C, et al. Brain swelling and ischaemia in Kenyans with cerebral malaria. Arch Dis Child. 1994;70(4):281–7.
70. Seydel KB, Kampondeni SD, Valim C, Potchen MJ, Milner DA, Muwalo FW, et al. Brain swelling and death in children with cerebral malaria. N Engl J Med. 2015;372(12):1126–37.
71. Brown H, Rogerson S, Taylor T, Tembo M, Mwenechanya J, Molyneux M, et al. Blood-brain barrier function in cerebral malaria in Malawian children. Am J Trop Med Hyg. 2001;64(3–4):207–13.
72. Dorovini-Zis K, Schmidt K, Huynh H, Fu W, Whitten RO, Milner D, et al. The neuropathology of fatal cerebral malaria in Malawian children. Am J Pathol. 2011;178(5):2146–58.
73. Beare NA, Harding SP, Taylor TE, Lewallen S, Molyneux ME. Perfusion abnormalities in children with cerebral malaria and malarial retinopathy. J Infect Dis. 2009;199(2):263–71.
74. Beare NA, Glover SJ, Lewallen S, Taylor TE, Harding SP, Molyneux ME. Prevalence of raised intracranial pressure in cerebral malaria detected by optic nerve sheath ultrasound. Am J Trop Med Hyg. 2012;87(6):985–8.
75. Beare NA, Kampondeni S, Glover SJ, Molyneux E, Taylor TE, Harding SP, et al. Detection of raised intracranial pressure by ultrasound measurement of optic nerve sheath diameter in African children. Tropical Med Int Health. 2008;13(11):1400–4.
76. Murphy S, Cserti-Gazdewich C, Dhabangi A, Musoke C, Nabukeera-Barungi N, Price D, et al. Ultrasound findings in Plasmodium falciparum malaria: a pilot study. Pediatr Crit Care Med. 2011;12(2):e58–63.
77. O'Brien NF, Mutatshi Taty T, Moore-Clingenpeel M, Bodi Mabiala J, Mbaka Pongo J, Ambitapio Musungufu D, et al. Transcranial Doppler ultrasonography provides insights into neurovascular changes in children with cerebral malaria. J Pediatr. 2018;203:116-24.e3.
78. Clavier N, Rahimy C, Falanga P, Ayivi B, Payen D. No evidence for cerebral hypoperfusion during cerebral malaria. Crit Care Med. 1999;27(3):628–32.
79. Newton CR, Marsh K, Peshu N, Kirkham FJ. Perturbations of cerebral hemodynamics in Kenyans with cerebral malaria. Pediatr Neurol. 1996;15(1):41–9.
80. Polder TW, Jerusalem CR, Eling WM. Morphological characteristics of intracerebral arterioles in clinical (Plasmodium falciparum) and experimental (plasmodium berghei) cerebral malaria. J Neurol Sci. 1991;101(1):35–46.
81. Cabrales P, Zanini GM, Meays D, Frangos JA, Carvalho LJ. Murine cerebral malaria is associated with a vasospasm-like microcirculatory dysfunction, and survival upon rescue treatment is markedly increased by nimodipine. Am J Pathol. 2010;176(3):1306–15.
82. Martins YC, Clemmer L, Orjuela-Sánchez P, Zanini GM, Ong PK, Frangos JA, et al. Slow and continuous delivery of a low dose of nimodipine improves survival and electrocardiogram parameters in rescue therapy of mice with experimental cerebral malaria. Malar J. 2013;12:138.
83. Potchen MJ, Kampondeni SD, Seydel KB, Haacke EM, Sinyangwe SS, Mwenechanya M, et al. 1.5 tesla magnetic resonance imaging to investigate potential etiologies of brain swelling in pediatric cerebral malaria. Am J Trop Med Hyg. 2018:98, 497.
84. Mohanty S, Benjamin LA, Majhi M, Panda P, Kampondeni S, Sahu PK, et al. Magnetic resonance imaging of cerebral malaria patients reveals distinct pathogenetic processes in different parts of the brain. mSphere. 2017;2(3)
85. Fugate JE, Rabinstein AA. Posterior reversible encephalopathy syndrome: clinical and radiological manifestations, pathophysiology, and outstanding questions. Lancet Neurol. 2015;14(9):914–25.
86. Bartynski WS. Posterior reversible encephalopathy syndrome, part 2: controversies surrounding pathophysiology of vasogenic edema. AJNR Am J Neuroradiol. 2008;29(6):1043–9.
87. Stockman JA, Nigro MA, Mishkin MM, Oski FA. Occlusion of large cerebral vessels in sickle-cell anemia. N Engl J Med. 1972;287(17):846–9.
88. Merkel KH, Ginsberg PL, Parker JC, Post MJ. Cerebrovascular disease in sickle cell anemia:

a clinical, pathological and radiological correlation. Stroke. 1978;9(1):45–52.
89. Boros L, Thomas C, Weiner WJ. Large cerebral vessel disease in sickle cell anaemia. J Neurol Neurosurg Psychiatry. 1976;39(12):1236–9.
90. Adams RJ, McKie VC, Carl EM, Nichols FT, Perry R, Brock K, et al. Long-term stroke risk in children with sickle cell disease screened with transcranial Doppler. Ann Neurol. 1997;42(5):699–704.
91. Adams R, McKie V, Nichols F, Carl E, Zhang DL, McKie K, et al. The use of transcranial ultrasonography to predict stroke in sickle cell disease. N Engl J Med. 1992;326(9):605–10.
92. Adams RJ, McKie VC, Hsu L, Files B, Vichinsky E, Pegelow C, et al. Prevention of a first stroke by transfusions in children with sickle cell anemia and abnormal results on transcranial Doppler ultrasonography. N Engl J Med. 1998;339(1):5–11.
93. Sarnaik SA, Lusher JM. Neurological complications of sickle cell anemia. Am J Pediatr Hematol Oncol. 1982;4(4):386–94.
94. Galadanci NA, Umar Abdullahi S, Vance LD, Musa Tabari A, Ali S, Belonwu R, et al. Feasibility trial for primary stroke prevention in children with sickle cell anemia in Nigeria (SPIN trial). Am J Hematol. 2018;93(3):E83.
95. Dewan MC, Rattani A, Mekary R, Glancz LJ, Yunusa I, Baticulon RE, et al. Global hydrocephalus epidemiology and incidence: systematic review and meta-analysis. J Neurosurg. 2018:1–15.
96. Collaborators GTBIaSCI. Global, regional, and national burden of traumatic brain injury and spinal cord injury, 1990-2016: a systematic analysis for the global burden of disease study 2016. Lancet Neurol. 2019;18(1):56–87.
97. Smart LR, Mangat HS, Issarow B, McClelland P, Mayaya G, Kanumba E, et al. Severe traumatic brain injury at a tertiary referral center in Tanzania: epidemiology and adherence to brain trauma foundation guidelines. World Neurosurg. 2017;105:238.
98. Chesnut RM, Temkin N, Carney N, Dikmen S, Rondina C, Videtta W, et al. A trial of intracranial-pressure monitoring in traumatic brain injury. N Engl J Med. 2012;367(26):2471–81.
99. Vora TK, Karunakaran S, Kumar A, Chiluka A, Srinivasan H, Parmar K, et al. Intracranial pressure monitoring in diffuse brain injury-why the developing world needs it more? Acta Neurochir. 2018;160(6):1291–9.
100. THET. Making It Work - A toolkit for medical equipment donations to low-resource settings. https://www.thet.org/wp-content/uploads/2017/08/THET_MakingItWork_Toolkit_Final_Online.pdf; 2013.

Part VII

Pathology and Clinical Applications: Specific Considerations

21 Pediatric Population (Pathology and Clinical Applications: Specific Considerations)

Llewellyn C. Padayachy

Contents

21.1 Introduction

The use of ultrasound in pediatric neurosurgery has gained increasing popularity in recent years. The improvement in image quality and the convenience of portable, bedside diagnostic capability, combined with the radiation-free benefit of ultrasound imaging, have all contributed to the resurgence of its use. In neonates especially, patency of the anterior fontanelle provides a sonographic window to the brain. In particular, children with conditions like hydrocephalus, congenital cystic lesions, intraventricular hemorrhage, vascular abnormalities, tumors, and intracranial infections can be imaged and followed up using transcranial sonography. Further, ultrasound guidance has been used to assist certain therapeutic interventions, like insertion of intracranial catheters and aspiration of intracranial collections. Intraoperative ultrasound guidance as a real-time navigation adjunct can provide valuable information to the neurosurgeon. Additionally transorbital imaging, specifically of the optic nerve sheath diameter (ONSD) and transcranial Doppler sonography, has been used as a noninvasive marker of intracranial pressure (ICP) in children (1-Padayachy, 2-Robba). These applications have been used mostly in the intensive care unit (ICU) for bedside diagnosis and for follow-up, post-treatment in patients with raised ICP. These techniques also have definite value in the emergency unit and prehospital emergency context as screening tools for raised ICP. The

L. C. Padayachy (✉)
Department of Neurosurgery, School of Medicine, Faculty of Health Sciences, University of Pretoria, Steve Biko Academic Hospital, Pretoria, South Africa
e-mail: l.padayachy@uct.ac.za

C. Robba, G. Citerio (eds.), *Echography and Doppler of the Brain*,
https://doi.org/10.1007/978-3-030-48202-2_21

applications of ultrasound in the pediatric population with neurological and neurosurgical disease therefore include diagnostic techniques, image-guided interventions, and even intraoperative navigation.

21.2 Diagnostic Techniques

21.2.1 Transcranial Doppler Sonography (TCD)

TCD measures the velocity of blood flow through major intracranial vessels by emitting high-frequency (>2 MHz) sound waves and detecting the frequency shift between the incident and reflected waves. This difference directly correlates with the speed of blood flow (the Doppler effect) [1, 2].

TCD has been used to measure cerebral blood flow (CBF) velocity in the circle of Willis and the vertebrobasilar system, both diagnostically and to adjust treatment strategies in neurovascular disease and raised ICP [3–5]. The parameters assessed include peak systolic and diastolic velocity, mean velocity, resistance index (RI), and pulsatility index (PI). The measurements are usually taken over regions of the skull with the thinnest bony windows, i.e., the temporal region, through the eye, and at the back of the head. A recent study in children found TCD to be an excellent first-line examination for identifying patients likely to need invasive ICP monitoring, while another study, also in children with severe traumatic brain injury, found the PI to be a less reliable indicator of absolute ICP values [6, 7]. TCD remains an attractive alternative to invasive ICP because of its ability to detect cerebral ischemia, relative cost-effectiveness, and widespread availability. It is however limited by the requirement for trained operators and user variability. Two-depth TCD assessment has also demonstrated a good relationship with ICP, but also has certain limitations in accurately reflecting ICP [8].

21.2.2 Transorbital Imaging

The early work by Helmke and Hansen [9] investigating transorbital ultrasound imaging of the optic nerve sheath (ONS) in children still remains fundamental to our understanding of this technique [10–12]. Despite several studies demonstrating a good relationship with ICP, a lack of consensus regarding the optimal age-related ONSD cutoff value in children has been a shortcoming of the technique [13]. Recommendations for the ONSD measurement cutoff values in children include the folowing:

- More than 5 mm in children older than 4 years and more than 4 mm in children under the age 4 years that are considered definitely enlarged have been widely used [9].
- Greater than 4 mm in children under 1 year and greater than 4.5 mm in older children should be considered abnormal [14].
- Normal ONSD values of 4.0 mm in children under the age of 1 year and 4.5 mm in children over the age of 1 year [15].
- A mean ONSD value of 5.6 ± 0.6 mm in symptomatic children compared to 3.3 ± 0.6 mm in a control group [16].
- A cutoff point of 4.2 mm with a sensitivity of 100% and specificity of 86%, as the upper limit of normal, with measurements ≥4.5 mm indicative of raised ICP [17]

McAuley et al. suggested that repeat ONSD measurements were more useful in detecting raised ICP, especially in children with hydrocephalus [18]. This approach appears to be very sensible given the inter-individual variation in baseline ONSD measurements and our limited understanding of the elastic properties of the ONS (Fig. 21.1a,b). Steinborn et al. recently reported higher ONSD cutoff values than previously reported, suggesting that better high-resolution ultrasound imaging provided a better understanding of the ultrastructure of the optic nerve sheath complex [19]. A distinct limitation with most of these studies has been the lack of comparison between ONSD and the gold standard of invasive ICP measurement.

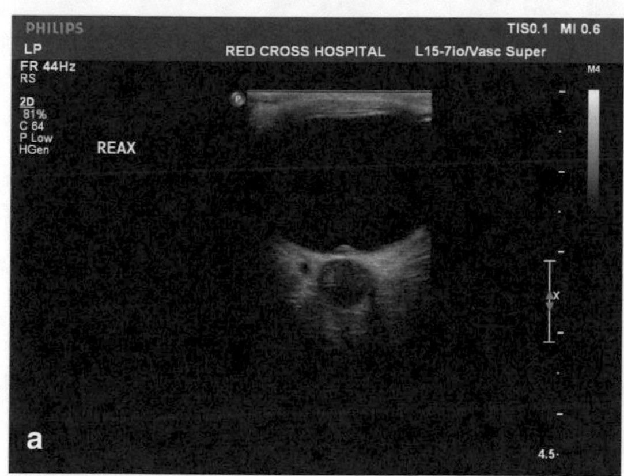

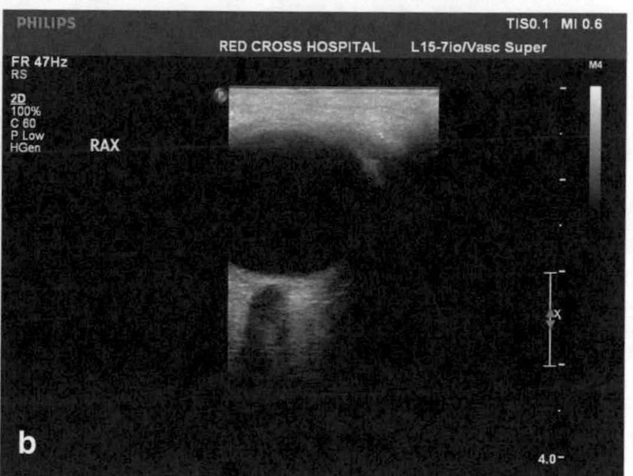

Fig. 21.1 (**a**) Axial image of the optic nerve sheath in a pediatric patient with raised intracranial pressure, demonstrating herniation of the optic nerve head into the globe, consistent with papilledema and a widened optic nerve sheath diameter. (**b**) Axial image of the optic nerve sheath in a pediatric patient after treatment for raised ICP, demonstrating resolution of the optic nerve head herniation, and reduction in the optic nerve sheath diameter

In the largest study to date in children, examining the relationship between ONSD measurement and invasive ICP readings, Padayachy et al. described the following ONSD values with the best diagnostic accuracy in children with a closed anterior fontanelle [20, 21]:

- ICP >5 mmHg: 5 mm,
- ICP >10 mmHg: 5.2 mm,
- ICP > 15 mmHg: 5.5 mm,
- ICP >20 mmHg: 5.8 mm [20, 21].

The current limitations of ONSD measurement in children relate to a lack of consistency in the literature [10, 14, 15, 19–21]. Most studies only compare ONSD measurement to other noninvasive, surrogate markers of ICP and as such make the recommendation for a standardised cut-off value for ONSD quite complicated. In children, the age-related variation further makes interpretation of the ONSD cut-off values even more challenging.

ONSD measurement has also demonstrated a poorer relationship with shunt failure prediction in pediatric hydrocephalus. Invasive ICP measurement using lumbar puncture CSF pressure also differs from direct intracranial ICP measurement, making comparison between noninvasive and invasive techniques in this context, quite difficult [22].

In an effort to address some of these limitations in diagnostic accuracy, recent studies have combined ONSD measurement with dynamic parameters like venous TCD [23] and deformability of the ONS as a marker of its stiffness [24, 25]. Improved diagnostic accuracy is essential for the widespread use of any noninvasive technique, and novel approaches to these issues are required.

21.2.3 Transcranial Imaging

Transcranial sonography provides an attractive imaging modality in the neonatal ICU, as it is less expensive, free from radiation, and portable. Access to magnetic resonance imaging (MRI) is not often limited, especially in resource-limited environments and for unstable and critically ill patients who cannot be transported from the ICU. Most centers have ultrasound machines, making access to this imaging modality widely available [26]. Linear-array, high-frequency probes are useful for scanning through the patent fontanelle, but require a detailed, multiplanar understanding of the intracranial anatomy, as well as the relevant intracranial pathology, particularly in the sagittal and coronal planes. Alternate sonographic windows include the temporal, mastoid, and lambdoid views. Exquisite

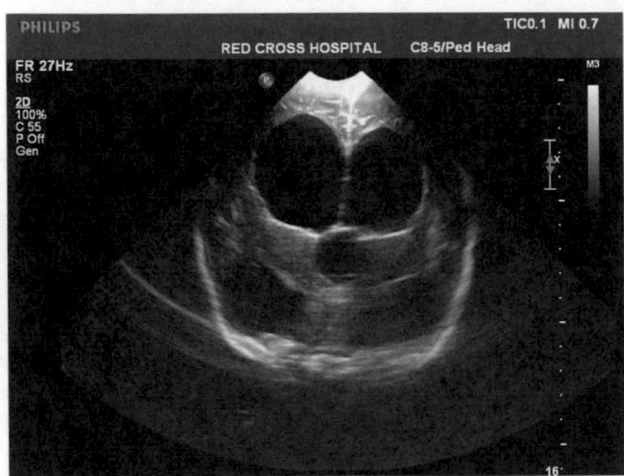

Fig. 21.2 Coronal image demonstrating marked ventriculomegaly, involving both lateral ventricles, frontal and occipital horns, as well as the third ventricle

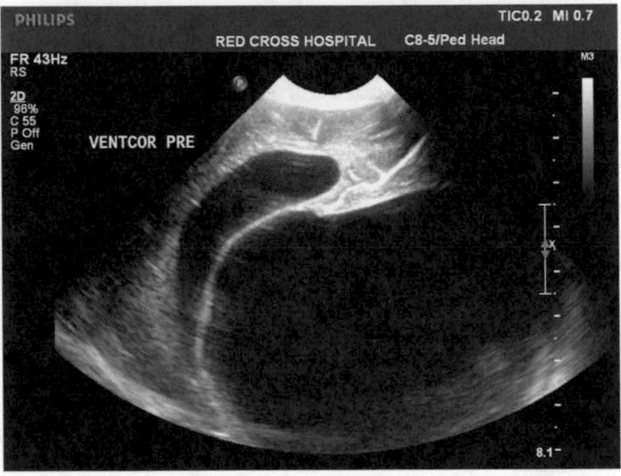

Fig. 21.3 Coronal image demonstrating a large intraventricular cyst displacing the midline and causing contralateral entrapment hydrocephalus

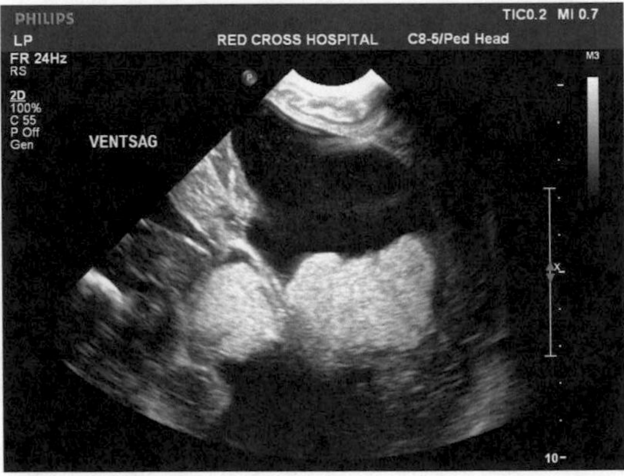

Fig. 21.4 Coronal image demonstrating a large, bilobar, hyperechogenic mass within the lateral ventricle, arising from the choroid plexus

detail and rapid diagnosis in conditions like hydrocephalus (Figs. 21.2 and 21.3), intracranial tumors (Fig. 21.4), hemorrhage, congenital anomalies, infections, hypoxic-ischemic damage, and vascular malformations underscore the value of transcranial ultrasound and Doppler as a bedside diagnostic tool [27, 28].

Published guidelines and the ALARA (as low as reasonably achievable) principle define thermal and mechanical indices which are generally accepted as safe [29]. The correct and most effective use of ultrasound in pediatric neurosurgery requires appropriate training and once the user is comfortable and more acquianted with the unique imaging techniques and the interpretation of these planes and images, ultrasound provides a very useful and safe imaging modality.

21.3 Image-Guided Therapeutic Interventions

Ultrasound provides exquisite image guidance at the bedside for diagnostic and therapeutic interventions, like insertion of ventricular catheters and drainage of accessible intracranial collections, and for monitoring of post-intervention progress. In conditions like hydrocephalus secondary to myelomeningocele, where serial measurement of ventricular size is required, and performing ventricular taps as a temporizing measure in case of infection, ultrasound provides an invaluable option for early management. Limiting the exposure of the developing brain to high doses of radiation from repeat CT scans is a further benefit in the pediatric population.

21.4 Intraoperative Navigation

Use of intraoperative ultrasound as a real-time navigation tool has also gained increased favor amongst neurosurgeons. Guidance and delineation of tumor resection margins, placement of ventricular catheters, endoscopic procedures, and surgery for vascular malformations are a few of the described indications. The improved quality of ultrasound images and ease of acquisition due to advances in probe technology have been important factors in the resurgence of this imaging modality. Further refinement of imaging quality and techniques through the development of higher resolution, purpose-designed probes, as well as advances in acoustic coupling fluid and techniques to sterilise and use certain probes will certainly make the widespread use of intraoperative ultrasound more attractive.

The diversity of applications for ultrasound as a bedside diagnostic and navigation tool in the pediatric population makes it very appealing indeed. A wide spectrum of intracranial pathology in the infant and neonatal group especially, can be well demonstrated through the patent anterior fontanelle. Image guidance for minor bedside therapeutic interventions as well as intraoperative guidance from real-time navigation further underscores the incredible value of this adjunctive imaging modality.

References

1. Lupetin AR, Davis DA, Beckham I, Dash N. Transcranial Doppler Sonography. Part 1. Principles, technique and normal appearances. Radiographics. 1995;15(1):179–91.
2. Aaslid R, Markwalder TM, Nornes H. Noninvasive intracranial Doppler ultrasound recording of flow velocity in the basal cerebral arteries. J Neurosurg. 1982;57:769–74.
3. Bellner J, Romner B, Reinstrup P, et al. Transcranial Doppler sonography pulsatility index (PI) reflects intracranial pressure (ICP). Surg Neurol. 2004;62(1):45–51.
4. Adams RJ. TCD in sickle cell disease: an important and useful test. Pediatr Radiol. 2005;35(3): 229–34.
5. Radolovich DK, Aries MJH, Castellani G, et al. Pulsatile intracranial pressure and cerebral autoregulation after traumatic brain injury. Neurocrit Care. 2011;15(3):379–86.
6. Melo JRT, Di Rocco F, Blanot S, et al. Transcranial Doppler can predict intracranial hypertension in children with severe traumatic brain injuries. Childs Nerv Syst. 2011;27(6):979–84.
7. Figaji A, Zwane E, Fieggen AG, Siesjo P, Peter JC. Transcranial Doppler pulsatility index is not a reliable indicator of intracranial pressure in children with severe traumatic brain injury. Surg Neurol. 2009;72(4):389–94.
8. Ragauskas A, Matijosaitis V, Zakelis R, et al. Clinical assessment of noninvasive intracranial pressure absolute value assessment method. Neurology. 2012;78(21):1684–91.
9. Helmke K, Hansen HC. Fundamentals of transorbital sonographic evaluation of optic nerve sheath expansion under intracranial hypertension. Pediatr Radiol. 1996;26(10):701–5.
10. Hansen HC, Helmke K. The subarachnoid space surrounding the optic nerves. An ultrasound study of the optic nerve sheath. Surg Radiol Anat. 1996;18(4):323–8.
11. Galetta S, Frazier BS, Smith JL. Echographic correlation of optic nerve sheath size and cerebrospinal fluid pressure. J Neuroophthalmol. 1989;9(2):79–82.
12. Ossoinig KC. Standardized echography: basic principles, clinical applications, and results. Int Ophthalmol Clin. 1979;19(4):127–210.
13. Padayachy LC. Non-invasive intracranial pressure assessment. Childs Nerv Syst. 2016;32(9):1587–97.
14. Ballantyne J, Hollman A, Hamilton R, et al. Transorbital optic nerve sheath ultrasonography in normal children. Clin Radiol. 1999;54(11):740–2.
15. Newman WD, Hollman AS, Dutton GN, Carachi R. Measurement of optic nerve sheath diameter by ultrasound: a means of detecting acute raised intracranial pressure in hydrocephalus. Br J Ophthalmol. 2002;86(10):1109–13.
16. Malayeri AA, Bavarian S, Mehdizadeh M. Sonographic evaluation of optic nerve diameter in children with raised intracranial pressure. J Ultrasound Med. 2005;24(2):143–7.
17. Beare NA, Kampondeni S, Glover SJ, et al. Detection of raised intracranial pressure by ultrasound measurement of optic nerve sheath diameter in African children. Trop Med Int Health. 2008;13(11):1400–4.
18. McAuley D, Paterson A, Sweeney L. Optic nerve sheath ultrasound in the assessment of paediatric hydrocephalus. Childs Nerv Syst. 2009;25(1):87–90.
19. Steinborn M, Fiegler J, Kraus V, et al. High resolution transbulbar sonography in children with suspicion of increased intracranial pressure. Childs Nerv Syst. 2016;32(4):655–60.
20. Padayachy LC, Padayachy V, Galal U, Grey R, Fieggen AG. The relationship between transorbital ultrasound measurement of the optic nerve sheath diameter (ONSD) and invasively measured ICP in children. Part I: repeatability, observer variability and general analysis. Childs Nerv Syst. 2016;32(10): 1769–78.
21. Padayachy LC, Padayachy V, Galal U, Pollock T, Fieggen AG. The relationship between transorbital ultrasound measurement of the optic nerve sheath diameter (ONSD) and invasively measured ICP in children. Part II: role of the anterior fontanelle. Childs Nerv Syst. 2016;32(10):1779–86.
22. Cartwright C, Igbaseimokumo U. Lumbar puncture opening pressure is not a reliable measure of intracranial pressure in children. J Child Neurol. 2015;30(2):170–3.
23. Robba C, Cardim D, Tajsic T, et al. Ultrasound non-invasive measurement of intracranial pressure

in neurointensive care: a prospective observational study. PLoS Med. 2017;14(7):e1002356.
24. Padayachy LC, Brekken R, Fieggen AG, Selbekk T. Pulsatile dynamics of the optic nerve sheath and intracranial pressure: an exploratory in vivo investigation. Neurosurgery. 2016;79(1):100–7.
25. Padayachy LC, Brekken R, Fieggen AG, Selbekk T. Noninvasive transorbital assessment of the optic nerve sheath in children: relationship between optic nerve sheath diameter, deformability index and intracranial pressure. Oper Neurosurg. 2018;16(6):726–33.
26. Diwakar RK, Khurana O. Cranial sonography in preterm infants with short review of literature. J Pediatr Neurosci. 2018;13:141–9.
27. Gupta P, Singh K, Kumar A, et al. Neonatal cranial sonography: a concise review for clinicians. J Pediatr Neurosci. 2016;1(1):7–13.
28. Ecury-Goosen GM, Camfferman FA, Leijser LM, et al. State of the art cranial ultrasound imaging in neonates. J Vis Exp. 2015;96:52238.
29. Toms DA. The mechanical index, ultrasound practices, and the ALARA principle. J Ultrasound Med. 2006;8:67–8.

Brain Ultrasound in the Critically Ill Pregnant and Puerperium Women

22

Pablo Blanco and Anselmo Abdo-Cuza

Contents

22.1 Introduction

In the pregnant and puerperium women, neurological diseases may contribute to substantial maternal morbidity and up to 20% of maternal deaths. Therefore, their timely recognition and management are crucial for improving outcomes [1].

P. Blanco (✉)
Intensive Care Unit, Clínica Cruz Azul, Necochea, Argentina

A. Abdo-Cuza
Intensive Care Unit, Centro de Investigaciones Médico Quirúrgicas, La Habana, Cuba
e-mail: aaabdo@infomed.sld.cu

The brain of the pregnant and puerperium women may be compromised in several general conditions, such as in low-flow states of peripartum cardiomyopathy or hypovolemia secondary to obstetric hemorrhage, sepsis-induced encephalopathy (e.g., puerperal sepsis), hepatic encephalopathy as may be observed in acute fatty liver of pregnancy, aortic dissection extending to the carotids—50% of all aortic dissections presenting in women younger than 40 years occur in pregnancy and puerperium [2], or ischemic stroke secondary to paradoxical thromboembolism or to cardioembolism as may occur in peripartum cardiomyopathy (Table 22.1). The occurrence of these presentations emphasizes the need to use a

C. Robba, G. Citerio (eds.), *Echography and Doppler of the Brain*,
https://doi.org/10.1007/978-3-030-48202-2_22

Table 22.1 Disorders involving the brain in the pregnant or puerperium women

Systemic conditions affecting the brain blood flow	Brain diseases common to non-obstetric young women	Brain diseases unique to pregnancy or puerperium
Low-flow states (e.g., peripartum cardiomyopathy, hypovolemia, acute cor pulmonale)	Hemorrhagic stroke: Subarachnoid hemorrhage: aneurysmal rupture; arteriovenous malformation rupture	Preeclampsia/eclampsia (PRES)
Sepsis-induced encephalopathy (e.g., puerperal sepsis)	Ischemic stroke: thrombophilia; paradoxical embolism; cardioembolism; aortic dissection with extension to carotids	Postpartum angiopathy
Hepatic encephalopathy (e.g., AFLP)		Cerebral venous sinus thrombosis

PRES posterior reversible encephalopathy syndrome, *AFLP* acute fatty liver of pregnancy

multiorgan ultrasound approach in this population (e.g., adding a transthoracic echocardiogram and/or leg vein compression ultrasound to brain ultrasound) [2]. Furthermore, there are unique entities that may occur in the obstetric patient that should always be considered by intensivists. These include preeclampsia/eclampsia, postpartum angiopathy, and cerebral venous sinus thrombosis [1, 2] (Table 22.1).

22.2 Brain Ultrasound

Multimodal diagnosis and monitoring are key in caring for every neurocritical care patient, including the pregnant and puerperium women. Brain ultrasound (BUS), as a noninvasive, widely available, repeatable, and nonionizing radiation technique, should be integrated within this approach and never be used as a stand-alone technique. Our approach is to perform BUS which includes transcranial Doppler (TCD), measurement of the optic nerve sheath diameter (ONDS), and finally complementing of the physical examination with a pupillary assessment by ultrasound (comparative dimension and consensual pupillary light reflex) (Fig. 22.1). Regarding TCD technique, we prefer to perform transcranial color-coded duplex sonography (TCCS) instead of blind TCD, since the former uses the same transducers and equipment common to general ultrasound in the intensive care unit (ICU) [3, 4]. In addition, TCCS aids in estimating velocities more accurately compared to blind TCD given that the blood flow is approached with a lower angulation or eventually performing angle correction [3–5]. Finally, TCCS may contribute in detecting intra- and extra-axial lesions such as hematomas, and also in evaluating the midline shift [2–4]. The ONSD is measured in both eyes in the usual manner and its values are averaged for obtaining a mean ONSD. Pupillary evaluation using US may be useful in this population in particular when there are generalized edemas as seen for example in preeclampsia, precluding an adequate opening of the eyes. For doing so, a linear probe is placed over each globe in a coronal position and the pupillary diameter is measured comparatively and best showed in a dual screen. Consensual pupillary light reflex is performed illuminating one pupil and observing in real time the pupillary contraction in the contralateral eye (Fig. 22.1).

22.3 Normal Cerebral Physiology in Pregnancy

According to physiologic changes of pregnancy (i.e., high cardiac output, low systemic vascular resistance, and a slight decrease in arterial blood pressure), cerebral blood flow (CBF) shows a trend to increase, although in a small amount (10% in average) compared to nonpregnant women [6, 7]. Studies using transcranial Doppler (TCD) have demonstrated a progressive decrease in CBF velocities and pulsatility index (PI) compared with non-pregnancy status [8], indicating an intact autoregulation mechanism which maintains the CBF within normal values [6]. Furthermore, there is observed in normal pregnancy a leftward shift on the lower limit and a

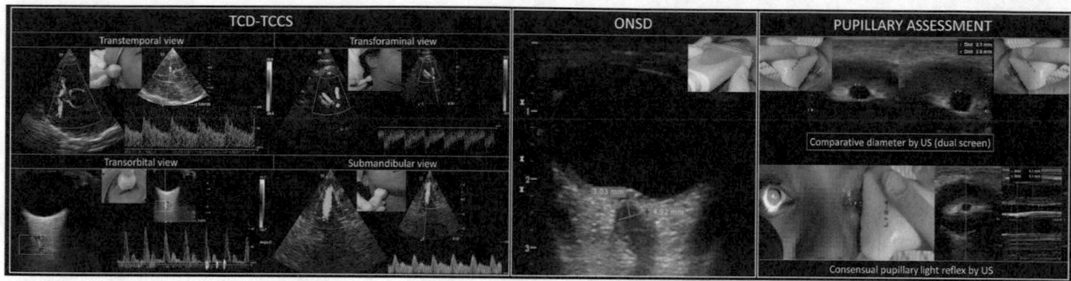

Fig. 22.1 The brain ultrasound approach in the critically ill pregnant or puerperium patient. *TCD* transcranial Doppler (blind technique), *TCCS* transcranial color-coded duplex sonography, *ONDS* optic nerve sheath diameter, *US* ultrasound

rightward shift on the upper limit of the autoregulation curve. This guarantees the perfusion of the brain at a lower and at higher mean arterial pressure, respectively [6]. The aforementioned changes resolve at the same timeframes of systemic hemodynamic changes, approximately 8 weeks after delivery.

22.4 Unique Brain Diseases of Pregnancy and Puerperium

As mentioned before, these include preeclampsia and eclampsia, postpartum angiopathy, and cerebral venous sinus thrombosis. Key findings in BUS are summarized in Table 22.2.

22.4.1 Preeclampsia and Eclampsia

Preeclampsia and eclampsia (P/E) are well-known complications of pregnancy and puerperium, occurring in approximately 6–8% of pregnancies [1]. Preeclampsia is defined as arterial hypertension and proteinuria appearing after 20 weeks of gestation, while eclampsia is characterized by new-onset seizures presenting in the setting of preeclampsia. Of note, some patients may present with eclampsia in the absence of a preeclampsia syndrome, as may be observed in late postpartum eclampsia [1].

Neurologic manifestations of this pregnancy-induced disease, such as headache, blurred vision, hyperreflexia, or seizures, are best explained by alterations in cerebral hemodynamics which induce vasogenic cerebral edema. This feature is very close to that observed in posterior reversible encephalopathy syndrome (PRES) [9–13]. In fact, 12% of preeclamptic patients and almost all eclamptic women have evidence of PRES on neuroimages [14]. In cerebral computed tomography (CT) or magnetic resonance (MR) imaging, PRES is typically manifested as focal regions of symmetric hemispheric brain edema, affecting more often the parietal and occipital lobes, followed by the frontal lobes, the inferior temporal-occipital junction, and the cerebellum [11]. Based on angiographic studies, PRES is associated with diffuse vasoconstriction, focal vasoconstriction, vasodilation, and even a “string-of-bead” appearance, the last finding typically observed in postpartum angiopathy (see below), indicating that both entities may coexist. There are two main theories regarding the mechanism leading to PRES: vasogenic brain edema secondary to hypertension/hyperperfusion (similar to hypertensive encephalopathy) versus vasogenic brain edema secondary to hypoperfusion (generalized vasoconstriction) and the subsequent disruption of the blood-brain barrier. The latter seems to be the most plausible explanation since PRES can also be observed in normotensive patients or in patients with moderate hypertension (i.e., within the normal limits of autoregulation) [13].

In contrast to normal pregnancy, studies using TCD showed that cerebral blood flow velocities are increased in P/E [8], and even reach the criteria of vasospasm; PI remains low.

Table 22.2 Main and additional findings in brain ultrasound for the three neurologic unique entities which can be observed in the pregnant or puerperium women

Neurologic disease	Brain ultrasound	
	Main findings	Additional findings—complications
Preeclampsia and eclampsia (PRES)	Increase in velocities (MCA mV > 80 cm/s) even reaching the criteria of vasospasm (LR > 3) Ophthalmic artery flow: peak velocity ratio >0.78 ONSD >5.8 mm may indicate a rise in the ICP	A decrease in arterial velocities (MCA mV < 30; dV < 20) and an increase in the PI (>1.4) may indicate a rise in the ICP/decrease in the CPP Intra-axial hematomas: hyperechoic lesion in brain parenchyma (TCCS) Midline shift (A – B/2): TCCS (secondary to hematomas or eventually to cerebral infarction) Pupillary assessment (may demonstrate anisocoria) Absent pupillary contraction: indicates compromise of the contralateral CN II (afferent) or ipsilateral CN III (efferent, e.g., cerebral herniation) Pupillary hippus (may indicate seizure activity)
Postpartum angiopathy	Multifocal vasospasm (mV > 80; LR > 3)	A decrease in arterial velocities (MCA mV < 30; dV < 20) and an increase in the PI (>1.4) may indicate a rise in the ICP/decrease in the CPP Intra-axial hematomas: hyperechoic lesion in brain parenchyma (TCCS) Midline shift (A – B/2): TCCS (secondary to hematomas or eventually to cerebral infarction) Pupillary assessment (may demonstrate anisocoria) Absent pupillary contraction: indicates compromise of the contralateral CN II (afferent) or ipsilateral CN III (efferent, e.g., cerebral herniation)
Cerebral venous sinus thrombosis	Indirect criteria: increased venous velocities (compensatory venous flow) Direct criteria: occlusion of a cerebral venous sinus (CE-TCCS) Optic disc elevation (papilledema) as an indicator of a subacute rise in the ICP	A decrease in arterial velocities (MCA mV < 30; dV < 20) and increase in the PI (>1.4) may indicate a rise in the ICP/decrease in the CPP Intra-axial hematomas: hyperechoic lesion in brain parenchyma (TCCS) Extra-axial hematoma (subdural hematoma, rare): hyperechoic lesion adjacent to the cranial bone (TCCS) Midline shift (A – B/2): TCCS (secondary to hematomas or eventually to venous infarction) Pupillary assessment (may demonstrate anisocoria) Absent pupillary contraction: indicates compromise of the contralateral CN II (afferent) or ipsilateral CN III (efferent, e.g., cavernous sinus thrombosis, cerebral herniation)

MCA middle cerebral artery, *mv* mean flow velocity, *LR* Lindegaard ratio, *dv* end-diastolic flow velocity, *PI* pulsatility index, *ICP* intracranial pressure, *CPP* cerebral perfusion pressure, *CVST* cerebral venous sinus thrombosis, *PRES* posterior reversible encephalopathy syndrome, *PPA* postpartum angiopathy, *TCCS* transcranial color-coded duplex sonography, *CN* cranial nerve

Autoregulation is often impaired, while CO2 reactivity may or may not be compromised in P/E [15–17]. Complications of PRES, such as cerebral infarction or cerebral hemorrhage, may be associated with the criteria of vasospasm in the former, and low velocities (in patients with high blood pressure) in the latter [18].

22.4.1.1 Role of BUS

TCD may aid in detecting the alterations in blood flow described above, distinguishing either hypoperfusion, vasospasm, or hyperemia (Fig. 22.2a,b), and monitoring the response to interventions. In addition, the cerebral autoregulation may be assessed with the transient hyper-

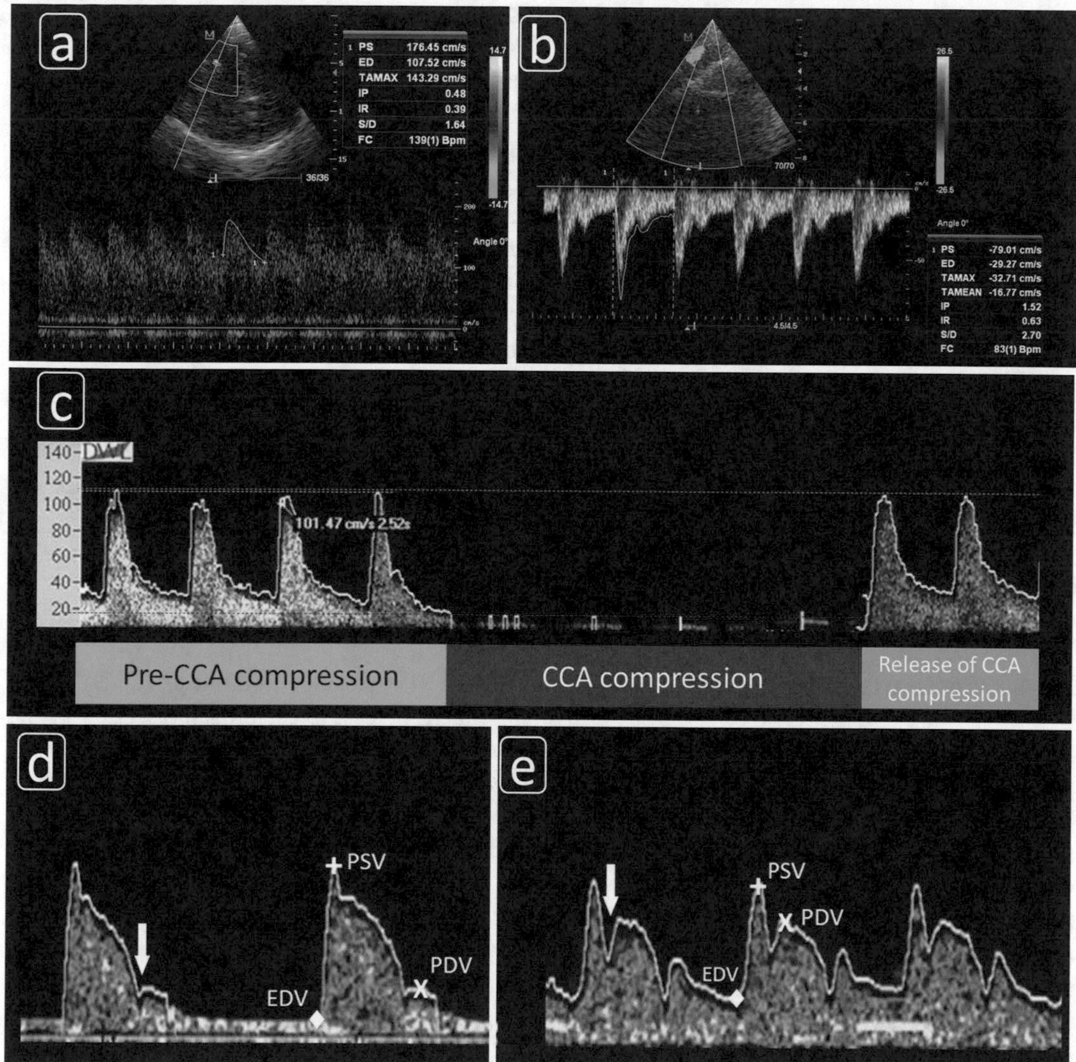

Fig. 22.2 Brain ultrasound in severe preeclampsia and eclampsia (P/E). (**a**) Transcranial color-coded duplex sonography (TCCS) showing grossly elevated velocities in the right middle cerebral artery (mV of 143 cm/s); (**b**) TCCS of the ipsilateral extracranial internal carotid artery (submandibular view), with mV of 33 cm/s. Lindegaard ratio is 4.3, corresponding to vasospasm in a patient with eclampsia and posterior reversible encephalopathy syndrome (PRES); (**c**) transient hyperemic response test showing an impaired cerebral autoregulation (<10% increase in peak systolic velocities after releasing the compression in the ipsilateral common carotid artery (CCA) in the neck); (**d**) ophthalmic artery flow in normal pregnancy and (**e**) in P/E. As noted, the resistive index ((PSV-EDV)/PSV) and pulsatility index are higher in normal pregnancy, but increase in P/E. PDV is also higher in P/E, with a higher ratio between PDV and PSV. White arrow: diastolic notch; PSV: peak systolic velocity; PDV: peak diastolic velocity (the first wave appearing immediately after the dicrotic notch); EDV: end-diastolic velocity

emic response test (Fig. 22.2c). TCCS may provide a way to detect and follow up intracranial hematomas and midline shift as complications of PRES in P/E [4].

Besides TCD-TCCS, measurement of the ONSD may aid in assessing noninvasively the intracranial pressure, having observed in P/E an increase in the ONDS, in contrast to normal pregnancy [19, 20]. Cutoff values above 5.8 mm may indicate an elevation of the ICP [20]. However, ONSD has not been compared directly with invasive ICP monitoring in studies, and thus further research is needed to validate this application in this population.

Ophthalmic artery flow, which in normal pregnancy shows a high-resistance velocity profile, in P/E typically shows a low resistive and pulsatility index. Peak diastolic velocity (PDV) and peak velocity ratio (PDV/peak systolic velocity (PSV)) are higher in P/E and chronic hypertension compared to normal pregnancy [21, 22]. Cutoff values are 0.657 for the resistive index, 1.318 for the PI, and 0.784 for the peak velocity ratio for discriminating severe preeclampsia or eclampsia versus mild preeclampsia or chronic hypertension (Fig. 22.2d,e) [22].

22.4.2 Postpartum Angiopathy

Postpartum angiopathy (PPA), also known as postpartum reversible vasoconstriction syndrome, is a clinical-angiographic syndrome appearing in the puerperium characterized by the abrupt onset of severe headaches ("thunderclap" type), seizures, focal neurological deficits, and segmental narrowing and dilatation of large- and medium-sized cerebral arteries ("string-of-bead" appearance in cerebral angiography). Incidence of PPA is as low as 0.11% or 1 case in every 900 women [23]. Pathophysiology is not clear, with disturbances in the control of the cerebral vascular tone seemed to be a critical element. These disturbances may be evoked by endogenous and/or exogenous factors, such as catecholamines, endocrine factors, or uncontrolled hypertension [24].

In contrast to aneurysmal subarachnoid hemorrhage, vasospasm is multifocal [24] in PPA, a datum that aids in distinguishing between both entities. As previously mentioned, PPA may coexist with PRES. The main complications of PPA are cerebral infarction and intracranial hemorrhage.

22.4.2.1 Role of BUS

TCD aids in diagnosing this disease when there are observed increased arterial blood flow velocities reaching the criteria of vasospasm. Involvement of several vessels aids in discriminating from vasospasm of subarachnoid hemorrhage, as mentioned before. Although TCD findings may raise suspicion for PPA, one requisite for this diagnosis is the exclusion of an aneurysmal subarachnoid hemorrhage and therefore obtaining a brain CT or MR imaging is mandatory [24]. TCD is also useful for monitoring the resolution of vasospasm as well as detecting complications such as cerebral hemorrhage and midline shift (TCCS).

22.4.3 Cerebral Venous Sinus Thrombosis

Cerebral venous sinus thrombosis (CVST) is an infrequent disease presenting most often in the puerperium [9], and having a remarkably wide spectrum of clinical signs and symptoms such as headache, nausea, seizures, focal neurological deficits, raised intracranial pressure, and coma [9] [25, 26]. Of note, this entity several times is left undiagnosed [27]. The incidence is 11.6 per 1,000,000 deliveries and strong risk factors associated with CVST are cesarean delivery, pregnancy-related hypertension, and anemia [28]. Involvement of the superior sagittal sinus and transverse sinus is most common, while the compromise of the cavernous sinus and deep cerebral veins is less frequent [1]. Papilledema, as an expression of a subacute increase in the ICP, is a frequent finding and should raise the suspicion of this disease. Venous infarctions and intracranial hemorrhages are common complications.

22.4.3.1 Role of BUS

Papilledema can be readily detected by US (Fig. 22.3a). In addition, signs of increased ICP can be recognized with TCD, such as low arterial flow velocities and elevation of the PI.

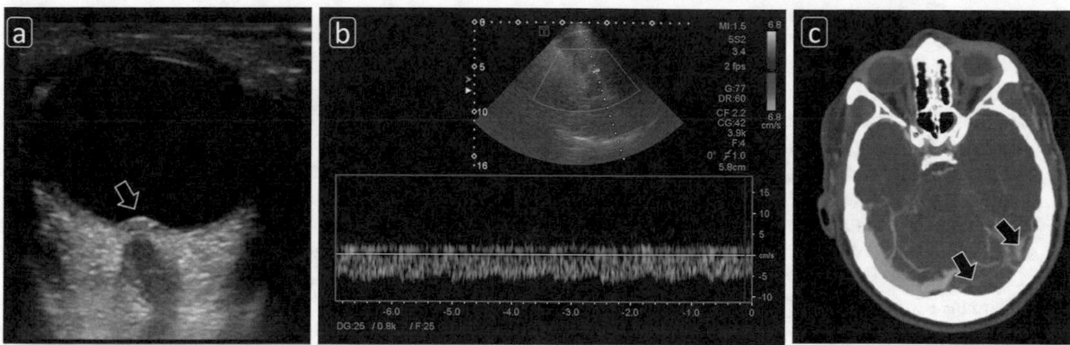

Fig. 22.3 Cerebral venous sinus thrombosis. (**a**) Eye ultrasound demonstrating papilledema (arrow); (**b**) TCCS. In this case, the insonated vessel is the left-sided basal vein of Rosenthal (deep venous system), a constant and bilateral vein often found around the P2 segment of the posterior cerebral artery. Velocities are not elevated as expected; (**c**) brain CT angiography in venous phase, showing the lack of visualization of the left transverse sinus (arrows), indicating a CVST

Complications such as intraparenchymal hemorrhage (extra-axial hematomas are also reported) and the resulting midline shift can also be detected by TCCS. The direct sign of CVST is the detection of the occluded vein in contrast-enhanced-TCCS (CE-TCCS); however, given that the detection rate of venous flow is variable, and that anatomical variations are not uncommon, CE-TCCS is far from perfect to confirm CVST, with a sensitivity that ranges between 73% and 100% and a specificity between 65% and 80% [25]. Indirect TCCS criterion (with or without US contrast agents) is the elevation in venous velocities, indicating compensatory venous flow [25] (Fig. 22.3b). Given that US contrast agents are not licensed for using in pregnant or puerperium patients, and given the poor availability of these agents in most ICUs, suspicion of CVST relies mainly on indirect TCCS findings or papilledema in eye ultrasound, and therefore CVST always requires confirmation by other imaging techniques, such as magnetic resonance venography or CT angiography in venous phase (Fig. 22.3c).

22.5 Conclusions

BUS may offer clues for diagnosing many neurologic diseases affecting the pregnant or puerperium patient, and is especially useful for monitoring purposes. For best using this method, BUS should be integrated within the multimodal neurologic monitoring and with general point-of-care ultrasound as well. In addition to general diseases affecting the brain, unique neurologic entities occurring in this population should also be taken into account. US contrast agents may have a role in improving the detection of arterial flow in difficult cases, as well as cerebral venous flow. However, these agents are not licensed to date for using in the pregnant or puerperium patient.

References

1. Hosley CM, McCullough LD. Acute neurological issues in pregnancy and the peripartum. Neurohospitalist. 2011;1(2):104–16.
2. Blanco P, Abdo-Cuza A. Point-of-care ultrasound in the critically ill pregnant or postpartum patient: what every intensivist should know. Intensive Care Med. 2019;45(8):1123–6.
3. Blanco P, Blaivas M. Applications of transcranial color-coded sonography in the emergency department. J Ultrasound Med. 2017;36(6):1251–66.
4. Blanco P, Abdo-Cuza A. Transcranial Doppler ultrasound in neurocritical care. J Ultrasound. 2018;21(1):1–16.
5. Martin PJ, Evans DH, Naylor AR. Measurement of blood flow velocity in the basal cerebral circulation: advantages of transcranial color-coded sonography over conventional transcranial Doppler. J Clin Ultrasound. 1995;23(1):21–6.

6. Johnson AC, Cipolla MJ. The cerebral circulation during pregnancy: adapting to preserve normalcy. Physiology (Bethesda). 2015;30(2):139–47.
7. Nevo O, Soustiel JF, Thaler I. Maternal cerebral blood flow during normal pregnancy: a cross-sectional study. Am J Obstet Gynecol. 2010;203(5):475.e1-6.
8. Sherman RW, Bowie RA, Henfrey MM, Mahajan RP, Bogod D. Cerebral haemodynamics in pregnancy and pre-eclampsia as assessed by transcranial Doppler ultrasonography. Br J Anaesth. 2002;89(5):687–92.
9. Plowman RS, Javidan-Nejad C, Raptis CA, Katz DS, Mellnick VM, Bhalla S, Cornejo P, Menias CO. Imaging of pregnancy-related vascular complications. Radiographics. 2017;37(4):1270–89.
10. Sudulagunta SR, Sodalagunta MB, Kumbhat M, Settikere NA. Posterior reversible encephalopathy syndrome (PRES). Oxf Med Case Reports. 2017;2017(4):omx011.
11. Bartynski WS. Posterior reversible encephalopathy syndrome, part 1: fundamental imaging and clinical features. AJNR Am J Neuroradiol. 2008;29(6):1036–42.
12. Belfort MA, Saade GR, Yared M, Grunewald C, Herd JA, Varner MA, Nisell H. Change in estimated cerebral perfusion pressure after treatment with nimodipine or magnesium sulfate in patients with preeclampsia. Am J Obstet Gynecol. 1999;181(2):402–7.
13. Brewer J, Owens MY, Wallace K, Reeves AA, Morris R, Khan M, LaMarca B, Martin JN Jr. Posterior reversible encephalopathy syndrome in 46 of 47 patients with eclampsia. Am J Obstet Gynecol. 2013;208(6):468.e1-6.
14. Wen Y, Yang B, Huang Q, Liu Y. Posterior reversible encephalopathy syndrome in pregnancy: a retrospective series of 36 patients from mainland China. Ir J Med Sci. 2017;186(3):699–705.
15. van Veen TR, Panerai RB, Haeri S, Griffioen AC, Zeeman GG, Belfort MA. Cerebral autoregulation in normal pregnancy and preeclampsia. Obstet Gynecol. 2013;122(5):1064–9.
16. van Veen TR, Panerai RB, Haeri S, Singh J, Adusumalli JA, Zeeman GG, Belfort MA. Cerebral autoregulation in different hypertensive disorders of pregnancy. Am J Obstet Gynecol. 2015;212(4):513.e1-7.
17. Riskin-Mashiah S, Belfort MA, Saade GR, Herd JA. Cerebrovascular reactivity in normal pregnancy and preeclampsia. Obstet Gynecol. 2001;98(5 Pt 1):827–32.
18. Costa A, Filipe JP, Santos R, Ferreira C, Abreu P, Azevedo E. The role of transcranial Doppler ultrasonography in posterior reversible encephalopathy syndrome. Cerebrovasc Dis. 2015;39(suppl 1):1–52.
19. Arteaga Favela CB, Ortega Salas J, Urías Romo del Vivar EG, Chacón Uraga EJ. Comparative study of the optic nerve sheath by transorbital ultrasound in healthy women, healthy pregnant ones, and those with preeclampsia-eclampsia. An Med (Mex). 2017;62(3):166–71.
20. Dubost C, Le Gouez A, Jouffroy V, Roger-Christoph S, Benhamou D, Mercier FJ, Geeraerts T. Optic nerve sheath diameter used as ultrasonographic assessment of the incidence of raised intracranial pressure in preeclampsia: a pilot study. Anesthesiology. 2012;116(5):1066–71.
21. Olatunji RB, Adekanmi AJ, Obajimi MO, Roberts OA, Ojo TO. Maternal ophthalmic artery Doppler velocimetry in pre-eclampsia in Southwestern Nigeria. Int J Women's Health. 2015;7:723–34.
22. de Oliveira CA, de Sá RA, Velarde LG, da Silva FC, doVale FA, Netto HC. Changes in ophthalmic artery Doppler indices in hypertensive disorders during pregnancy. J Ultrasound Med. 2013;32(4):609–16.
23. Anzola GP, Brighenti R, Cobelli M, Giossi A, Mazzucco S, Olivato S, Pari E, Piras MP, Padovani A, Rinaldi F, Turri G. Reversible cerebral vasoconstriction syndrome in puerperium: a prospective study. J Neurol Sci. 2017;375:130–6.
24. Calabrese LH, Dodick DW, Schwedt TJ, Singhal AB. Narrative review: reversible cerebral vasoconstriction syndromes. Ann Intern Med. 2007;146(1):34–44.
25. Stolz EP. Role of ultrasound in diagnosis and management of cerebral vein and sinus thrombosis. Front Neurol Neurosci. 2008;23:112–21.
26. Wardlaw JM, Vaughan GT, Steers AJ, Sellar RJ. Transcranial Doppler ultrasound findings in cerebral venous sinus thrombosis. Case report. J Neurosurg. 1994;80(2):332–5.
27. Dangal G, Thapa LB. Cerebral venous sinus thrombosis presenting in pregnancy and puerperium. BMJ Case Rep. 2009;2009:bcr0620092045.
28. Sharma N, Sharma SR, Hussain M. An audit of cerebral venous thrombosis associated with pregnancy and puerperium in teaching hospital in North Eastern India. J Family Med Prim Care. 2019;8(3):1054–7.

Part VIII

Pathology and Clinical Applications: Intraoperative Applications

Intraoperative Application of Brain Ultrasound in Non-cardiac Surgery

23

Rita Bertuetti

Contents

23.1 Introduction

Ultrasound machines have nowadays gained their place in the operating theatre: as a tool not only for surgeons and cardiologists but also for anaesthetists.

Although the application of ultrasounds for central vein cannulation, nerve blocks and cardiac function monitoring represents a cornerstone for the daily practice of anaesthetists, the purpose of using brain ultrasound (BUS) and transcranial Doppler (TCD) during surgery may not seem so straightforward.

Leaving cardiac surgery aside, transcranial (colour coded) Doppler (TCD/TCCD) in operating theatre can assess the adequacy of cerebral blood flow, identify cerebral embolism and estimate intracranial pressure (ICP) and cerebral perfusion pressure (CPP).

Regardless of the type of surgery, alteration of cerebral perfusion is associated with post-operative delirium and even post-operative cognitive disorders; moreover there are cases in which surgery itself can worsen situations of borderline ICP.

R. Bertuetti (✉)
Department of Anesthesiology, Critical Care Medicine and Emergency, Division of Neurocritical Care, ASST Spedali Civili di Brescia, University Hospital, Brescia, Italy

C. Robba, G. Citerio (eds.), *Echography and Doppler of the Brain*,
https://doi.org/10.1007/978-3-030-48202-2_23

23.2 Techniques and Methods

Key Points

- Global CBF is affected by MAP, ICP and vascular resistance.
- Flow velocity of cerebral vessels acts as a surrogate of CBF as long as the cross-sectional area of a vessel is kept constant.
- Reduction in mean and diastolic FV can reflect drops in ABP below the lower limit of autoregulation or in a state of deranged autoregulation, as well as it can reflect increased ICP.
- Cerebral perfusion pressure (CPP) and ICP estimation is feasible in patients undergoing general anaesthesia through the application of the diastolic flow velocity formula of Czosnyka, pulsatility index (PI) and ultrasound measurement of the optic nerve sheath diameter (ONSD).

23.2.1 Assessment of CBF: TCD and TCCD

Global *CBF* is affected by:

- MAP
- ICP
- Vascular resistance

CBF can be assessed through the use of TCD or TCCD by insonating the vessels of the circle of Willis. Pulsed Doppler mode measures flow velocity; it follows that adequacy of flow itself can be only estimated: flow velocity acts as a surrogate of CBF as long as the cross-sectional area of a vessel is kept constant:

$$\mathrm{CBF} \propto (\mathrm{MAP} - \mathrm{ICP}) * r^4$$

TCD/TCCD provide information on CBF in either a quantitative or a qualitative way:

(a) Quantitative assessment of CBF:

Reduction in regional CBF is translated into a reduction in flow velocities at TCCD/TCD; mean flow velocity (MFV) is mostly related to CBF. In order to monitor and identify CBF alterations in a subject anaesthetised, undergoing surgery is fundamental to have a reference baseline examination before any pharmacological intervention or surgical manoeuvre could alter haemodynamic parameters. In order to assess hemispheric perfusion, basal cerebral arteries are insonated bilaterally and flow velocities are taken before induction of general anaesthesia; arterial blood pressure (ABP) must be simultaneously monitored (as flow is being dependent on the driving pressure of the system).

As standard, when there is no surgical manipulation of supra-aortic vessels (as in vascular surgery) MCA flow velocities are monitored throughout the duration of surgery by means of either a continuous TCD monitoring or a repeated freehand intonation any time necessary.

Reduction in mean and diastolic FV can reflect drops in ABP below the lower limit of autoregulation or in a state of deranged autoregulation, as well as it can reflect increased ICP [1].

Unfortunately, in literature, a clear cut-off percentage drop value in mean/diastolic FV has not been described yet; only in a couple of studies investigating the use of TCD during type A aortic dissection repair and one during carotid endarterectomy authors report as significative a reduction of at least 50% from the baseline of mean FV [2, 3]. However, any sensitive reduction in FV can imply a reduction in CBF; whether this might be detrimental is yet to be clarified (especially in an anaesthetised brain where metabolic demand is low): recent studies are exploring the association between variation in cerebral perfusion, oxygenation and cerebral electrical activity (EEG) during anaesthesia and post-operative delirium, post-operative cognitive disorder (POCD) and stroke [4].

Another way to assess how significative can be the alteration of flow velocity is by evaluating cerebral vascular autoregulation: when the cerebrovascular system approaches the lower limit of autoregulation, at that point, there is no more vascular tone compensation and hypoperfusion becomes an issue. If a continuous TCD monitoring is available, mean flow velocity index (Mx) can be used for cerebral autoregulation assessment [5, 6]; otherwise THRT is not advisable in a condition of already reduced flow.

(b) Qualitative assessment of CBF:

Colour Doppler mode (TCCD only) can provide a qualitative assessment of CBF: when CBF is extremely low especially in a situation of increased ICP, the colorimetric map that normally displays the vessels will appear during systole and disappear during diastole, so that the operator will perceive a flashing image of the Willis circle (Fig. 23.1 a,b).

23.2.2 Estimation of CPP and ICP

Just like the application in other clinical situations, cerebral perfusion pressure (CPP) and ICP estimation are feasible in patients undergoing general anaesthesia for non-cardiac surgery. CPP can estimated by application of the diastolic flow velocity formula of Czosnyka:

$$\text{Estimated CPP} = \text{MAP} \times \text{Diastolic FV} / \text{Mean FV} + 14.$$

From CPP we then can easily derive estimated ICP [7, 8].

Pulsatility index (PI) and ultrasound measurement of the optic nerve sheath diameter (ONSD) are also feasible in operating theatre (techniques are described in dedicated chapters in the book).

23.2.3 Embolism Detection

TCD/TCCD allows the identification of both gaseous and thrombotic microemboli in the cerebral circulation: classically used by neurologists in order to assess paradoxical embolism through the patent oval foramen, TCD can diagnose a right-to-left cardiac shunt with almost 100% concordance with a transoesophageal cardiac echography (TEE) through the detection of gaseous microemboli in the cerebral arteries after

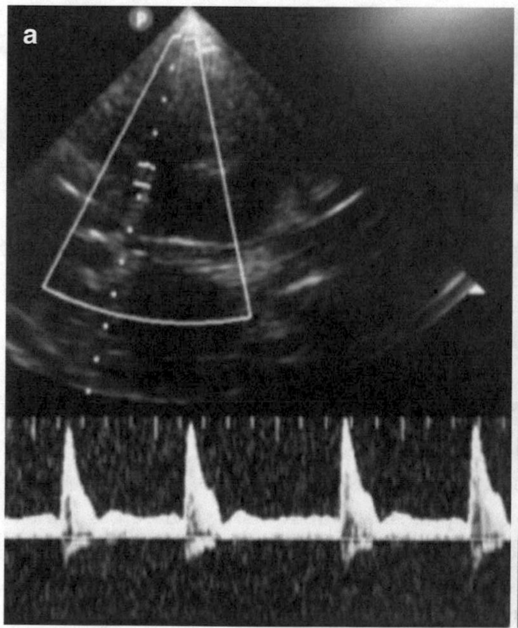

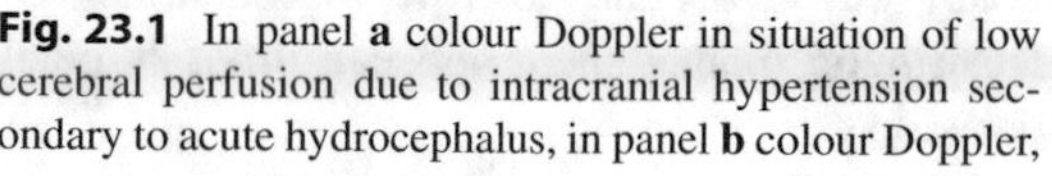

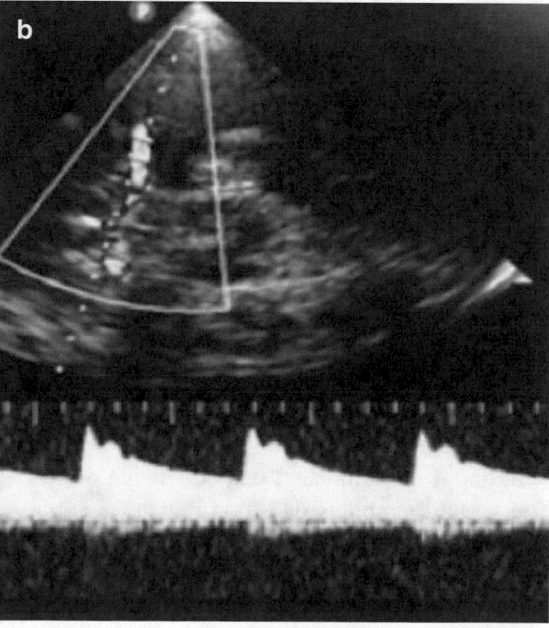

Fig. 23.1 In panel **a** colour Doppler in situation of low cerebral perfusion due to intracranial hypertension secondary to acute hydrocephalus, in panel **b** colour Doppler, in the same patient after external ventricular deviation positioning and restoration of good cerebral perfusion

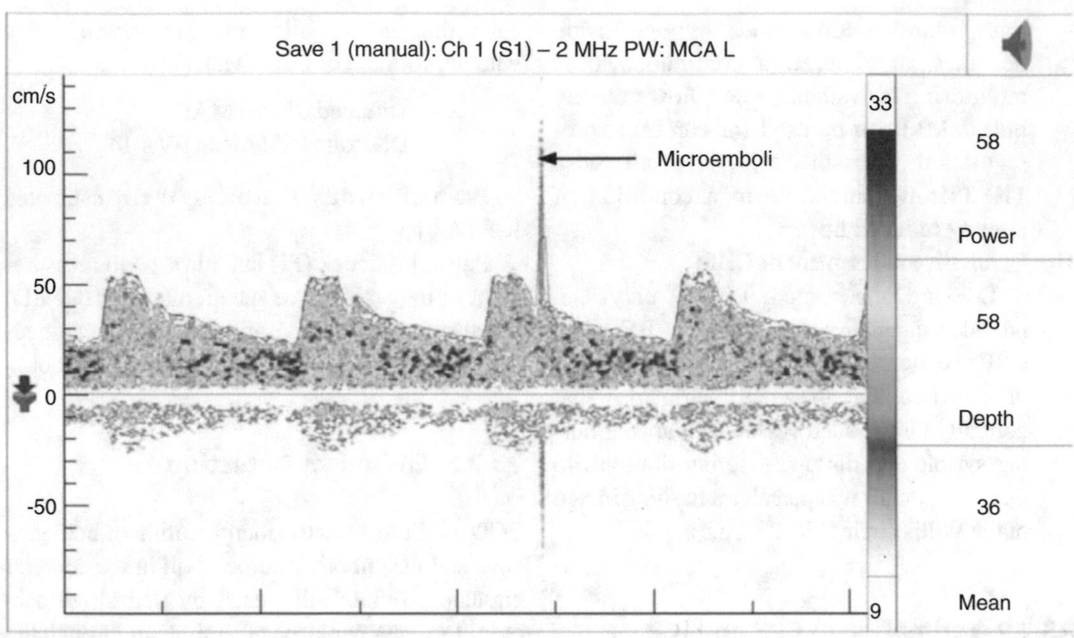

Fig. 23.2 Detection of a single hyperintensity thromboembolic signal on the spectrum of TCD waveform

injection of contrast medium ("bubble test") [9]. Specifically, the technique is based on the injection of 9 ml of physiological solution mixed with 1 ml of air through a three-port tap into one of the large forearm veins. If there is right-to-left shunt, gaseous microemboli are seen 5–15 s after the injection as "interference" in the normal Doppler flow pattern (hyperintensity thromboembolic signal) of MCA (Fig. 23.2).

In operating theatre detection of microembolic signal (MES) requires continuous or subcontinuous TCD monitoring through a specific headset or helmet allowing continuous bilateral MCA intonation. TCD engineers have developed multi-frequency TCD device and specific software for MES detection that both reject artifact and differentiate between gaseous and solid emboli (Fig. 23.3).

Without an automated embolic signal detection system, embolus detection remains a cumbersome process, unsuitable for clinical practice. In order to separate artefacts from emboli, the use of a dual-gate TCD is suggested; this system consists of tracing the embolus at two different depths in the same artery taking advantage of the time delay which is observed in case of emboli detection while not in case of artefacts (reported sensitivity 50–80% and specificity 80–98% depending on the applied algorithm). Gaseous versus solid emboli present with different frequencies/amplitudes and symmetry of the envelope encasing the signal (Fig. 23.4) [10–12].

Assessment of both gaseous and solid embolism is quite established in cardiac surgery; in non-cardiac surgery this application of TCD finds a role in vascular surgery: carotid endarterectomy, aortic arch surgery and supra-aortic vessel bypass, but also in orthopaedic surgery.

23.3 Clinical Applications

The need of assessing cerebral blood flow during surgery is related to either the type of surgical procedure or the characteristics of the patient.

Despite in literature there is no clear indication to the use of TCD or TCCD in patients under anaesthesia undergoing surgical intervention, there are situations in which monitoring the adequacy of CBF can lead to optimisation of anaesthetic management and can drive surgical decision.

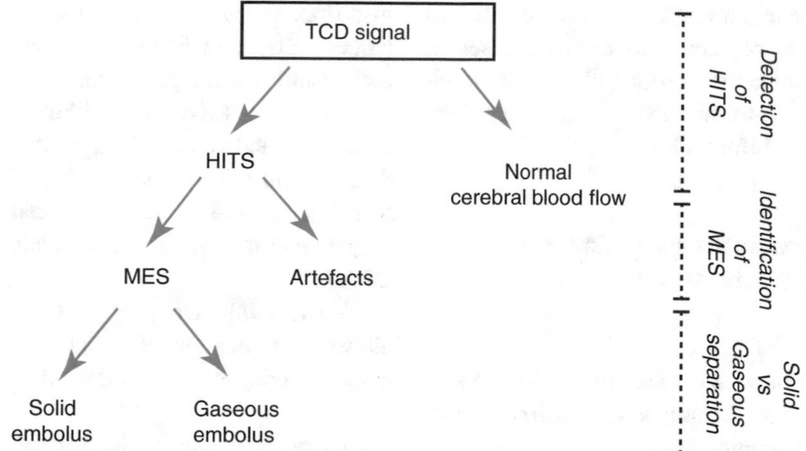

Fig. 23.3 Decision tree with the three steps of transcranial Doppler (TCD) signal analysis: (1) detection of high-intensity signals (HITS), i.e. differentiation between HITS and background Doppler signal; (2) identification of microembolic signals (MES), i.e. differentiation between MES and artefacts; and (3) MES classification, i.e. separation between solid and gaseous emboli

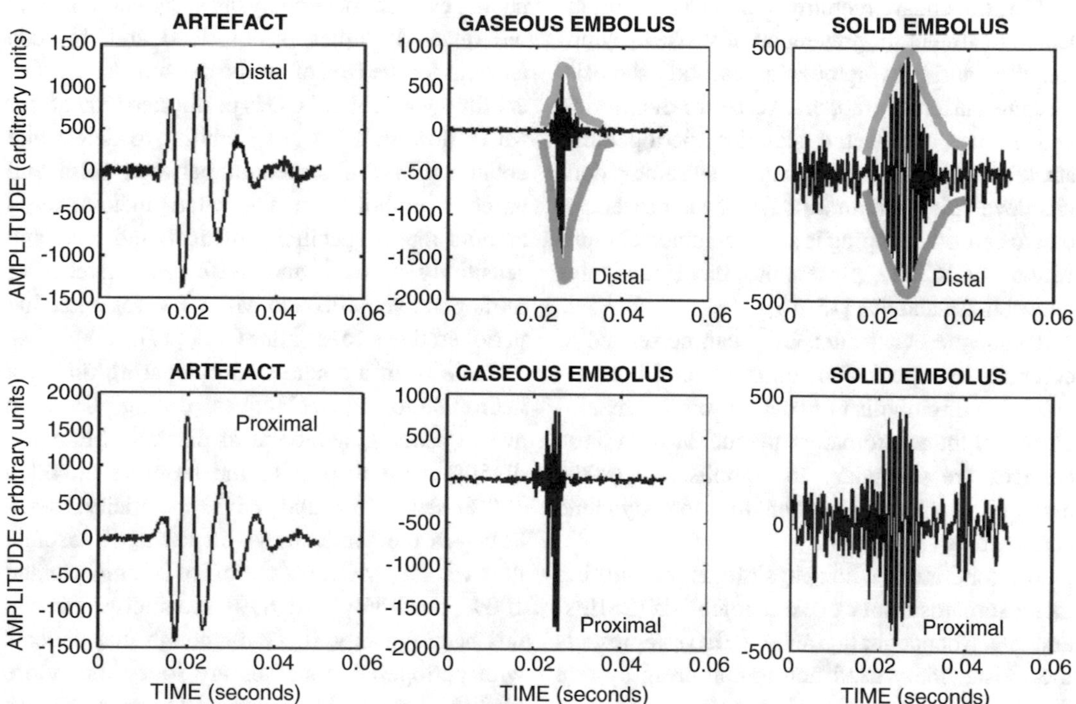

Fig. 23.4 Differentiation of artefact vs. gaseous/solid emboli in frequency and time domain

Knowledge and awareness of such conditions may allow the physician to evaluate cases in which the introduction of brain ultrasound monitoring may add useful and potential decision-making clinical information.

23.3.1 Vascular Surgery: Carotid Endarterectomy

Key Points

- 80% of ischaemic events after CEA are secondary to embolisation and just a 20% to haemodynamic components.
- In CEA, the role of TCD is to pair neurophysiological monitoring in order to help differentiate neuronal suffering due to hypoperfusion (drop in MCA FV), rather than secondary to embolism (detection of MES).

Carotid endarterectomy (CEA) is an established treatment for prevention of stroke in symptomatic and asymptomatic carotid stenosis. Despite current intraoperative neuro-monitoring and the use of selective shunting, perioperative stroke, i.e. transient or persistent neurologic deficits developing within 30 days of the procedure, due to carotid clamping is still a common complication of CEA, presenting incidence rates between 2% and 4% [13–15].

Ischaemic event after CEA can be related to cerebral hypoperfusion during carotid cross-clamping or embolisation due to surgical manipulation of the atheromatous plaque. Most of these changes are secondary to embolisation (80%) and just a small proportion to haemodynamic components (20%) [16].

Intraoperative neurophysiologic monitoring using somatosensory evoked potentials (SSEPs) and electroencephalography (EEG) represents the most widely used neuromonitoring system during CEA when general anaesthesia is necessary or indicated, and therefore neurological clinical monitoring is not feasible. SSEPs and EEG alterations are used to identify cerebral hypoperfusion secondary to carotid clamping and guide insertion of intraluminal shunting; nevertheless literature shows that despite shunt insertion, there is a percentage of patients in whom SSEP and EEG alterations do not normalise and develop preoperative stroke (patients are 14 and 6 times more likely to develop a stroke after substantial changes in intraoperative SSEPs and EEG, respectively). In fact, although SSEPs and EEG identify neuronal "suffering", they cannot identify embolic phenomena during CEA [17].

Transcranial Doppler (TCD) monitoring allows identification of either haemodyamic or embolic complications by detecting:

(a) Drop in cerebral blood flow reflected by reduction in the middle cerebral artery flow velocity (MCA FV)
(b) Cerebral microembolic signal (MES)

Reported accuracy for MCA FV and MES in detecting perioperative stroke is quite heterogeneous; even in meta-analysis, great variability in the selected studies is described and this can account for the lack of uniform results (i.e. different timing at which TCD is performed, cut-off for MCA flow velocity (FV), ability to detect and count MES, differentiation between solid and gaseous emboli); in the cited meta-analysis authors report specificity of 56% and 84% and sensitivity of 61% and 49%, respectively, for intraoperative MES and MCA FV for detecting perioperative strokes after CEA [17].

Instead, in a single trial comparing different neuromonitoring techniques during CEA in awake patients, reduction of diastolic MCA FV of 50% with respect to the baseline provided 100% sensitivity and 86% specificity; similarly—in the same study—in terms of absolute flow velocity MCA FV cut-off of 25 cm/s yielded 100% sensitivity and 69% specificity. Despite this heterogeneity, it seems though that patients with perioperative strokes are four times more likely to have had transcranial Doppler changes (either MCA FV or MES) [3].

It seems reasonable to think that the role of TCD in this kind of surgery is to pair neurophysiological monitoring in order to help differentiate neuronal suffering due to hypoperfusion, rather than secondary to embolism.

23.3.2 Pneumoperitoneum and Prone Position

Key Points

- Pneumoperitoneum institution, CO_2 rise, Trendelenburg position, prone position and PEEP application can increase ICP.
- Currently no indication to invasive ICP monitoring during laparoscopy exists.
- PI, ONSD and diastolic flow velocity formula for ICP estimation seem to have a good concordance in the detection of ICP relative changes during laparoscopic procedures, and during prone position.
- Application of non-invasive techniques should be taken into consideration in selected patients in whom cerebral compliance is reduced because of masses or hydrocephalus, and therefore ICP changes, induced by increased CO2 and reduced cerebral venous return, can realistically affect neurological recover after anaesthesia.

During laparoscopic surgery ICP can increase because of pneumoperitoneum institution, CO_2 rise and necessity of Trendelenburg position.

In spinal surgery, prone positioning can as well affect changes in ICP; finally application of a positive end-expiratory pressure (PEEP) can contribute to ICP changes.

Intra-abdominal pressure rise caused by insufflation of pneumoperitoneum determines decreased venous return and therefore decreased cardiac output, hypercapnia and consequent respiratory acidosis. On top of this, for surgical reason, Trendelenburg position further worsens cerebral blood volume congestion by obstructing venous return on an already vasodilated cerebral vascular bed because of hypercapnia. Analogously, PEEP contributes to rise in intrabdominal pressure and reduction in cardiac preload as well as creates further impediment to cerebral venous outflow [18, 19].

Some authors have documented rare severe neurological complications during laparoscopy related to cerebral ischaemia and cerebral oedema. Generally, neurological complications are rare: more frequently, minor clinical symptoms, such as nausea and headache, which could be associated with transitory increased ICP, have been reported after laparoscopy.

The overall low incidence of neurological complications after laparoscopy makes it difficult to recommend more extensive screening procedures for intracranial hypertension in general population; in patients at risk of developing an increased ICP as a result of head injury or of space-occupying lesions, peritoneal insufflation could induce abrupt and detrimental intracranial hypertension and therefore it should probably be used with special caution and close monitoring [20].

Because currently no indication to invasive ICP monitoring during laparoscopy exists, in humans the only studies reporting the trend of ICP during pneumoperitoneum are few, and confined to patients undergoing ventriculo-peritoneal shunt placement; here a sustained increase in ICP of more than 12 mmHg above the baseline is described in one study while in another a linear increase of ICP up to 25 mmHg during pneumoperitoneum is demonstrated [21, 22].

All the nICP methods seem to have a good concordance in the detection of ICP changes during laparoscopic procedures. All of them showed a significant increase of estimated ICP after the institution of PP and the TP. Only ICPFVd increased significantly after PP alone.

Animal models show that ICP increases significantly above 15 mmHg of IAP, reaching 150% over control values with intra-abdominal pressure above 16 mmHg during Trendelenburg [23].

23.3.2.1 How Can We Monitor ICP?

Invasive techniques are the gold standard, although neurosurgeons are reluctant at applying such techniques in these situations because of possible complications and because current literature does not provide any specific indication. Ultrasound-based techniques for ICP monitoring have been tested during laparoscopic surgery and spinal surgery in few studies in order to assess whether they could reliably identify alleged ICP changes associated with pneumoperitoneum and Trendelenburg position or prone positioning. PI, ONSD and diastolic flow velocity formula for

ICP (ICP_FVd) estimation seem to have a good concordance in the detection of ICP changes during laparoscopic procedures. All of them show a significant increase of estimated ICP after the institution of pneumoperitoneum and Trendelenburg position while only ICP_FVd seems to increase significantly after pneumoperitoneum alone. Similarly the same non-invasive techniques show increased estimated ICP after prone positioning for spinal surgery [24, 25]. Despite speculative studies trying to demonstrate that an increase in ICP does happen during the mentioned surgical procedures, the fact that intracranial hypertension may become a major issue in patients undergoing laparoscopic cannot be predicted in general population. Rather, application of such non-invasive techniques should be taken into consideration in selected patients in whom cerebral compliance is reduced because of masses or hydrocephalus, and therefore ICP changes, induced by increased CO2 and reduced cerebral venous return, can realistically affect neurological recover after anaesthesia; alternatively cerebral oedema may represent a problem in healthy subjects undergoing very prolonged laparoscopic procedure in Trendelenburg position.

23.3.3 Beach Chair Position and Orthopaedic Surgery

Key Points

- Beach chair/sitting position increases the risk of significative hypotension during general anaesthesia and the risks of neurologic complications secondary to haemodynamic derangement.
- Reduction of estimated CPP, in critical closing pressure (secondary to blood pressure decrease), and a deterioration of the autoregulation index Mxa above the autoregulatory limit can occur during hypotensive phase.

Beach chair and sitting position offers several advantages for shoulder surgery (and in some cases for neurosurgery of the posterior fossa); however it also greatly increases the risk of significative hypotension during general anaesthesia and the risks of neurologic complications secondary to haemodynamic derangement [26]. Although the incidence remains unknown (a survey describes an alleged incidence of around 0.0004% for major stroke, though it is likely that these complications are left mostly unreported), in literature few cases are reported of severe neurologic events occurring during sitting position [27, 28].

While in awake healthy people upright position increases systemic vascular resistance and systemic blood pressure through sympathetic nervous system activation [29], in anaesthetised patients baroreflex is altered making challenging the haemodynamic optimisation. Adverse neurologic events reported after shoulder surgery in beach chair position were mainly attributed to inadequate cerebral perfusion at least in part because of systemic hypotension and gravitational effect of positioning the head above the level of the heart. Such hypotensive episodes, even more pronounced in chronic hypertensive patients under specific medications, require prompt correction with boluses of fluid or vasopressors.

Available studies actually describe a moderate transient reduction in flow velocity in MCA from supine to beach chair position under general anaesthesia [30], a reduction of estimated CPP, a reduction in critical closing pressure (secondary to blood pressure decrease) and a deterioration of the autoregulation index Mxa (correlation coefficient between mean flow velocity in MCA and MAP) above the autoregulatory limit [31]. These findings suggest that there are situations when ABP falls below the lower limit of cerebral autoregulation (despite interventions aiming to correct hypotension): in fact, targeting ABP may be challenging for the anaesthetist, being a compromise between perfusion and prevention of bleeding in the surgical site.

Monitoring autoregulation and critical closing pressure could represent a potential tool for guiding haemodynamic management and avoiding undetected cerebral hypoperfusion.

In major orthopaedic surgery, i.e. hip replacement, knee replacement, shoulder replacement and femur fixation, there is also a reported increase of microembolisation detectable by means of new-generation multi-frequency TCD machine. Available study has shown so far that a great majority of MES observed during orthopaedic surgery seems to be of gaseous nature, attributing a role to anaesthesia and iv infusions to such a result. More studies are needed to explore this field and also to assign, to detected MES, a role too in terms of neurological complication/ outcome after surgery (i.e. delirium, postoperative cognitive disorder) [32].

References

1. Ursino M, Giuglioni M, Lodi CA. Relationships among cerebral perfusion pressure, autoregulation, and transcranial Doppler waveform: a modeling study. J Neurosurg. 1998;89:255–66.
2. Estrera AL, Garami Z, Miller CC III. Cerebral monitoring with transcranial Doppler ultrasonography improves neurologic outcome during repairs of acute type A aortic dissection. J Thorac Cardiovasc Surg. 2005;129(2):277–85.
3. Moritz S, Kasprzak P, Arlt M, Taeger K, Metz C. Accuracy of cerebral monitoring in detecting cerebral ischemia during carotid endarterectomy: a comparison of transcranial Doppler sonography, near-infrared spectroscopy, stump pressure, and somatosensory evoked potentials. Anesthesiology. 2007;107:563–9.
4. Goettel N, Burkhart CS, Rossi A, Cabella BCT, Berres M, Monsch AU, Czosnyka M, Steiner LA. Associations between impaired cerebral blood flow autoregulation, cerebral oxygenation, and biomarkers of brain injury and postoperative cognitive dysfunction in elderly patients after major noncardiac surgery. Anesth Analg. 2017;124:934–42.
5. Czosnyka M, Smielewski P, Piechnik S, Schmidt EA, Seeley H, al-Rawi P, Matta BF, Kirkpatrick PJ, Pickard JD. Continuous assessment of cerebral autoregulation- clinical verification of the method in head injured patients. Acta Neurochir Suppl. 2000;76:483–4.
6. Hori D, Nomura Y, Ono M, et al. Optimal blood pressure during cardiopulmonary bypass defined by cerebral autoregulation monitoring. J Thorac Cardiovasc Surg. 2017;154(5):1590–8.
7. Czosnyka M, Matta B, Smielewski P, et al. Cerebral perfusion pressure in head-injured patients: a noninvasive assessment using transcranial Doppler ultrasonography. Neurosurgery. 1998;88:802–8.
8. Schmidt EA, Czosnyka M, Matta BF, Gooskens I, Piechnik S, Pickard JD. Non-invasive cerebral perfusion pressure (nCPP): evaluation of the monitoring methodology in head injured patients. Acta Neurochir Suppl. 2000;76:451–2.
9. Droste DW, Lakemeier S, Wichter T, et al. Optimizing the technique of contrast transcranial Doppler ultrasound in the detection of right-to-left shunts. Stroke. 2002;33:221–6.
10. Devuyst G, Darbellay GA, Vesin JM, et al. Automatic classification of HITS into artifacts or solid or gaseous emboli by a wavelet representation combined with dual-gate TCD. Stroke. 2001;32:2803–9.
11. Darbellay GA, Duff R, Vesin JM, et al. Solid or gaseous circulating brain emboli: are they separable by transcranial ultrasound? J Cereb Blood Flow Metab. 2004;24(8):860.
12. Markus HS, Punter M. Can transcranial Doppler discriminate between solid and gaseous microemboli? Assessment of a dual-frequency transducer system. Stroke. 2005;36:1731–4.
13. Randomised trial of endarterectomy for recently symptomatic carotid stenosis: final results of the MRC European carotid surgery trial (ECST). Lancet. 1998;351:1379–87.
14. Halliday A, Harrison M, Hayter E, et al. 10-year stroke prevention after successful carotid endarterectomy for asymptomatic stenosis (ACST- 1): a multicentre randomised trial. Lancet. 2010;376:1074–84.
15. Hill MD, Brooks W, Mackey A, et al. Stroke after carotid stenting and endarterectomy in the carotid revascularization endarterectomy versus stenting trial (CREST). Circulation. 2012;126:3054–61.
16. Krul JM, van Gijn J, Ackerstaff RG, Eikelboom BC, Theodorides T, Vermeulen FE. Site and pathogenesis of infarcts associated with carotid endarterectomy. Stroke. 1989;20:324–8.
17. Udesh R, Natarajan P, Thiagarajan K, Wechsler LR, Crammond DJ, Balzer JR, Thirumala PD. Transcranial Doppler monitoring in carotid endarterectomy. J Ultrasound Med. 2017;36:621–30.
18. Bloomfield GL, Ridings PC, Blocher CR, Marmarou A, Sugerman HJ. A proposed relationship between increased intra-abdominal, intrathoracic, and intracranial pressure. Crit Care Med. 1997;25(3):496–503.
19. Citerio G, Vascotto E, Villa F, Celotti S, Pesenti A. Induced abdominal compartment syndrome increases intracranial pressure in neurotrauma patients: a prospective study. Crit Care Med. 2001;29(7):1466–71.
20. Mobbs RJ, Yang MO. The dangers of diagnostic laparoscopy in the head injured patient. J Clin Neurosci. 2002;9(5):592–3.
21. Uzzo RG, Bilsky M, Mininberg DT, Poppas DP. Laparoscopic surgery in children with ventriculoperitoneal shunts: effect of pneumoperitoneum on intracranial pressure—preliminary experience. Urology. 1997;49(5):753–7.
22. Kamine TH, Papavassiliou E, Schneider BE. Effect of abdominal insufflation for laparoscopy on intracranial pressure. JAMA Surg. 2014;149(4):380–2.
23. Rosenthal RJ, Hiatt JR, Phillips EH, Hewitt W, Demetriou AA, Grode M. Intracranial pressure.

Effects of pneumoperitoneum in large-animal model. Surg Endosc. 1997;11(4):376–80.
24. Robba C, Cardim D, Donnelly J, Bertuccio A, Bacigaluppi S, Bragazzi N, Cabella B, et al. Effects of pneumoperitoneum and Trendelenburg position on intracranial pressure assessed using different non-invasive methods. Br J Anaesth. 2016;117(6):783–91.
25. Robba C, Bragazzi NL, Bertuccio A, Cardim D, Donnelly J, Sekhon M, Lavino A, et al. Effects of prone position and positive end-expiratory pressure on noninvasive estimators of ICP: a pilot study. J Neurosurg Anesthesiol. 2017;29(3):243–50.
26. Peruto CM, Ciccotti MG, Cohen SB. Shoulder arthroscopy positioning: lateral decubitus versus beach chair. Arthrosc J Arthrosc Relat Surg. 2009;25:891–6.
27. Pohl A, Cullen DJ. Cerebral ischemia during shoulder surgery in the upright position: a case series. J Clin Anesth. 2005;17:463–9.
28. Morandi X, Riffaud L, Amlashi SF, Brassier G. Extensive spinal cord infarction after posterior fossa surgery in the sitting position: case report. Neurosurgery. 2004;54:1512–5.
29. Smith JJ, Porth CM, Erickson M. Hemodynamic response to the upright posture. J Clin Pharmacol. 1994;34:375–86.
30. Hanouz JL, Fiant AL, Gérard Jl. Middle cerebral artery blood flow velocity during beach chair position for shoulder surgery under general anesthesia. J Clin Anesth. 2016;33:31–6.
31. Cardim D, Robba C, Matta B, Tytherleigh-Strong G, Kang N, Schmidt B, Donnelly J, et al. Cerebrovascular assessment of patients undergoing shoulder surgery in beach chair position using a multiparameter transcranial Doppler approach. J Clin Monit Comput. 2019;33(4):615–25.
32. Kietaibl C, Engel A, Horvat Menih I, Huepfl M, Erdoes G, Kubista B, Ullrich R, et al. Detection and differentiation of cerebral microemboli in patients undergoing major orthopaedic surgery using transcranial Doppler ultrasound. Br J Anaesth. 2017 Mar 1;118(3):400–6.

Cardiac Surgery

24

Massimo Lamperti, Amit Jain, and Vinay Byrappa

Contents

M. Lamperti (✉) · A. Jain · V. Byrappa
Anesthesiology Institute, Cleveland Clinic Abu Dhabi, Abu Dhabi, United Arab Emirates
e-mail: lamperm@clevelandclinicabudhabi.ae

C. Robba, G. Citerio (eds.), *Echography and Doppler of the Brain*,
https://doi.org/10.1007/978-3-030-48202-2_24

24.1 Introduction

Preserving cerebral perfusion during cardiac surgery represents a challenge due to the baseline characteristics of patients with cardiovascular diseases who often have coexisting peripheral vessel disease, impaired cerebral circulation, and altered autoregulation of cerebral blood flow (CBF). Cardiopulmonary bypass (CPB) can further impair CBF due to the inflammatory process that happens during hypothermia and low flow during retrograde perfusion [1].

Neurological complications are common after cardiac surgery or establishment of extracirculatory mechanical oxygenation (ECMO) when cerebral ischaemia can occur due to inadequate perfusion pressure or microemboli. Stroke has been reported in 6–10% of high-risk cardiac surgical patients [2] and more frequently postoperative delirium can affect up to 75% of patients after cardiac surgery [3].

Point-of-care brain ultrasound (POCUS-B) can be a useful perioperative tool to investigate neurologic complications during the intraoperative phase and to predict major post-operative neurological complications [4]. POCUS-B should be used as a stepwise tool starting from a black-and-white 2D imaging to more complex monitoring as transcranial colour-coded duplex sonography (TCCD) to visualise the vessels and then to transcranial Doppler (TCD) to analyse the flow in the main cerebral arteries during cardiac procedures or in states where the CBF can be altered. The main goal of this section is to show the possible use of POCUS-B in cardiac surgery during the perioperative setting both in adult and paediatric patients.

24.2 Basic POCUS-B in Cardiac Surgery

Cardiac patients or patients on ECMO are at risk of cerebral accidents due to the need to keep them anticoagulated. An early detection of an intracerebral problem caused by excessive anticoagulation during the surgical procedure can be helpful to drive the need for a neurosurgical consult and eventual intervention.

TCCD [5–7] offers a non-invasive bedside alternative to radiologic methods to detect intracerebral haemorrhage (ICH). It can be helpful for the detection and monitoring of midline shift (MLS) that correlates to unfavourable neurological outcome [8]. The main transcranial window suggested for TCCD is the temporal window with a phased-array probe 2–2.5 MHz high frame-to-frame averaging.

The use of intraoperative POCUS-B can be suggested whenever there are sudden changes in the neuromonitoring signals as sudden drop of the cerebral oximetry in one cerebral lobe or altered electroencephalographic signal with appearance of burst suppression without increase of the sedative agents.

24.3 Brain Ultrasound Monitoring in Paediatric Cardiac Surgery

With the introduction of CPB in 1960s the repair of CHD was made possible. However, initially the mortality was high in infants and neonates with CHD. In the 1970s, Murphy and colleagues [9] and Barratt-Boyes and colleagues [10, 11] used deep hypothermic circulatory arrest (DHCA) for the performance of heart surgery in neonates and small infants which was associated with a significant improvement in short-term survival. But, with improved survival, the recognition of neurodevelopmental abnormalities among the survivors of successful cardiac repair also increased suggesting a multiple impact theory [12–15].

The neurological injury in CHD surgical patients is thus multifactorial and any one single monitoring modality is unlikely to detect all possible threats. Using a combination of various currently available neuro-monitoring modalities may allow for early detection and possible intervention and thus help to improve neurological outcome in CHD surgeries.

24.3.1 Usefulness of Preoperative Brain Ultrasonography in Paediatric Cardiac Surgery

In few centres performing CHD surgeries in infants, preoperative head ultrasound scans (HUSs) are routine, although the utility of HUS in detecting pre-existing brain injury in CHD is not established. The incidence of brain injury on MRI in patients with CHD is found to be between 25 and 40% in various studies [16–18]. A prospective study comparing the utility of preoperative HUSs with MRI in 167 infants with CHD found preoperative brain injury in 5 infants (3%) on HUS and on MRI in 44 infants (26%); authors concluded that in asymptomatic newborns and young infants undergoing CHD surgery routine HUS is not indicated [19].

24.3.2 Usefulness of Intraoperative Brain Ultrasonography in Paediatric Cardiac Surgery

During intraoperative period, CBF is best determined using transcranial Doppler (TCD) but conventional TCD devices are not routinely available in theatres, and it may be cumbersome to measure blood flow velocities by trans-temporal window in infants during surgery. Point-of-care trans-fontanellar cerebral ultrasound (TFCU) can be used in paediatric patients whose fontanelles have not closed yet [20]. The anterior fontanelle generally closes between 4 and 24 months of age. Some of the advantages of using TFCU are the following:

- Intraoperative application using a conventional cardiac ultrasound machine equipped with a sector probe (S12–4 sector probe; S3–8 sector probe)
- Easy adjustment of the Doppler beam angle parallel to the blood flow direction in internal carotid artery (ICA) and peri-callosal part of anterior cerebral artery (pACA)
- Detection of brain lesions such as intracerebral haemorrhage and hydrocephalus

A study done to evaluate the feasibility of intraoperative point-of-care TFCU in 35 infants showed that intraoperative TFCU can effectively measure the CBF at the ICA and pACA during paediatric cardiac surgery. Thus, TFCU can be a practical CBF monitoring modality when rSO2 on cerebral oximetry changes without any specific reason in infants [20].

24.3.2.1 Transcranial Doppler in Paediatric CHD Surgery

TCD has been used extensively in paediatric CHD surgery research to examine cerebral physiology in response to CPB, hypothermia, DHCA, low-flow bypass, and regional low-flow perfusion (RLFP). Multiple researchers have described the role of TCD in detecting cerebral emboli and CBF velocities during CPB in children undergoing CHD surgeries [21–23].

24.3.2.2 Role of TCD During Deep Hypothermic Cardiopulmonary Bypass (DHCPB), Deep Hypothermic Circulatory Arrest (DHCA) and Low-Flow Cardiopulmonary Bypass

In complex aortic arch repair surgeries, the introduction of DHCPB and DHCA has improved the operating conditions and decreased cardiac morbidity. Continuous low-flow CPB with profound hypothermia hypothetically provides an indefinite period of cerebral perfusion and has been suggested as being superior to DHCA in preventing neurological damage [24, 25]. However, cerebral autoregulation (CA) defined as the maintenance of constant CBF despite changes in cerebral perfusion pressure (CPP) is deeply affected by temperature. Autoregulation is preserved during normothermic CPB; it begins to alter at temperature less than 25 °C, and it is lost at temperature less than 20 °C [26]. TCD pattern consistent with increased cerebral vascular resistance in the early post-operative period is seen in patients treated with profound hypothermia and low-flow CPB or circulatory arrest, whereas this pattern is not present in patients treated with moderately hypothermic CPB. This pattern of cerebrovascular changes occurred with greater frequency in patients who had a period of circulatory arrest [27]. The CBF remains decreased even after CPB rewarming whereas it returned to baseline in normothermic CPB [28]. A study which used TCD as an indicator of perfusion during repair of congenital heart defects requiring moderate or profound hypothermia and low-flow CPB found that there was an immediate loss of detectable CBFV in the middle cerebral artery (MCA) when CPP decreased below 9 mmHg suggesting that CPP is a crucial parameter, rather than pump flow rate, in impacting brain perfusion [23]. Similarly a study by Zimmermann et al. [29] performed on 28 neonates undergoing the arterial switch operation with α-stat acid-base management showed that cerebral perfusion is detected by TCD in the MCA in some neonates at bypass flow as low as 10 ml/kg per minute. But a minimum bypass flow rate of 30 ml/kg per minute was needed to detect cerebral perfusion in all neonates. All patients with a mean arterial pressure (MAP) of 19 mmHg or greater, regardless of pump flow rate, had detectable cerebral perfusion by TCD but correlation between MAP and CPB pump flow rates was minimal, confirming the conclusions of Taylor et al. [26] that MAP alone is a poor indicator of CPP.

TCD is also useful in identifying the "ductal steal phenomenon", which is described as a sharp decrease in diastolic flow velocity and an increase in pulse amplitude in the anterior communicating artery (ACA) in the presence of a large unrestricted patent ductus arteriosus (PDA) [30]. End-diastolic block in the absence of end-diastolic blood flow is cranial Doppler waveforms for at least 20 consecutive cardiac cycles in the ACA or basilic artery (BA). The occurrence of end-diastolic block in either ACA or BA, a MAP <30 mmHg and a PDA appear to correlate with the development of an intraventricular haemorrhage in infants with a birthweight <1000 gm [31].

24.3.2.3 Role of TCD During Regional Low-Flow Perfusion (RLFP) for Neonatal Aortic Arch Reconstruction

Regional low-flow perfusion is a technique where the brain is perfused via the right innominate artery in neonates undergoing aortic arch reconstruction surgeries. When unilateral near-infrared spectroscopy (NIRS) was used to assess the unilateral cerebral oxygen saturation during RLFP, the mean regional cerebral oxygen saturation (rSO2) was 6.3% lower on the left side, and about half of the patients had a difference of 10% in the absolute values of rSO2 during RLFP. When perfusion was initiated through carotid arteries before or after RLFP/with or without bypass, bilateral rSO2 values agreed closely [32]. However, NIRS is able to detect only inadequate CBF but not excessive CBF. TCD can be a very useful monitoring tool to identify excessive cerebral flow and aid in maintaining adequate CBF to prevent cerebral oedema and haemorrhage.

24.3.2.4 Role of TCD for Detecting Cerebral Emboli

Emboli can be easily detected using TCD. True emboli produce characteristic audio and visual signals known as high-intensity transient signals (HITS) which can be counted by the TCD software. Although emboli can be detected by TCD, false-positive artefacts due to electrocautery and physical contact with the transducer probe can occur [33]. The TCD counter can accurately detect the number of emboli in the artery of study but it will not be able to distinguish from the false-positive artefacts and if a large number of artefacts are detected in a short period of time, the number counted is meaningless. There are a number of limitations of TCD in cerebral embolus detection. The number of emboli detected in the carotid artery during paediatric congenital heart surgery does not appear to correlate with acute post-operative neurological deficits [33] and the emboli are detected when already it has occurred.

24.4 Brain Ultrasound Monitoring in Adult Cardiac Surgery

TCD has been used extensively both as a sole modality and as a part of multimodal approach in studies looking into the neurological complications associated with adult cardiac surgery.

24.4.1 Preoperative Transcranial Doppler

However, usefulness of multimodal preoperative risk stratification strategies using preoperative neurophysiological examination and imaging modalities has not yet been established. Few researchers used TCD to identify at-risk patients [34].

24.4.1.1 Preoperative Transcranial Doppler and Short-Term POCD

Reduced preoperative CBF velocity in the left MCA detected on TCD represents an independent risk factor for short-term POCD in patients who underwent cardiac surgery [35]. However, CBF velocity in the right MCA was unrelated to short-term POCD [35]. Specifically, a reduction in left-sided blood flow velocity of 1 cm/s was related to roughly a 10% greater likelihood of exhibiting cognitive decline 1 week after cardiac surgery.

24.4.1.2 Preoperative Transcranial Doppler and Long-Term POCD

In an extension study by Benvenuti et al. [36], a reduced preoperative CBF velocity in left MCA but not in the right MCA was associated with the development of POCD at 3 months after cardiac surgery and this association was independent to years of education and EuroSCORE. As the short-term POCD following cardiac surgery has been associated with higher incidence of long-term cognitive dysfunction in recent studies, predicting risk of short-term POCD with preoperative reduced left CBF velocity that may indirectly identify the patients at risk of longer term cognitive dysfunctions.

24.4.1.3 Preoperative Transcranial Doppler and Cerebral Autoregulation Before Cardiac Surgery

CA is the intrinsic ability of cerebral vasculature to maintain adequate CBF over a wide range of cerebral perfusion pressure despite fluctuations in blood pressures. Cardiac surgery may result in alterations in CA and methods to determine CA at the baseline, during, and after the cardiac surgery may help in understanding the effects of CPB on CA as well as in understanding the pathogenesis of neurological complications in these patients [1].

A few researchers used TCD to assess CA through static methods. Two studies analysed dynamic CA using autoregulation index and rate of dynamic autoregulation recovery indices [37]. None of the study identified impaired CA before surgery. But impairment of CA during surgery was a common finding; there exists a significant relationship between impaired CA and adverse clinical outcomes including stroke, acute kidney injury, delirium, and mortality [38].

Understanding the significance of impaired preoperative CA therefore has considerable potential to improve models for the prediction of brain damage after cardiac surgery and warrants further investigation.

24.4.1.4 Preoperative Transcranial Doppler and Right-to-Left Intra-cardiac Shunt

For detection of right-to-left shunt (RLS), TCD monitoring is performed during the intravenous injection of agitated saline or contrast medium and patient performance of a Valsalva manoeuvre to enhance flow across the shunt.

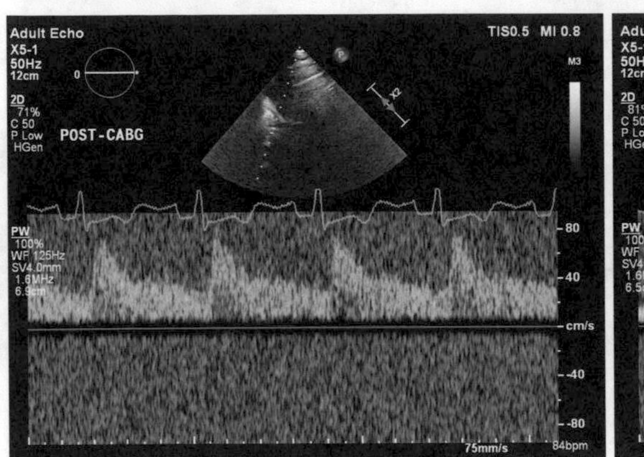

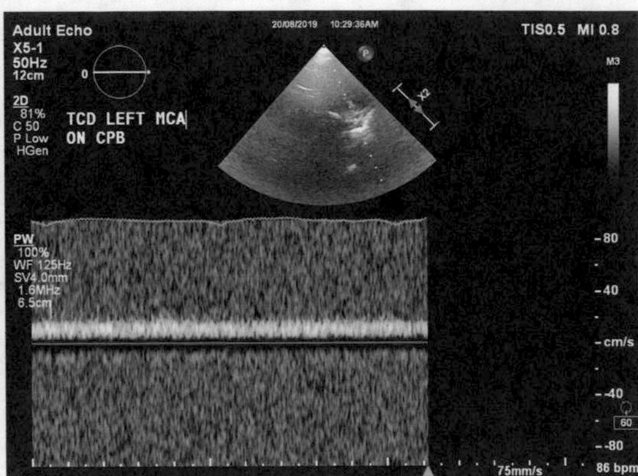

Fig. 24.1 Showing TCD in left MCA in an adult patient

TCD with "bubble test" appears as the best screening test for the detection of RLS in young and middle-aged adults. In a recent study by Palazzo et al. [39] when comparing TCD with "bubble test" to transoesophageal echocardiography (TEE), sensitivity and specificity were both 100%. In patients with cryptogenic acute cerebral ischaemic events, TCD can help to select patients potentially suitable for closure procedure after TEE confirmation.

24.4.2 Intraoperative Use of Transcranial Doppler

TCD is the only clinically useful brain ultrasound modality that has been evaluated for use in adult cardiac surgery. Typically, prior to surgery a baseline TCD evaluation is performed bilaterally in all basal arteries. However, during the cardiac surgery, initial segment (M1) of MCA is monitored through trans-temporal acoustic window. The key elements that can be evaluated using TCD during cardiac surgery are described in detail:

24.4.2.1 Transcranial Doppler for Evaluation of Cerebral Autoregulation (CA)

As highlighted above, TCD has a potential role in determining CA. TCD provides greater flexibility and accuracy than more classical techniques to measure CBF such as 133Xe. With a greater focus on the impairment of CA during cardiac surgery and its potential role in post-operative neurological complications, interest has been created in studying the role of TCD in the evaluation of CA during and after cardiac surgeries. Figure 24.1 shows TCD in patients before and during CPB.

Few researchers utilised TCD to evaluate CA (both static and dynamic models) during CPB as a sole monitoring modality as well as in combination with NIRS and ultrasound-tagged NIRS. TCD-derived indices of static CA (sCA) are defined as change in cerebral vascular resistance index (CVRi) related to change in CPP during the Trendelenburg manoeuvre. TCD indices of dynamic CA that were variably used in these studies include [40]:

- Autoregulation index (ARI)
- Coherence: fraction of CBFV power, linearly explained by MAP at each frequency
- Phase: transfer function analysis phase lag between CBFV and MAP at each frequency
- Gain: transfer function analysis amplitude between CBFV and BP at each frequency
- Rate of dynamic autoregulation recovery (RoR): ratio of slope of CBFV recovery normalised by BP after thigh cuff release

During CPB, as many as 10–30% of the patients have impaired CA (ARI lower than pre-bypass values). CA parameters are adversely affected by haemodilution and hypercapnia and during rewarming. Most studies demonstrated better preserved average CA after surgery with return of pulsatile flow.

Ono et al. [41] reported higher incidence of perioperative stroke in patients with impaired CA. In a study by Joshi et al. [42] all seven strokes that occurred perioperatively were in patients with impaired CBF autoregulation during CPB rewarming. Other researchers identified impaired CA during CPB as a risk factor for postoperative delirium but not for stroke. Hori et al. [43] reported fourfold higher frequency of delirium in patients whom MAP exceeded upper limit of autoregulation, but not with lower limit of autoregulation.

Changes in CA following DHCA have been demonstrated in adults. In a study of 67 patients undergoing aortic arch surgery, Neri and colleagues [44] compared the influence of intraoperative DHCA ($n = 23$), selective antegrade cerebral perfusion (SACP; $n = 25$), and retrograde cerebral perfusion (RCP; $n = 19$). Dynamic CA was assessed using bilateral thigh compression to produce a step decrease in arterial pressure. Autoregulation was preserved only in patients managed with SACP. In the other two groups, impaired autoregulation persisted in some of the patients until the seventh postoperative day.

Overall, the excellent temporal resolution of TCD is particularly suitable to be combined with dynamic models of CA, but it is important to be aware of the diversity of modelling techniques that have been proposed. Moreover, there is need for extensive validation and further research to improve the reliability and usefulness of TCD for monitoring CA.

24.4.2.2 Transcranial Doppler to Monitor Cerebral Perfusion During Cardiac Surgery

Detection of Cerebral Hypotension During Off-Pump Versus On-Pump CABG

TCD determination of systolic and diastolic flow velocity baselines prior to surgical manipulation will allow for determining an intervention threshold. Both cerebral hypoperfusion and hyperperfusion can be diagnosed. Generally, a reduction of mean systolic velocity by 60% or absence of diastolic velocity is considered a sign of hypoperfusion. Marked hypoperfusion during off-pump CABG is usually observed during manipulation and cardiac verticalisation [45]. Often, TCD flow velocity spectrum normalises upon stabilising the heart in proper position. During non-pulsatile flow, a velocity reduction of 80% is considered an ischaemic threshold. Changes in flow velocities can be related to head position, cannula position or insufficient pump flow/blood pressure during CPB.

Detection of Cerebral Hyperperfusion During Cardiac Surgery

Cerebral hyperperfusion during CPB may also increase the risk of neurological injury. In a study by Brillman et al. [46], five patients undergoing CABG had more than a 50% increase in MCA mean flow velocity during the initial phase (10–120 s) of CPB. Four of these five patients developed neurological complications including stroke and encephalopathy. Hyperaemia would result in elevation of CBF velocities in both the MCA and ICA with Lindegaard ratios <3.

Detection of Efficacy of Selective Cerebral Perfusion During Deep Hypothermic Circulatory Arrest

TCD can be used to monitor the efficacy of selective cerebral perfusion during DHCA. It can detect both antegrade and retrograde flow in the MCA. In a study of 32 consecutive adults undergoing thoracic aortic aneurysm repair, Tanoue et al. [47] used TCD to monitor low-flow cerebral perfusion during DHCA. MCA blood flow could only be detected in 20% of patients managed with RCP (15–25 mmHg). In contrast, MCA blood flow was detected in 16/17 patients managed with SACP (500 ml/min). Patients managed with RCP had significant cerebral hyperaemia in the early post-operative period. It is suggested that the use of RCP pressures higher than those usually recommended (≥40 mmHg) may improve cerebral protection [48].

24.4.2.3 Transcranial Doppler to Detect Cerebral Emboli During Cardiac Surgery

Traditionally, cerebral embolism has been recognised as one of the most important mechanisms for perioperative stroke in cardiac patients. However, a few studies have shown a robust correlation between the embolic load and cognitive dysfunction [49]. Furthermore, a recently published study failed to demonstrate a significant relation between neurological complications and presence, size, or number of new lesions on MRI [50]. Whatsoever the mechanism, TCD remains the most common modality to determine the presence, size (macro or micro), and number and nature (solid or gaseous) of embolic phenomenon during cardiac surgeries.

Technique

Cerebral microemboli (MES) can be diagnosed by non-imaging TCD monitoring through the detection of HITS, and are defined by the following criteria:

- HITS usually lasting less than 300 ms
- Doppler amplitude exceeding background Doppler frequency spectrum signal by at least 3 dB
- Unidirectional signal within the Doppler velocity spectrum
- A characteristic "moaning" or "chirping" sound

Bilateral or unilateral monitoring of a targeted intracranial vessel is recorded for a minimum of 30 min. TCD systems equipped with automated HITS detection software that counts the number of microemboli and measures microembolic signal intensity are useful. However, for a reliable diagnosis, both visual and auditory inspection and confirmation of each detected HITS are required.

TCD Versus TEE for Detection of Cerebral Embolism

TCD detection of emboli has been compared with TEE [51]. TEE has an advantage over TCD as it allows assessment of aorta for atheroma and evaluation of cardiac functions for clinical decision-making. The numbers of emboli detected by TEE are usually substantially higher than with TCD, reflecting the fact that only a fraction of the aortic emboli enter the cerebral circulation. Also, the rates of embolisation on a second-by-second basis after clamp release are better delineated with TEE monitoring. However, TCD is non-invasive, less bulky, and less expensive. Several studies have demonstrated associations between TCD-detectable cerebral emboli and presence of significant aortic atheromatous disease that may be the factor responsible for adverse cerebral outcomes in cardiac surgery [52].

TCD-Detectable Cerebral Embolism and Aortic Atheroma

Atherosclerosis of the aortic arch has also been correlated with an increased risk of stroke after cardiac surgery [53]. The greater incidence of left-hemispheric (possibly due to the tendency of arch-generated emboli to move in the direction of blood flow to the downstream carotid vessel) strokes is an indirect evidence of the importance of aortic arch atherosclerosis [54].

TCD has helped us to further understand the factors responsible for cerebral embolism during CPB and non-bypass cardiac surgeries. A study by Mackensen et al. [52] supports the potential causal role of atheroma burden in the ascending aorta and the arch, but not in the descending aorta, genesis of TCD-detectable cerebral embolisation, and consequent neurological injury.

TCD-Detectable Emboli and Timing of Embolic Events During Cardiac Surgery

During cardiac surgery, cerebral emboli can be detected in virtually every patient regardless of whether CPB is used or not. Although cerebral embolism may occur during stable CPB, they are more frequently associated with distinct surgical and perfusion events. Several TCD-based studies have demonstrated that embolisation occurs primarily as a result of aortic manipulation during palpation, cannulation, cross-clamping, proximal coronary anastomosis, release of aortic clamping, start of cardiac ejection after open-heart surgery, and decannulation, and possibly as a result of a "sandblasting" effect from the high-velocity jet exiting the aortic cannula [55]. The highest number of microemboli is evident during aortic clamping and subsequent to the aortic declamping, especially for open-heart surgeries.

TCD-Detectable Cerebral Emboli and CPB Techniques During Cardiac Surgery and ECMO

There exists substantial role of circuits and devices in determining the microembolic incidence and the need for introducing adequate improvements to minimise microembolism during CPB and ECMO [56, 57]. Zanatta et al. [58] compared three different surgical procedures assisted by CPB (i.e. open-heart surgery, closed-heart surgery, and minimally invasive surgery) to characterise their emboligenic potential by monitoring blood flow velocity in the MCAs using the multi-frequency TCD system. Authors detected microemboli in every surgical procedure analysed, discovering the highest number of microembolic events in CPB with vacuum-assisted venous drainage, followed by open CPB and closed CPB. The higher number of microemboli in the open versus closed procedures is due to the entrapment of air in the heart chambers and pulmonary veins after the heart is closed. The higher number of microembolic load in CPB with vacuum-assisted venous drainage compared with open CPB, although rather limited, may be related to the vacuum-assisted venous drainage. Not surprisingly, the avoidance of CPB appears to reduce, but not entirely eliminate, cerebral embolism.

Membrane oxygenators appear to generate fewer cerebral microemboli than bubble oxygenators [59]. In comparison to alpha-stat, pH-stat arterial blood gas management during CPB is associated with greater delivery of microemboli to the cerebral circulation and worse neuropsychological outcome [60].

TCD evaluation of embolic events during bypass has helped to modify CPB techniques. This involves evaluation of procedure modifications, perfusion techniques, and novel devices that may reduce cerebral emboli. Numerous technical and procedural solutions, such as the application of double-venous cannulation, the cannulation of the distal aortic arch instead of the ascending aorta, the employment of arterial filters or air bubble traps in the arterial line, the use of membrane oxygenator, the application of an appropriate de-airing technique, the avoidance of aortic side clamping, the use of clampless devices, and the administration of drugs by a continuous infusion instead of bolus injection, seem to decrease the number of microemboli [57].

More widespread use of TCD monitoring in combination with TEE would allow individual teams of surgeons and perfusionists to refine their technique based on the results of their own practice.

TCD and Cerebral Embolus Differentiation (Particulate or Gaseous)

Despite significant advancement in the techniques of CPB, it remains a source for both particulate and gaseous emboli.

The issue of differentiating air and particulate emboli using TCD is important and is the subject of ongoing research. Based on acoustic signals on TCD, it is possible to distinguish gas from particulate emboli [61]. Due to greater density difference between blood and air, air emboli are usually loud and penetrate the Doppler spectral envelope, whereas particulate emboli are frequently contained within the envelope. Blood flow velocity, embolus size, and Doppler frequency also influence the differentiation of embolic signals. Higher frequencies give better resolution of the blood velocity, but lower frequencies allow better embolus recognition. Detailed analysis of Doppler ultrasound data can be used to provide an estimate of bubble diameter, total volume of air, and likely impact of embolic showers on cerebral blood flow [62]. Automated systems for embolus counting and identification are being developed.

Differentiation between solid and gaseous emboli is important not only to determine appropriate measures that need to be considered to reduce the load, but theoretically also to determine the nature of neurological complications [61]. Solid microemboli preferentially distribute in the right, rather than in the left, brain hemisphere, especially during aortic clamping and

Table 24.1 A systematic intervention plan initiated by EEG slowing[a] and/or cerebral venous oxygen desaturation[b]

	Temp	BP	TCD	Conclusion	Action
Pre-bypass	No change	No change	Peak velocity ↓	Aorta obstructed	Adjust aortic cannula
	No change	No change	Diastolic velocity ↓	Cava obstructed	Adjust venous cannula
	No change	No change	Solid emboli	Aortic atheroma dislodgement	Careful handling of aortic cannula
Cardiopulmonary bypass	No change	No change	Peak velocity ↑	Hyperaemia	↓pump flow
	No change	No change	Gas emboli	Gas emboli	De-air, repair circuit
	↑	No change	Peak velocity ↓	Flow-metabolism uncoupling	↑BP and ↓metabolic demand
	No change	No change	Peak velocity ↓	Cerebral flow low	Adjust cannula/clamp; ↑pump flow
Post-bypass	No change	No change	Diastolic velocity ↓	Cerebral oedema	Mannitol, ultrafiltration
Anytime	No change	↓	Peak velocity ↓	Dysautoregulation	↑BP; neuroprotectant
With increased EEG frequency	No change	No change/↑	No change or peak velocity ↑	Insufficient anaesthesia	↑Anaesthesia depth

[a]A suppressed EEG was defined as an amplitude of less than 10 pW or 50 dB (i.e. signal-to-noise ratio of <10:1) in more than 30% of epochs per minute. Excessive EEG slowing was defined as the relative delta (1.5–3.5 Hz) power band comprising more than 80% of the total power in the EEG signal

[b]Desaturation signifying cerebral ischaemia was defined as a regional cerebral venous oxygen saturation decrease of more than 20% of the baseline established just before aortic cannulation, which persisted for more than 3 min

declamping. The opposite was observed in the behaviour of the gaseous emboli during aortic clamping in CPB with vacuum-assisted venous drainage, presumably because of the different cannulation applied, femoral versus aortic. As the cognitive functions most investigated are attention, concentration, memory, and learning (typical of the left-brain functions), whereas right hemisphere dysfunction correlates with nonverbal memory decline, the higher distribution of the emboli in the right brain should not be considered as a minor problem [61].

24.5 Multimodal Neurologic Monitoring in Cardiac Surgery

Intraoperative monitoring of the brain can be challenging as there are multiple variables affecting the brain physiology (i.e. hypothermia, reduced pulse flow) and the patient is under general anaesthesia. Ultrasound with its basic POCUS-B findings and TCD provides good information on brain haemodynamic and brain content; this needs to be integrated with other information as electroencephalography and NIRS that inform regarding brain electrophysiology and global oxygenation. One such intervention algorithm based on the principles of integrated neuromonitoring is proposed by Austin et al. (Table 24.1) [63]. More complex integrated neurophysiological monitoring as evoked potentials can be useful for the early detection of brainstem- or spinal cord-related injuries during aortic arch repair.

24.6 Limitations of Transcranial Doppler in Cardiac Surgery

TCD requires adequate training and competences [64] and its application is still dedicated to complex cases or patients with a pre-existing neurological disorder who can benefit from a continuous monitoring of the CBF.

24.7 Conclusions

TCD can be extremely helpful in detecting brain complications related to cardiac surgery both in paediatric and adult patients. This technique is easy to perform during cardiac surgery and it can be considered as a good non-invasive tool for CBF monitoring and titrating perfusion flow both during cardiac surgery and when patients are under ECMO. Further research should be considered in this field given the new indications to put patients on ECMO when affected by acute lung injury.

References

1. Caldas JR, Haunton VJ, Panerai RB, Hajjar LA, Robinson TG. Cerebral autoregulation in cardiopulmonary bypass surgery: a systematic review. Interact Cardiovasc Thorac Surg. 2018;26:494–503.
2. Salazar JD, Wityk RJ, Grega MA, Borowicz LM, Doty JR, Petrofski JA, et al. Stroke after cardiac surgery: short- and long-term outcomes. Ann Thorac Surg. 2001;72:2.
3. Scolletta S, Taccone FS, Donadello K. Brain injury after cardiac surgery. Minerva Anestesiol. 2015;81:662–77.
4. Robba C, Goffi A, Geeraerts T, Cardim D, Via G, Czosnyka M, Park S, Sarwal A, Padayachy L, Rasulo F, Citerio G. Brain ultrasonography: methodology, basic and advanced principles and clinical applications. A narrative review. Intensive Care Med. 2019; https://doi.org/10.1007/s00134-019-05610-4. [Epub ahead of print]
5. Llompart Pou J, Abadal Centellas J, Palmer Sans M, et al. Monitoring midline shift by transcranial color-coded sonography in traumatic brain injury. Intensive Care Med. 2004;30:1672–5.
6. Stolz E, Gerriets T, Fiss I, Babacan SS, Seidel S, Kaps M. Comparison of transcranial color-coded duplex sonography and cranial CT measurements for determining third ventricle midline shift in space-occupying stroke. Am J Neuroradiol. 1999;20:1567–71.
7. Tang SC, Huang SJ, Jeng JS, Yip KP. Third ventricle midline shift due to spontaneous supratentorial intracerebral hemorrhage evaluated by transcranial color-coded sonography. J Ultrasound Med. 2006;5:203–9.
8. Voigt LP, Pastores SM, Raoof ND, Thaler HT, Halpern NA. Review of a large clinical series. Intrahospital transport of critically ill patients: outcomes, timing, and patterns. J Intensive Care Med. 2009;24:108–15.
9. Murphy JD, Freed MD, Keane JF, Norwood WI, Castaneda AR, As N. Hemodynamic results after intracardiac repair of tetralogy of Fallot by deep hypothermia and cardiopulmonary bypass. Circulation. 1980;62(2 Pt 2):1168.
10. Barratt-Boyes BG. Corrective surgery for congenital heart disease in infants with the use of profound hypothermia and circulatory arrest technique. Aust N Z J Surg. 1977;47:737–44.
11. Barratt-Boyes BG, Neutze JM. Primary repair of tetralogy of Fallot in infancy using profound hypothermia with circulatory arrest and limited cardiopulmonary bypass: a camparison with conventional two stage management. Ann Surg. 1973;178:406–11.
12. Boneva RS, Botto LD, Moore CA, Yang Y, Correa A, Erickson JD. Mortality associated with congenital heart defects in the United States: trends and racial disparities, 1979–1997. Circulation. 2001;103:2376–81.
13. Majnemer A, Limperopoulos C, Shevell M, Rosenblatt B, Rohlicek C, Tchervenkov C. Long term neuromotor outcome at school entry of infants with congenital heart defects requiring open heart surgery. J Pediatr. 2006;148:72–7.
14. Limperopoulos C, Majnemer A, Shevell MI, Rosenblatt B, Rohlicek C, Tchervenkov C. Neurodevelopmental status of newborns and infants with congenital heart defects before and after open heart surgery. J Pediatr. 2000;137:638–45.
15. Fuller S, Nord AS, Gerdes M, Wernovsky G, Jarvik GP, Bernbaum J, et al. Predictors of impaired neurodevelopmental outcomes at one year of age after infant cardiac surgery. Eur J Cardiothorac Surg. 2009;36:40–7.
16. Mahle WT, Tavani F, Zimmerman RA, et al. An MRI study of neurological injury before and after congenital heart surgery. Circulation. 2002;106(S1):I109–14.
17. Petit CJ, Rome JJ, Wernovsky G, et al. Preoperative brain injury in transposition of the great arteries is associated with oxygenation and time to surgery, not balloon atrial septostomy. Circulation. 2009;119:709–16.
18. Block AJ, McQuillen PS, Chau V, et al. Clinically silent preoperative brain injuries do not worsen with surgery in neonates with congenital heart disease. J Thorac Cardiovasc Surg. 2010;140:550–7.
19. Rios DR, Welty SE, Gunn JK, Beca J, Minard CG, Goldsworthy M, Coleman L, Hunter JV, Andropoulos DB, Shekerdemian LS. Usefulness of routine head ultrasound scans before surgery for congenital heart disease. Pediatrics. 2013;131:e1765–70.
20. Park YH, Song IK, Lee JH, Kim HS, Kim CS, Kim JT. Intraoperative trans-fontanellar cerebral ultrasonography in infants during cardiac surgery under cardiopulmonary bypass: an observational study. J Clin Monit Comput. 2017;31:159–65.
21. Van der Linden J, Priddy R, Ekroth R, et al. Cerebral perfusion and metabolism during profound hypothermia in children. A study of middle cerebral artery ultrasonic variables and cerebral extraction of oxygen. J Thorac Cardiovasc Surg. 1991;102:103–14.
22. Van der Linden J, Wesslen O, et al. Transcranial Doppler-estimated versus thermodilution-estimated cerebral blood flow during cardiac

operations. Influence of temperature and arterial carbon dioxide tension. J Thorac Cardiovasc Surg. 1991;102:95–102.
23. Burrows FA, Bissonnette B. Cerebral blood flow velocity patterns during cardiac surgery utilizing profound hypothermia with low-flow cardiopulmonary bypass or circulatory arrest in neonates and infants. Can J Anaesth. 1993;40:298–307.
24. Fox LS, Blackstone EH, Kirkling JW, Bishop SP, Bergdahl LA, Bradley EL. Relationship of brain blood flow and oxygen consumption to perfusion flow rate during profoundly hypothermic cardiopulmonary bypass. An experimental study. J Thorac Cardiovasc Surg. 1984;87:658–64.
25. Rebeyka IM, Coles JG, Wilson GJ, Watanabe T, Taylor MJ, Adler SF, Mickle DA, Romaschin AD, Ujc H, Burrows F. The effect of low flow cardiopulmonary bypass on cerebral function: an experimental study and clinical study. Ann Thorac Surg. 1987;43:391–6.
26. Taylor R, Burrows F, Bissonnette B. Cerebral pressure-flow velocity relationship during hypothermic cardiopulmonary bypass in neonates and infants. Anesth Analg. 1992;74:636–42.
27. Jonassen A, Quaegebeur J, Young W. Cerebral blood flow velocity in pediatric patients is reduced after cardiopulmonary bypass with profound hypothermia. J Thorac Cardiovasc Surg. 1995;110:934–43.
28. Greeley W, Ungerlider R, Kern F, Brusino G, Smith R, Reves J. Effect of cardiopulmonary bypass on cerebral blood flow in neonates, infants and children. Circulation. 1989;80(suppl I):209–15.
29. Zimmerman A, Burrows F, Jonas R, Hickey P. The limits of detectable cerebral perfusion by transcranial Doppler sonography in neonates undergoing deep hypothermic low-flow cardiopulmonary bypass. J Thorac Cardiovasc Surg. 1997;114:594–600.
30. Perlman JM, Hill A, Volpe JJ. The effect of patent ductus arteriosus on flow velocity in the anterior cerebral arteries: ductal steal in the premature newborn infant. J Pediatr. 1981;99:767–71.
31. Julkunen M, Parviainen T, Janas M, et al. End-diastolic block in cerebral circulation may predict intraventricular hemorrhage in hypotensive extremely low birth weight infants. Ultrasound Med Biol. 2008;34:538–45.
32. Andropoulos DB, Diaz LK, Fraser CD Jr, et al. Is bilateral monitoring of cerebral oxygen saturation necessary during neonatal aortic arch reconstruction? Anesth Analg. 2004;98:1267–72.
33. O'Brien JJ, Butterworth J, Hammon JW, et al. Cerebral emboli during cardiac surgery in children. Anesthesiology. 1997;87:1063–9.
34. Anastasiadis K, Karamitsos TD, Velissaris I, Makrygiannakis K, Kiskinis D. Preoperative screening and management of carotid artery disease in patients undergoing cardiac surgery. Perfusion. 2009;24:257–62.
35. Messerotti Benvenuti S, Zanatta P, Longo C, Mazzarolo AP, Palomba D. Preoperative cerebral hypoperfusion in the left, not in the right, hemisphere is associated with cognitive decline after cardiac surgery. Psychosom Med. 2012;74:73–80.
36. Messerotti Benvenuti S, Zanatta P, Valfrè C, Polesel E, Palomba D. Preliminary evidence for reduced preoperative cerebral blood flow velocity as a risk factor for cognitive decline three months after cardiac surgery: an extension study. Perfusion. 2012;27:486–92.
37. Severdija EE, Vranken NPA, Simons AP, Gommer ED, Heijmans JH, Maessen JG, et al. Hemodilution combined with hypercapnia impairs cerebral autoregulation during normothermic cardiopulmonary bypass. J Cardiothorac Vasc Anesth. 2015;29:1194–9.
38. Christiansen CB, Berg RM, Plovsing R, Ronit A, Holstein-Rathlou NH, Yndgaard S, et al. Dynamic cerebral autoregulation after cardiopulmonary bypass. Thorac Cardiovasc Surg. 2015;64:569–74.
39. Palazzo P, Ingrand P, Agius P, Belhadj Chaidi R, Neau JP. Transcranial Doppler to detect right-to-left shunt in cryptogenic acute ischemic stroke. Brain Behav. 2019;9:e01091.
40. Preisman S, Marks R, Nahtomi-Shick O, Sidi A. Preservation of static and dynamic cerebral autoregulation after mild hypothermic cardiopulmonary bypass. Br J Anaesth. 2005;95:207–11.
41. Ono M, Joshi B, Brady K, Easley RB, Zheng Y, Brown C, et al. Risks for impaired cerebral autoregulation during cardiopulmonary bypass and postoperative stroke. Br J Anaesth. 2012;109:391–8.
42. Joshi B, Brady K, Lee J, Easley B, Panigrahi R, Smielewski P, et al. Impaired autoregulation of cerebral blood flow during rewarming from hypothermic cardiopulmonary bypass and its potential association with stroke. Anesth Analg. 2010;110:321–8.
43. Hori D, Brown C, Ono M, Rappold T, Sieber F, Gottschalk A, et al. Arterial pressure above the upper cerebral autoregulation limit during cardiopulmonary bypass is associated with postoperative delirium. Br J Anaesth. 2014;113:1009–17.
44. Neri E, Sassi C, Barabesi L, et al. Cerebral autoregulation after hypothermic circulatory arrest in operations on the aortic arch. Ann Thorac Surg. 2004;77:72–9.
45. Kosir G, Tetickovic E. Intraoperative transcranial doppler ultrasonography monitoring of cerebral blood flow during coronary artery bypass grafting. Acta Clin Croat. 2011;50:5–11.
46. Brillman J, Davis D, Clark RE, et al. Increased middle cerebral artery flow velocity during the initial phase of cardiopulmonary bypass may cause neurological dysfunction. J Neuroimaging. 1995;5:135–41.
47. Tanoue Y, Tominaga R, Ochiai Y, et al. Comparative study of retrograde and selective cerebral perfusion with transcranial Doppler. Ann Thorac Surg. 1999;67:672–5.
48. Ganzel BL, Edmonds HL Jr, Pank JR, Goldsmith LJ. Neurophysiologic monitoring to assure delivery of retrograde cerebral perfusion. J Thorac Cardiovasc Surg. 1997;113:748–55.
49. Van der Linden J. Cerebral hemodynamics after low flow versus no-flow procedures. Ann Thorac Surg. 1995;59:1321–5.

50. Patel N, Horsfield MA, Banahan C, Janus J, Masters K, Morlese J, et al. Impact of perioperative infarcts after cardiac surgery. Stroke. 2015;46:680–6.
51. Barbut D, Yao FS, Hager DN, Kavanaugh P, Trifiletti RR, Gold JP. Comparison of transcranial Doppler ultrasonography and transesophageal echocardiography to monitor emboli during coronary artery bypass surgery. Stroke. 1996;27:87–90.
52. Mackensen GB, Ti LK, Phillips-Bute BG, Mathew JP, Newman MF, Grocott HP. Neurologic outcome research group (NORG). Cerebral embolization during cardiac surgery: impact of aortic atheroma burden. Br J Anaesth. 2003;91:656–61.
53. Roach G, Kanchuger M, Mora Mangano C, Newman M. Adverse cerebral outcomes after coronary bypass surgery. N Engl J Med. 1996;335:1857–63.
54. Marschall K, Kanchuger M, Kessler K, et al. Superiority of transesophageal echocardiography in detecting aortic arch atheromatous disease: identification of patients at increased risk of stroke during cardiac surgery. J Cardiothorac Vasc Anesth. 1994;8:5–13.
55. Arrowsmith JE, Maruthi SSRG. Intraoperative brain monitoring in cardiac surgery. In: Bonser RS, Pagano D, Haverich A, editors. Brain protection in cardiac surgery. London: Springer-Verlag; 2011.
56. MacLennan N, Lam AM. Intraoperative neurological monitoring with transcranial Doppler ultrasonography. Semin Anesthesiol. 1997;16:56–68.
57. Groom RC, Quinn RD, Lennon P, et al. Detection and elimination of microemboli related to cardiopulmonary bypass. Circ Cardiovasc Qual Outcomes. 2009;2:191–19.
58. Zanatta P, Forti A, Minniti G, Comin A, Mazzarolo AP, Chilufya M, et al. Brain emboli distribution and differentiation during cardiopulmonary bypass. J Cardiothorac Vasc Anesth. 2013;27:865–75.
59. Padayachee TS, Parsons S, Theobold R, Linley J, Gosling RG, Deverall PB. The detection of microemboli in the middle cerebral artery during cardiopulmonary bypass: a transcranial Doppler ultrasound investigation using membrane and bubble oxygenators. Ann Thorac Surg. 1987;44(3):298–302.
60. Murkin JM. Con: blood gases should not be corrected for temperature during hypothermic cardiopulmonary bypass: alpha-stat mode. J Cardiothorac Anesth. 1988;2:705–7.
61. Darbellay GA, Duff R, Vesin JM, Despland PA, Droste DW, Molina C, et al. Solid or gaseous circulating brain emboli: are they separable by transcranial ultrasound? J Cereb Blood Flow Metab. 2004;24:860–8.
62. Banahan C, Hague JP, Evans DH, Patel R, Ramnarine KV, Chung EM. Sizing gaseous emboli using Doppler embolic signal intensity. Ultrasound Med Biol. 2012;38:824–33.
63. Austin EH, Edmonds HL Jr, Auden SM, et al. Surgery for congenital heart disease: benefit of neurophysiologic monitoring for pediatric cardiac surgery. J Thorac Cardiovasc Surg. 1997;114:707–17.
64. Robba C, Poole D, Citerio G, Taccone FS, Rasulo FA. Consensus on brain ultrasonography in critical care group. Brain ultrasonography consensus on skill recommendations and competence levels within the critical care setting. Neurocrit Care. 2019; https://doi.org/10.1007/s12028-019-00766-9.

Part IX

Clinical Cases

25 Case 1: Vasospasm Treated with Intra-Arterial Nimodipine

Rita Bertuetti, Maurizio Saini, Davide Savo, Francesca Simonassi, Kartika Chandrapatham, and Tarek Senussi

A 46-year-old woman was admitted to A&E for poor-grade aSAH from ruptured left MCA aneurysm associated with intracranial haematoma (ICH) and intraventricular haemorrhage (IVH) (Fig. 25.1a–c). After surgical clipping and EVD positioning she was admitted to ICU. Between days 7 and 10 after bleeding, TCCD examination revealed increasing flow velocity in the left MCA M1 (Fig. 25.2a–h); therefore decision was taken then to perform an angio-CT and CT perfusion. CT showed severe vasospasm in the left MCA associated to prolonged mean transit time (MTT) in left fronto-temporo-parietal regions despite induced arterial hypertension (systolic ABP >200 mmHg) (Fig. 25.3a–c). Digital Subtraction Angiography (DSA) confirmed severe vasospasm and the neuroradiologist decided to start intra-arterial nimodipine infusion through the insertion of a catheter into the left internal carotid artery (Fig. 25.4a–f). After the treatment with intra-arterial vasodilators was started both TCD flow velocities progressive decrease and angiographic response were both observed (Fig. 25.5a–c).

R. Bertuetti (✉)
Department of Anesthesiology, Critical Care Medicine and Emergency, Division of Neurocritical Care, ASST Spedali Civili di Brescia, University Hospital, Brescia, Italy

M. Saini · D. Savo
Department of Emergency, Perioperative Medicine and Intensive Care, Neuroanesthesia and Neurointensive Care Unit, San Gerardo Hospital, ASST-Monza, Monza, Italy

F. Simonassi · K. Chandrapatham
Anesthesia and Intensive Care, Ospedale Policlinico San Martino – IRCCS for Oncology and Neurosciences, Genoa, Italy

T. Senussi
Department of Surgical Sciences and Integrated Diagnostics, University of Genoa, Genoa, Italy

C. Robba, G. Citerio (eds.), *Echography and Doppler of the Brain*,
https://doi.org/10.1007/978-3-030-48202-2_25

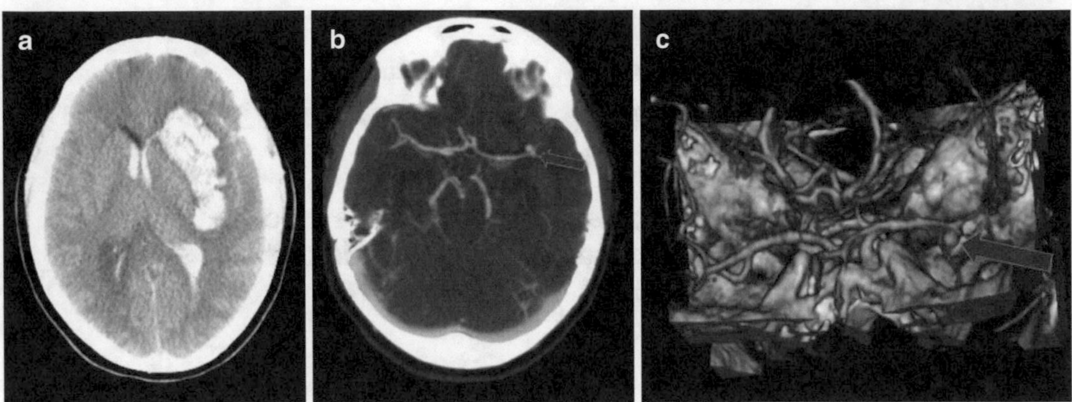

Fig. 25.1 (**a–c**) In panel **a** on the left: CT head showing right fronto parietal heamatoma, SAH and IVH. In panels **b** and **c**: CT angio points out aneurysm of the left MCA at its bifurcation

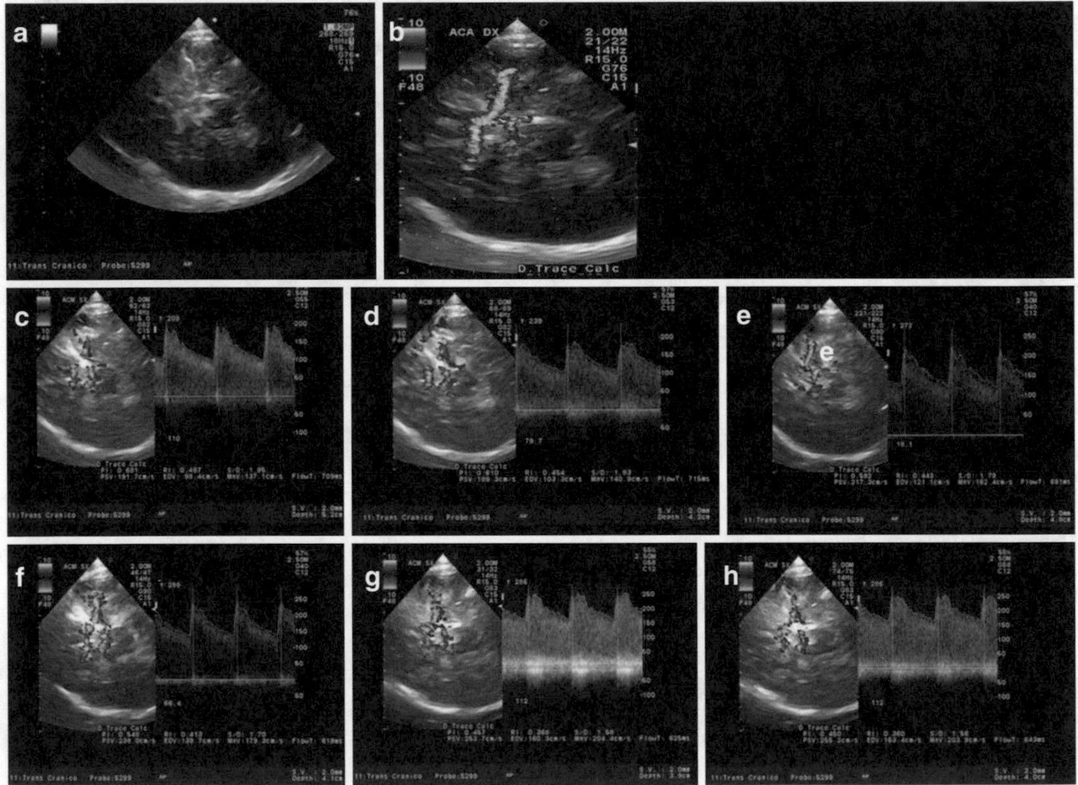

Fig. 25.2 (**a–h**) Brain ultrasound in B mode in panel **a** shows midbrain and basal cysterns, color doppler allows visualization of the vessels of the circle of willis (panel **b**). Application of pulsed doppler on left MCA (panels **c–h**) allows measurement of increased blood flow velocity consistent with probable vasospasm

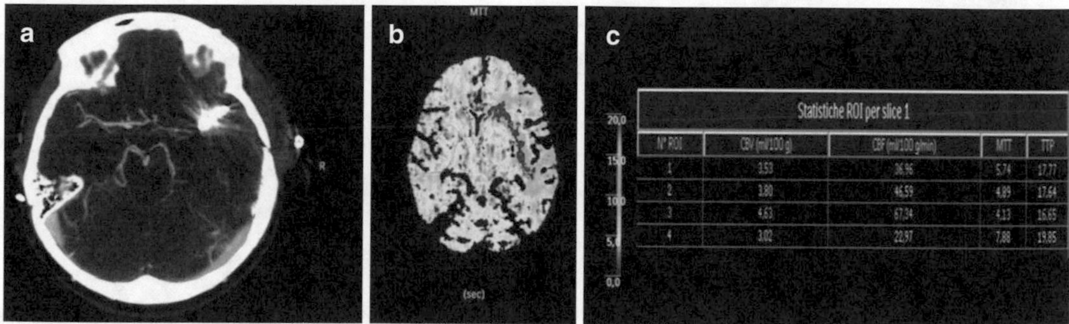

Fig. 25.3 (a–c) CT perfusion after the coiling of the aneurysm confirms the narrowing of the left MCA (panel **a**) and increased MTT (panels **b** and **c**) in the brain territories thereby supplied

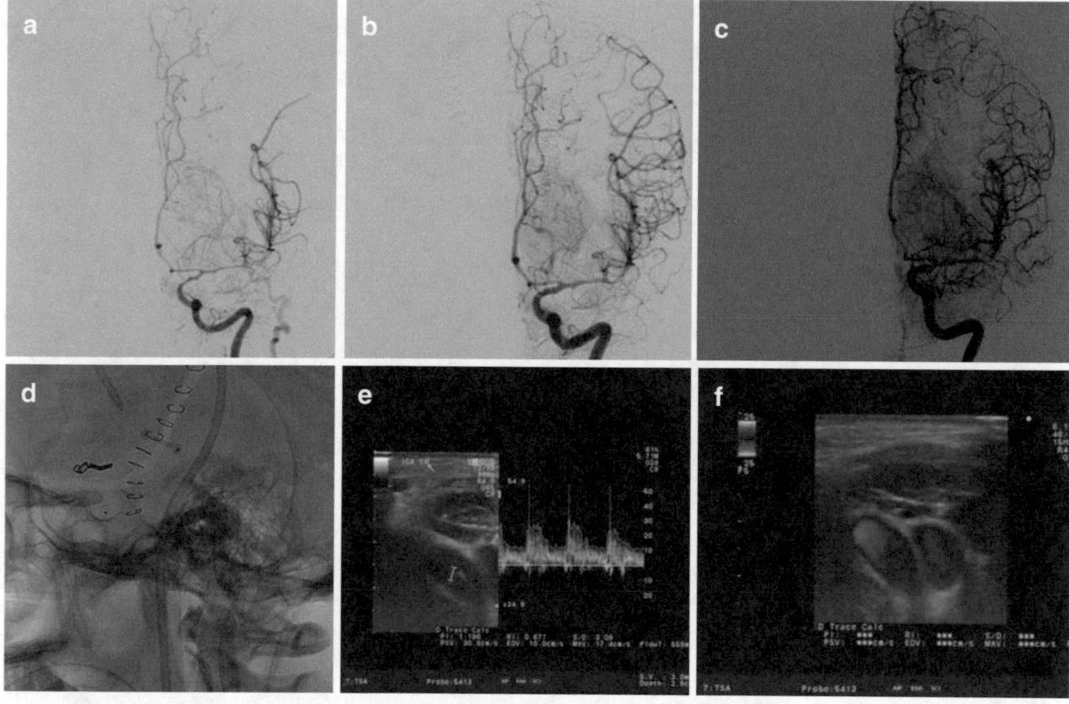

Fig. 25.4 (a–f) DSA frame images during the angiographic procedure for the insertion of a catheter in the left ICA for intra arterial nimodipine infusion

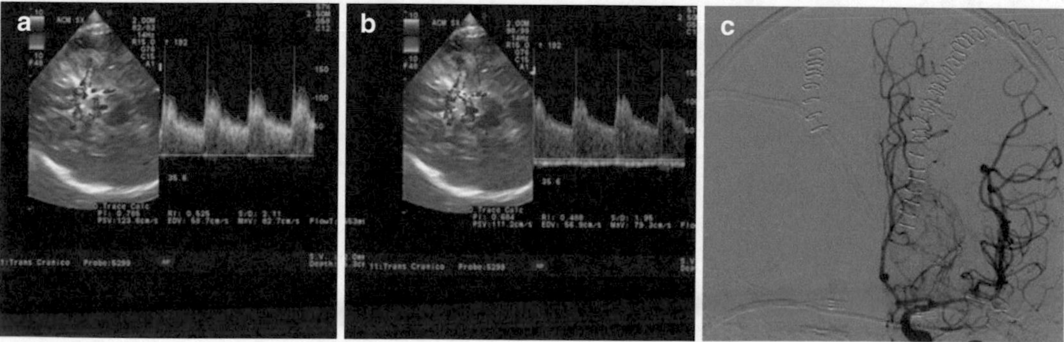

Fig. 25.5 (a–c) TCCD of left MCA during and after intra arterial nimodipine infusion shows normalization of blood flow velocity

26 Case 2: Vasospasm Treated with Ballooning Angioplasty

Rita Bertuetti, Maurizio Saini, Davide Savo, Francesca Simonassi, Kartika Chandrapatham, and Tarek Senussi

A 55-year-old woman was hospitalized for aSAH from ruptured right posterior communicating artery (PcomA) aneurysm (Fig. 26.1a, b): GCS 8 on admission, Fisher grade 4 with a clot in the fourth ventricle, and initial dilation of ventricle temporal horns (Fig. 26.2a–c). TCCD performed after the initial CT head scan showed an increased pulsatility index (PI) (Fig. 26.3a–c) confirming that an obstructive hydrocephalus was inducing a state of intracranial hypertension. After external ventricular drain (EVD) insertion, TCCD flow velocities improved and PI decreased: the patient promptly recovered her neurology up to a GCS of 14 (Fig. 26.4a, b) and successfully underwent aneurism coiling (Fig. 26.5a, b). On day 6 after bleeding, although completely asymptomatic and with normal brain CT perfusion, an increasing trend in flow velocity in the right MCA was noted (Figs. 26.6a, b and 26.7a, b) at the TCCD examination. On day 10 acute left hemiparesis and VII left cranial nerve palsy associated with a significative increase in mean flow velocity in the right MCA over 160 cm/s with evidence of turbulent flow (Fig. 26.7a–d) were noted; this time, plain CT head did not show hypodensity but CT perfusion was diagnostic for prolonged right frontotemporal MTT. Induced arterial hypertension with vasopressors and hemodynamic optimization (SABP > 200 mmHg and MAP > 100 mmHg) effectively restored perfusion in the suffering frontotemporal regions—as demonstrated by regression of neurological deficits—until day 12 when a relapse of clinical symptoms prompted an upgrading in the treatment strategy: the patient underwent a new DSA confirming severe vasospasm in the right M1 segment that was immediately treated with balloon angioplasty and intraprocedural arterial nimodipine infusion (Fig. 26.8a–c). After the angiographic procedure, TCCD velocities and motor deficits resolved (Fig. 26.9a–d).

R. Bertuetti (✉)
Department of Anesthesiology, Critical Care Medicine and Emergency, Division of Neurocritical Care, ASST Spedali Civili di Brescia, University Hospital, Brescia, Italy

M. Saini · D. Savo
Department of Emergency, Perioperative Medicine and Intensive Care, Neuroanesthesia and Neurointensive Care Unit, San Gerardo Hospital, ASST-Monza, Monza, Italy

F. Simonassi · K. Chandrapatham
Anesthesia and Intensive Care, Ospedale Policlinico San Martino – IRCCS for Oncology and Neurosciences, Genoa, Italy

T. Senussi
Department of Surgical Sciences and Integrated Diagnostics, University of Genoa, Genoa, Italy

C. Robba, G. Citerio (eds.), *Echography and Doppler of the Brain*,
https://doi.org/10.1007/978-3-030-48202-2_26

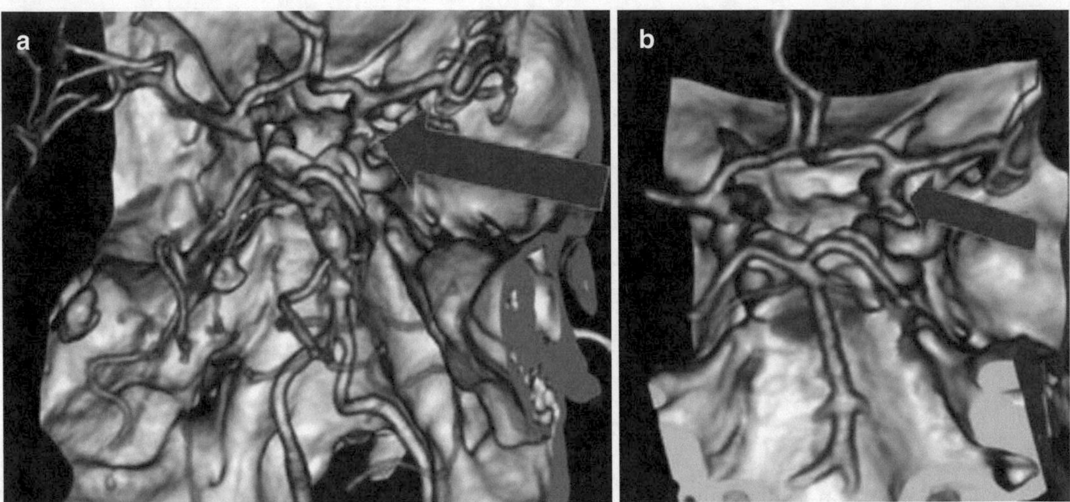

Fig. 26.1 (**a**, **b**) CT head angiography 3D rendering: the red arrow points out the aneurysm of the right PcomA, responsible of the bleeding

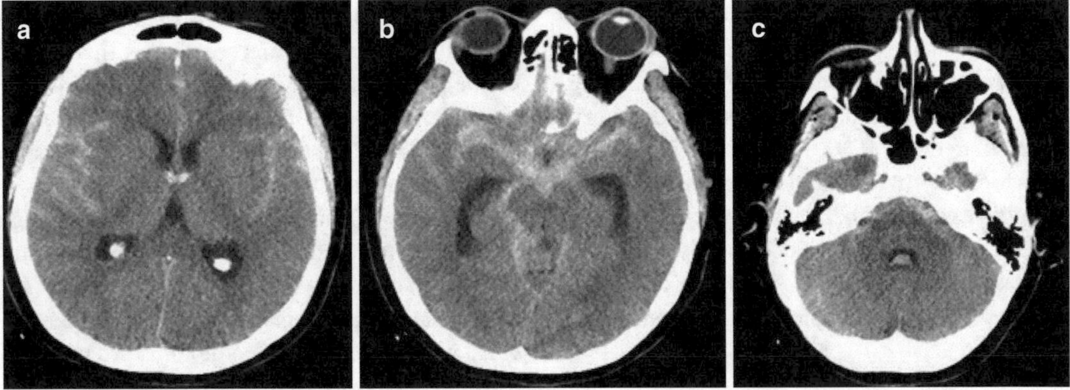

Fig. 26.2 (**a**-**c**) CT head shows SAH fisher grade 4: blood around sulcis (**a**), basal cisterns (**b**) and clot in the fourth ventricle (**c**). In panel b. initial dilation o temporal horns of the lateral ventricles can also be appreciated

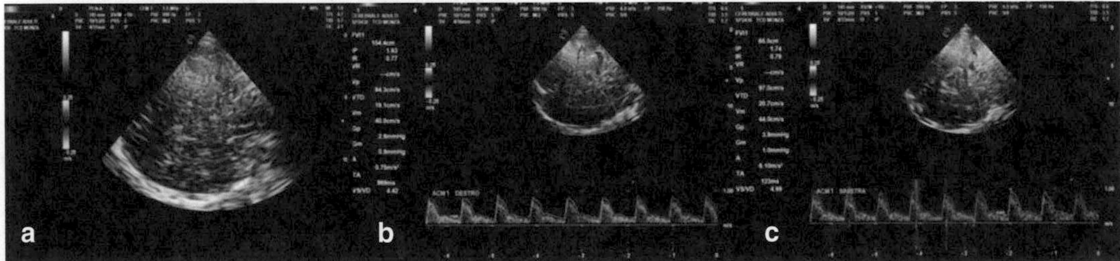

Fig. 26.3 (**a**-**c**) TCCD before EVD positioning: bilateral MCAs insonation demonstrates elevated PI and reduced diastolic flow as in a state of intracranial hypertension

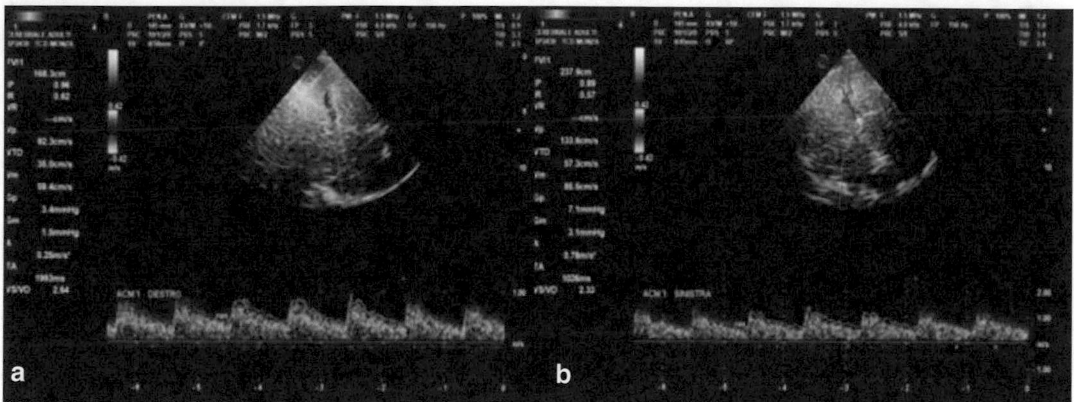

Fig. 26.4 (**a**, **b**) TCCD of bilateral MCAs after EVD positioning: a normalization of the PI and a restored diastolic flow can be appreciated

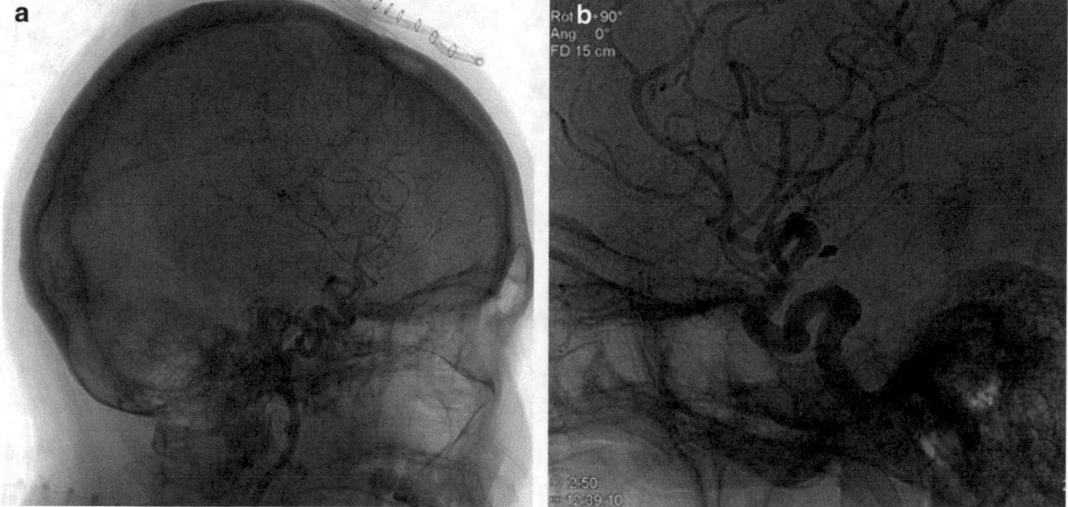

Fig. 26.5 (**a**, **b**) DSA frame images during the coiling of the aneurysm

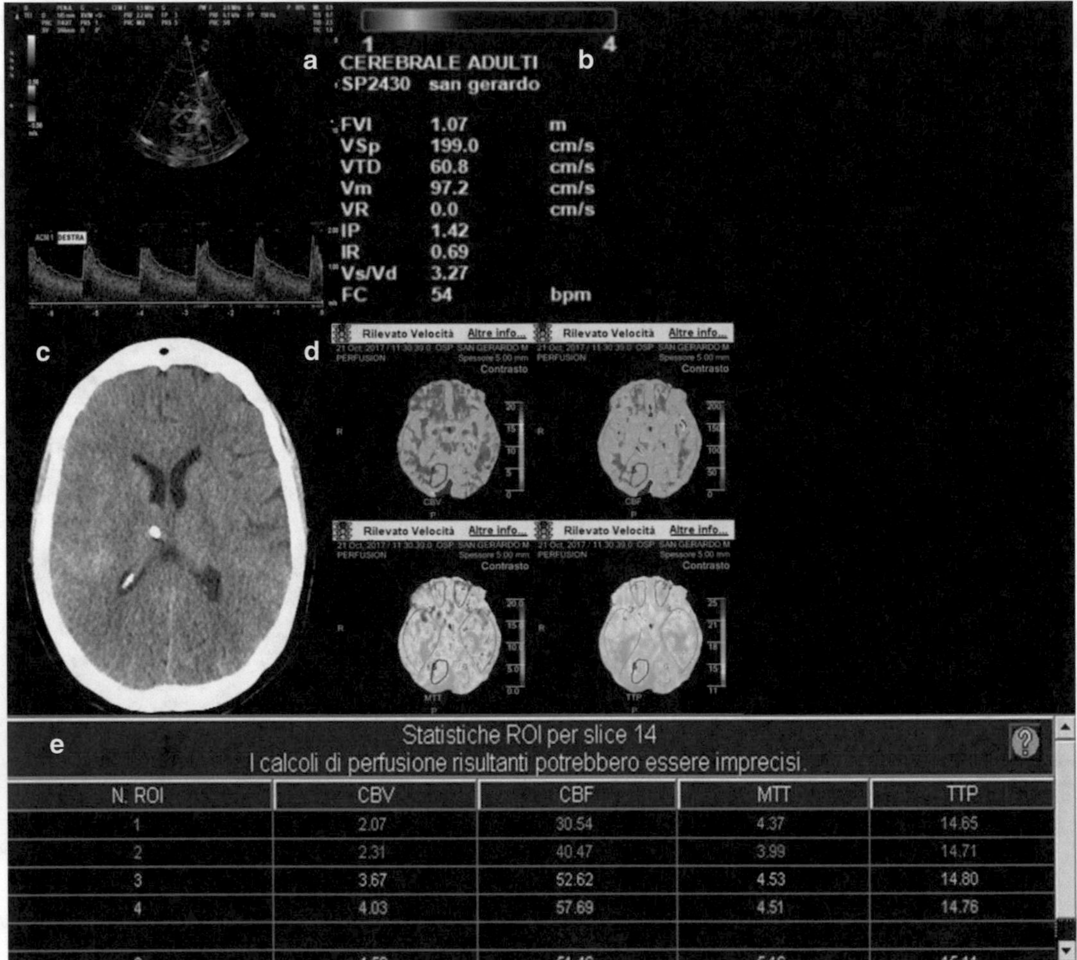

Fig. 26.6 (**a–e**) TCCD of MCA (panels a. and b.) shows a trending increase in mean flow velocity (97 cm/sec) although not yet fully pathological, in fact CT perfusion does not highlight any significative perfusive deficit consistent with vasospasm (c. and d.)

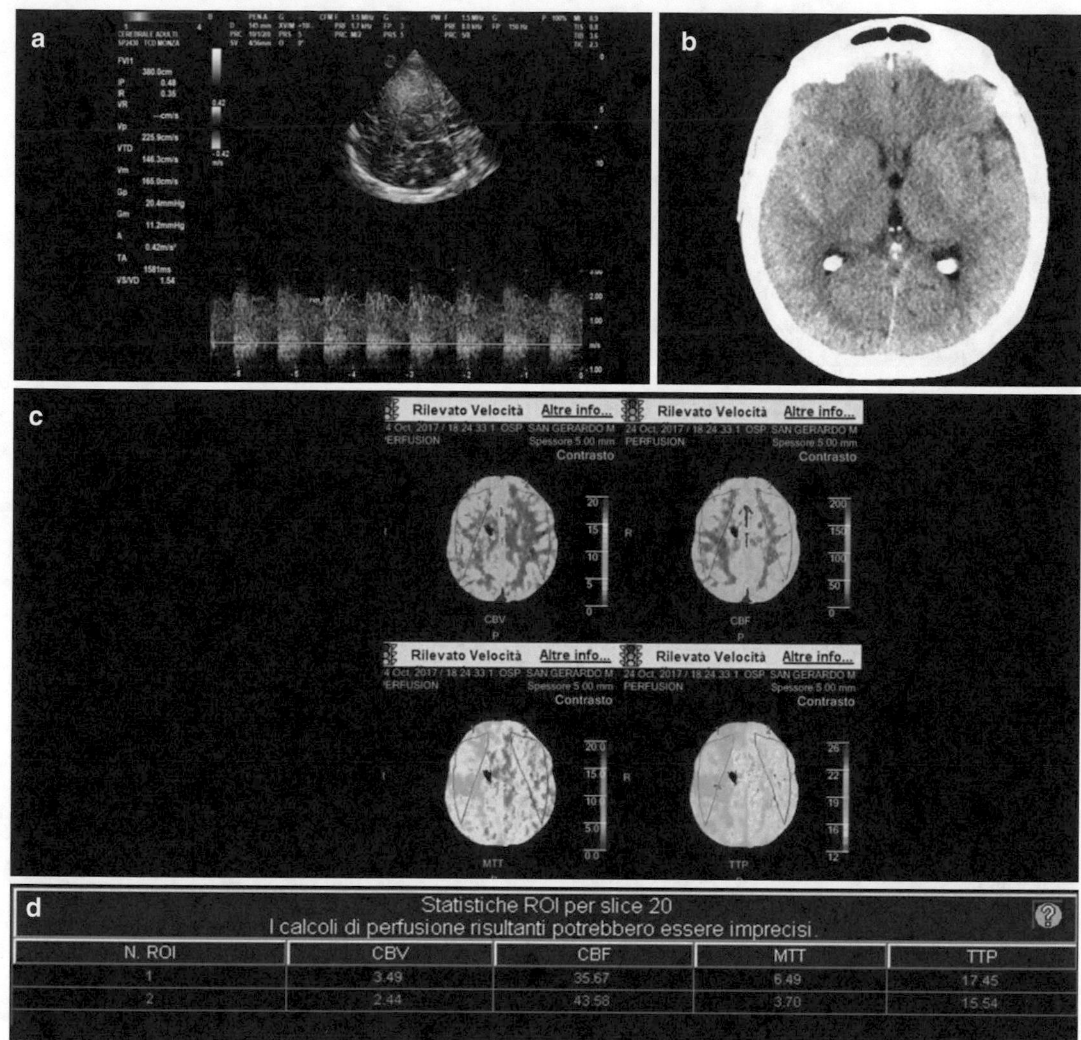

Statistiche ROI per slice 20
I calcoli di perfusione risultanti potrebbero essere imprecisi.

N. ROI	CBV	CBF	MTT	TTP
1	3.49	35.67	6.49	17.45
2	2.44	43.58	3.70	15.54

Fig. 26.7 (**a–d**) TCCD of MCA flags up a turbolent flow, in this case CT perfusion higlights hypoperfusion of the right hemisphere as shown by a decreased CBF and an increased MTT on the colorimetric map

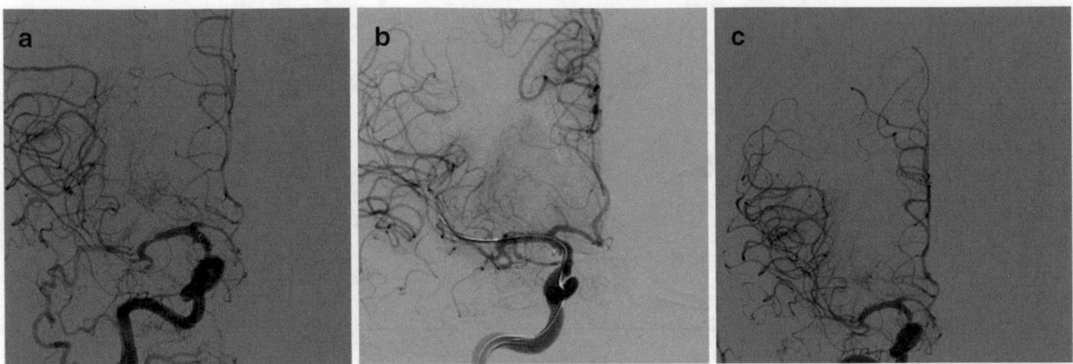

Fig. 26.8 (**a–c**) DSA image frames during baloon angioplasty

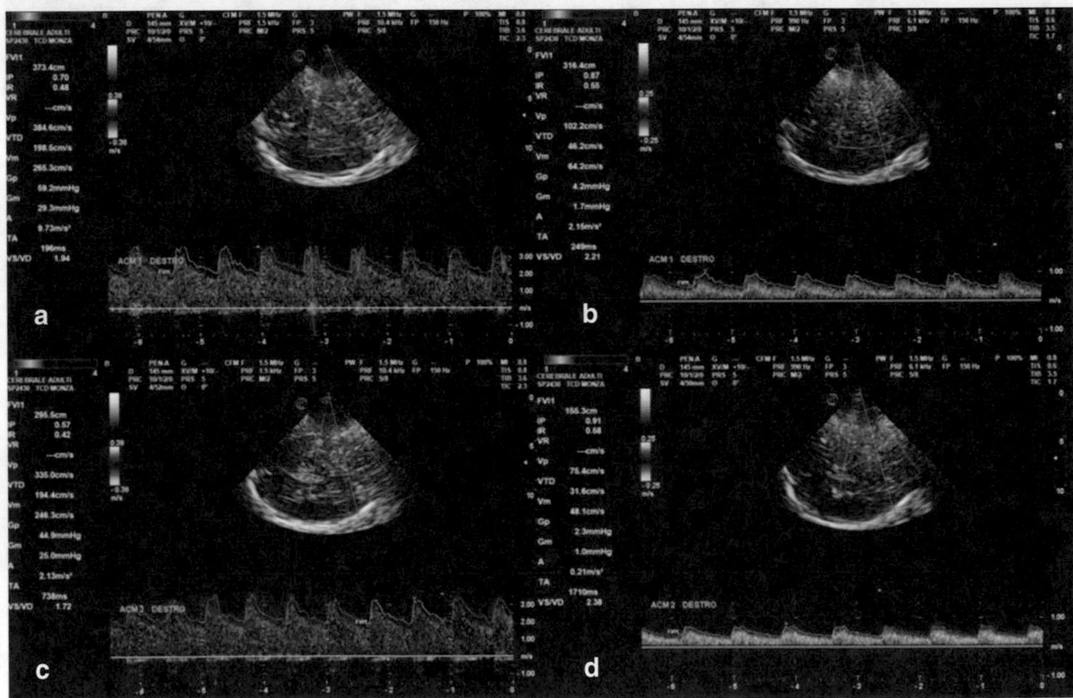

Fig. 26.9 (**a–d**) TCCD of MCAs after baloon angioplasty and intra arterial nimodipine infusion shows normalization of flow velocities

27 Case 3: Vasospasm Treated with Ballooning Angioplasty

Rita Bertuetti, Maurizio Saini, Davide Savo, Francesca Simonassi, Kartika Chandrapatham, and Tarek Senussi

A 40-year-old man presented to the emergency department for severe headache; head CT scan revealed aSAH from ruptured anterior communicating artery (ACA) aneurysm (Fig. 27.1a–c). Aneurysm was secured with angiographic coiling on day 1 (Fig. 27.2a–c) and patient neurological evolution was monitored by means of clinical evaluation and daily TCCD examinations. Since day 6 after coiling a progressive asymptomatic increase in flow velocity (Fig. 27.3a–f) was observed up to the eighth day when the patient presented right hemiparesis and confusion associated with extremely high mean flow velocity and turbulent flow in the left MCA (Fig. 27.4a–l). Severe vasospasm in left MCA was confirmed with DSA and treated with balloon angioplasty after which TCCD velocities started to normalize as well as neurological deficits disappeared.

R. Bertuetti (✉)
Department of Anesthesiology, Critical Care Medicine and Emergency, Division of Neurocritical Care, ASST Spedali Civili di Brescia, University Hospital, Brescia, Italy

M. Saini · D. Savo
Department of Emergency, Perioperative Medicine and Intensive Care, Neuroanesthesia and Neurointensive Care Unit, San Gerardo Hospital, ASST-Monza, Monza, Italy

F. Simonassi · K. Chandrapatham
Anesthesia and Intensive Care, Ospedale Policlinico San Martino – IRCCS for Oncology and Neurosciences, Genoa, Italy

T. Senussi
Department of Surgical Sciences and Integrated Diagnostics, University of Genoa, Genoa, Italy

C. Robba, G. Citerio (eds.), *Echography and Doppler of the Brain*,
https://doi.org/10.1007/978-3-030-48202-2_27

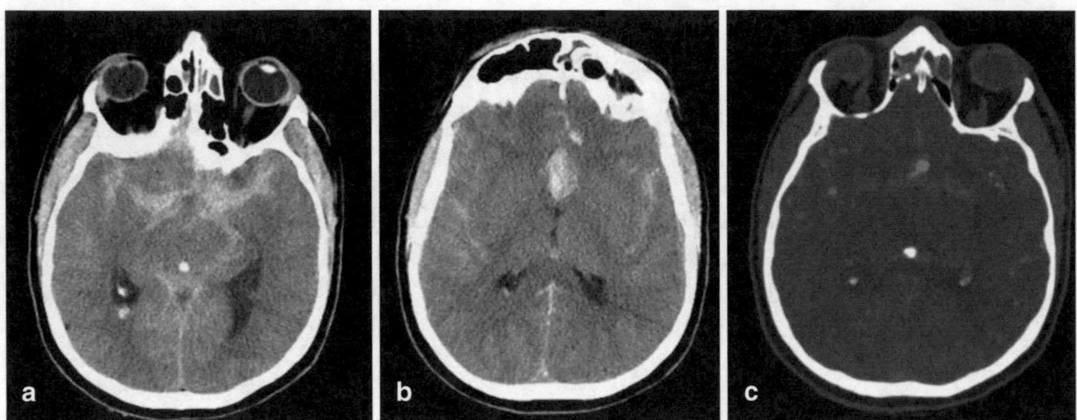

Fig. 27.1 (**a**–**c**) Head CT images showing thick aSAH and the ruptured aneurysm (panel **c**) of the ACA

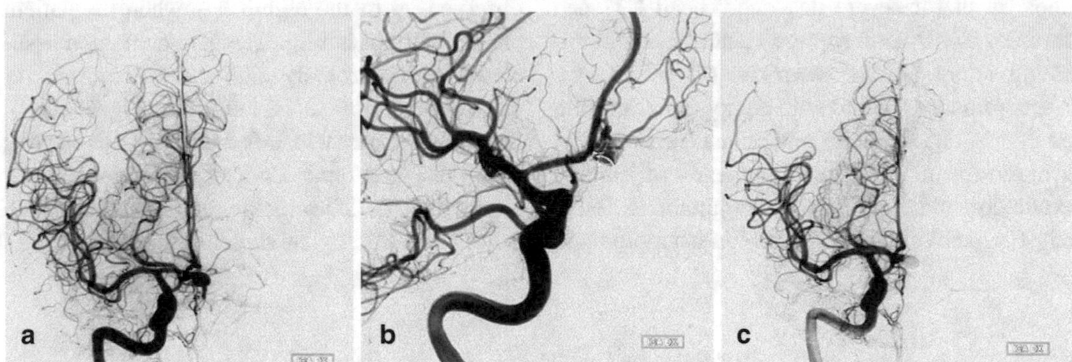

Fig. 27.2 (**a**–**c**) DSA image frames during the aneurysm coiling procedure: in panel **a**. and **b**. the aneurysm is recognizable, in panel **c**. it is secured with coils

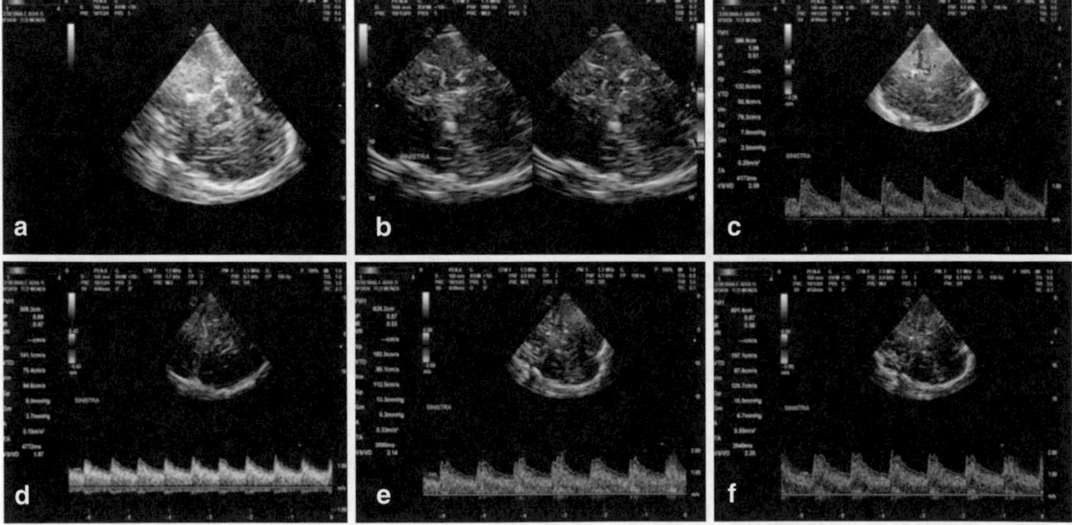

Fig. 27.3 (**a**–**f**) Brain ultrasound and TCCD showing increasing velocity in the left MCA

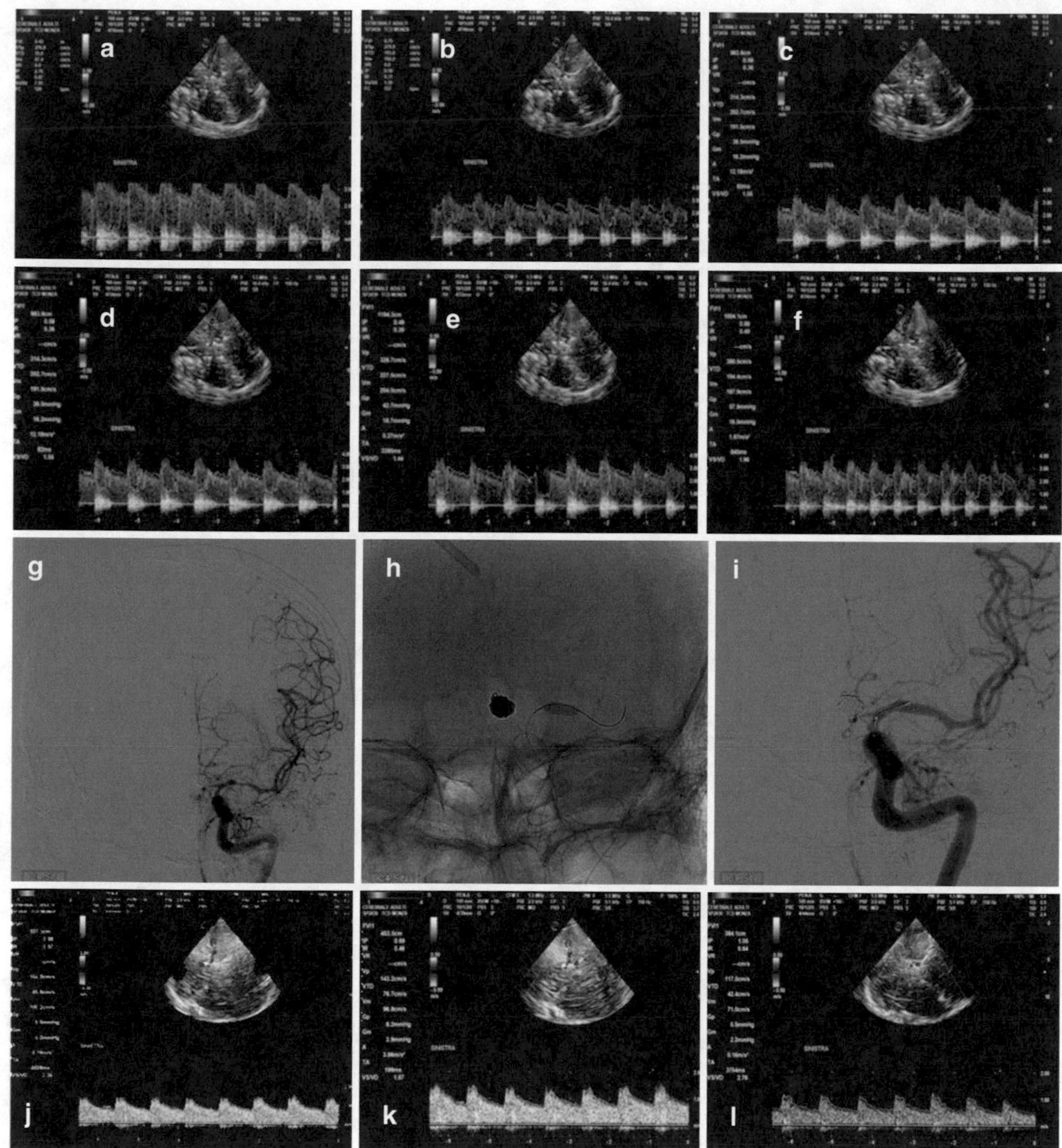

Fig. 27.4 In panels (**a–f**) TCCD of left MCA showing elevated flow velocities consistent with vasospasm. In panels (**g–i**) images frame of the DSA during baloon angioplasty. In panels (**j–l**), normalization of flow velocities after baloon angioplasty

Case 4: aSAH during Pregnancy

28

Rita Bertuetti, Maurizio Saini, Davide Savo, Francesca Simonassi, Kartika Chandrapatham, and Tarek Senussi

A 36-year-old pregnant woman (25th week) presented to the emergency department after loss of consciousness following severe headache and vomiting; head CT scan and angio-CT showed aSAH from ruptured right ICA aneurysm and hydrocephalus (HCP) (Fig. 28.1a–f). Aneurysm was then secured with coils (Fig. 28.2a–c) on day 1 after the neurosurgeon had inserted an EVD. Procedures were uneventful and the patient woke up fully recovering (GCS 15) right after. In the following day the young woman developed upper left limb weakness associated with elevated flow velocities detected in the right MCA (Fig. 28.3a–f). Induced arterial hypertension up to a CPP over 100 mmHg using vasopressors and fluid boluses was initiated and titrated by means of ultrasound monitoring of either placental vessel flow velocities and fetal transcranial vessel flow velocities in order to prevent blood flow impairment during vasopressor infusion (Fig. 28.4a–f).

R. Bertuetti (✉)
Department of Anesthesiology, Critical Care Medicine and Emergency, Division of Neurocritical Care, ASST Spedali Civili di Brescia, University Hospital, Brescia, Italy

M. Saini · D. Savo
Department of Emergency, Perioperative Medicine and Intensive Care, Neuroanesthesia and Neurointensive Care Unit, San Gerardo Hospital, ASST-Monza, Monza, Italy

F. Simonassi · K. Chandrapatham
Anesthesia and Intensive Care, Ospedale Policlinico San Martino – IRCCS for Oncology and Neurosciences, Genoa, Italy

T. Senussi
Department of Surgical Sciences and Integrated Diagnostics, University of Genoa, Genoa, Italy

C. Robba, G. Citerio (eds.), *Echography and Doppler of the Brain*,
https://doi.org/10.1007/978-3-030-48202-2_28

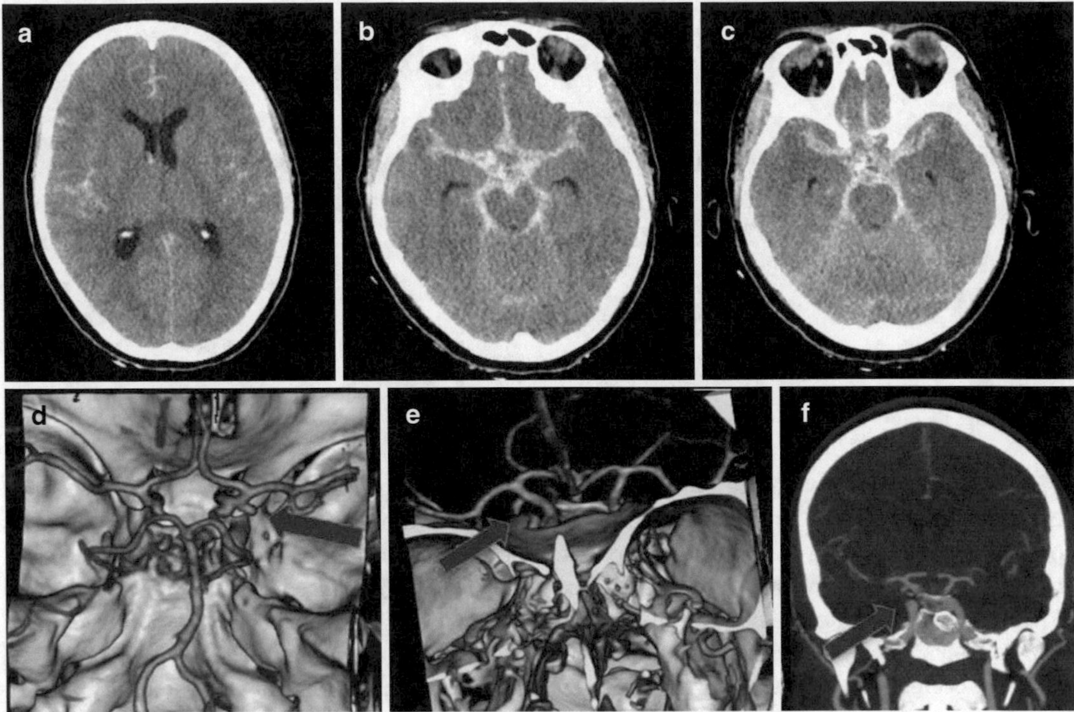

Fig. 28.1 (**a–f**) Plain CT head (a. to c.) shows thick SAH in the basal cysterns and around sulcis and initial HCP. CT angiography (d. to f.) points out (red arrow) the ruptured aneurysm (top of right ICA)

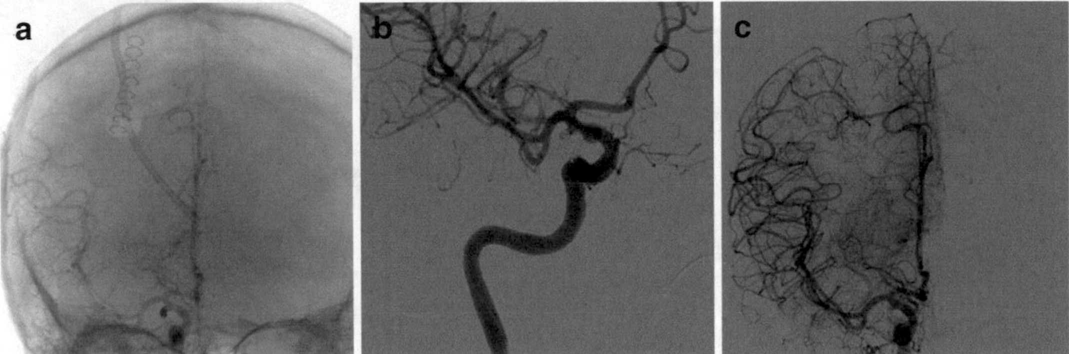

Fig. 28.2 (**a–c**) DSA frame images during the coiling of the aneurysm

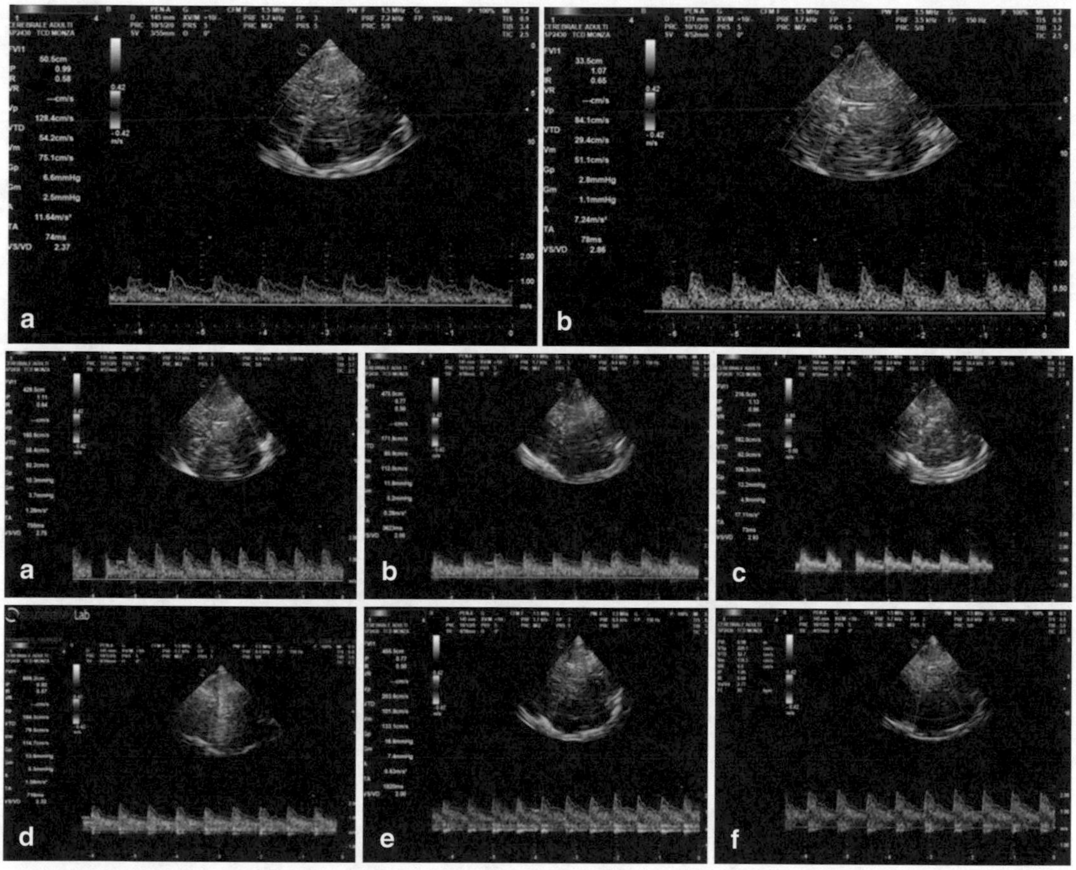

Fig. 28.3 (**a–f**) TCCD of the right MCA showing trending increasing velocities

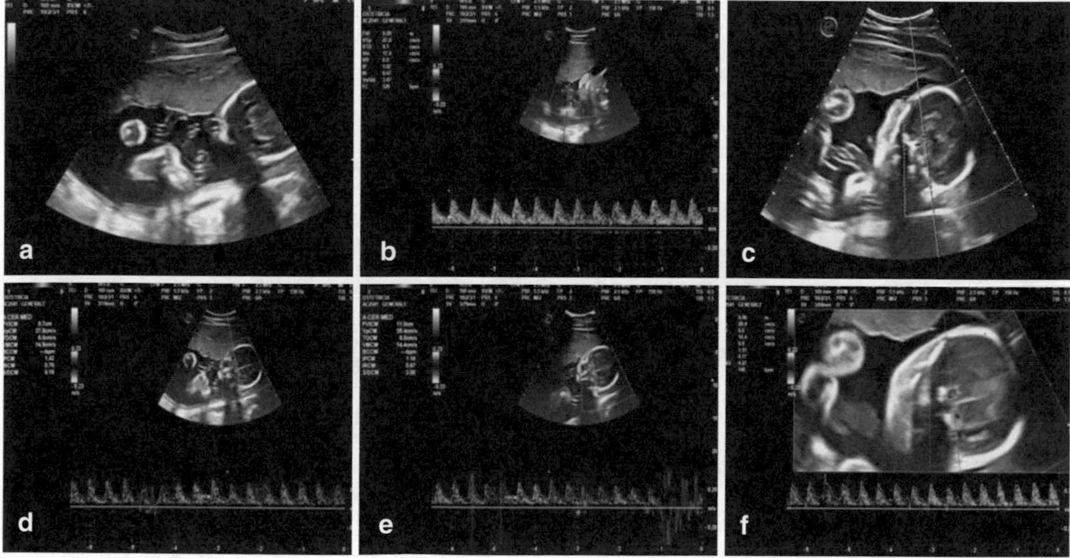

Fig. 28.4 (**a–f**) Fetal transcranial blood flow velocities

Case 5: Intracranial Hypertension and Decompressive Craniectomy in Severe aSAH

29

Rita Bertuetti, Maurizio Saini, Davide Savo, Francesca Simonassi, Kartika Chandrapatham, and Tarek Senussi

A 33-year-old man, cocaine abuser, was admitted to ICU for loss of consciousness; head CT and angio-CT showed aSAH Fisher 4 grade from ruptured anterior communicating artery aneurysm and lateral ventricles enlargement (Fig. 29.1a–e). Despite urgent EVD insertion and coiling of the ruptured aneurysm (Fig. 29.2a–d), the patient developed untreatable intracranial hypertension secondary to diffuse brain swelling, and bilateral frontal lobe infarctions. Neurosurgeons decided to perform a decompressive bifrontotemporal craniectomy in order to save the patient (Figs. 29.3a–c and 29.4a–d). On day 7 (Fig. 29.5), an increase in flow velocities was bilaterally detected in both ACAs and MCAs (Fig. 29.6a–b) and confirmed at the DSA as angiographic severe vasospasm that was then treated with multiple ballooning angioplasties (Figs. 29.7a–h and 29.8a–d). Moreover, after decompressive craniectomy, we were able to follow up the resolving hydrocephalus (HCP) and weaning from the EVD by means of brain ultrasound: a good correlation between ventricle sizes measured with the ultrasound and with the routine CT scans was observed (Fig. 29.9a–n).

R. Bertuetti (✉)
Department of Anesthesiology, Critical Care Medicine and Emergency, Division of Neurocritical Care, ASST Spedali Civili di Brescia, University Hospital, Brescia, Italy

M. Saini · D. Savo
Department of Emergency, Perioperative Medicine and Intensive Care, Neuroanesthesia and Neurointensive Care Unit, San Gerardo Hospital, ASST-Monza, Monza, Italy

F. Simonassi · K. Chandrapatham
Anesthesia and Intensive Care, Ospedale Policlinico San Martino – IRCCS for Oncology and Neurosciences, Genoa, Italy

T. Senussi
Department of Surgical Sciences and Integrated Diagnostics, University of Genoa, Genoa, Italy

C. Robba, G. Citerio (eds.), *Echography and Doppler of the Brain*,
https://doi.org/10.1007/978-3-030-48202-2_29

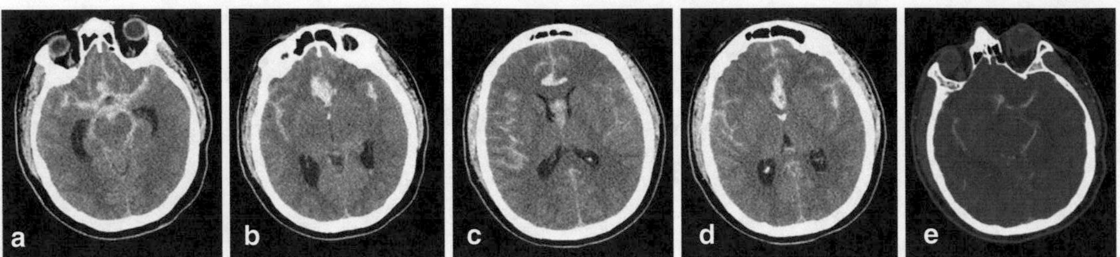

Fig. 29.1 (**a–e**) Head CT and angio-CT showed aSAH Fisher 4 grade from ruptured anterior communicating artery and lateral ventricle enlargement

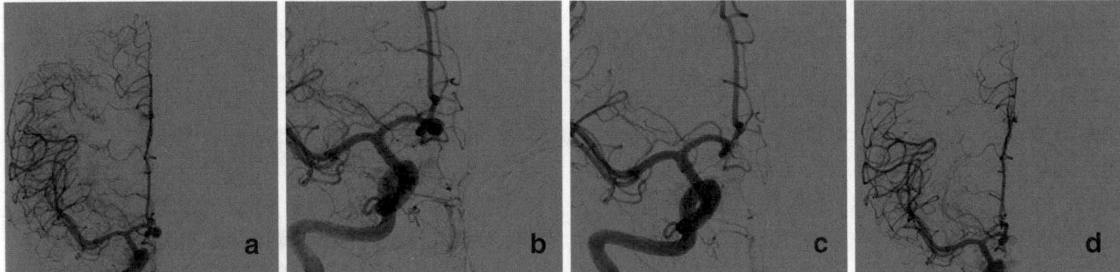

Fig. 29.2 (**a–d**) DSA (Digital subtraction angiography) images during aneurysm coiling

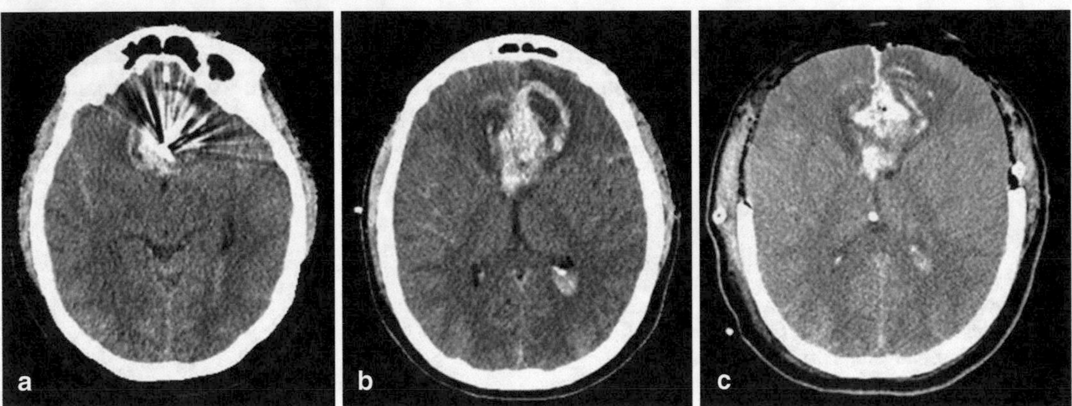

Fig. 29.3 (**a–c**) Head CT scan images before (left and middle panels) and after (right) decompressive craniectomy

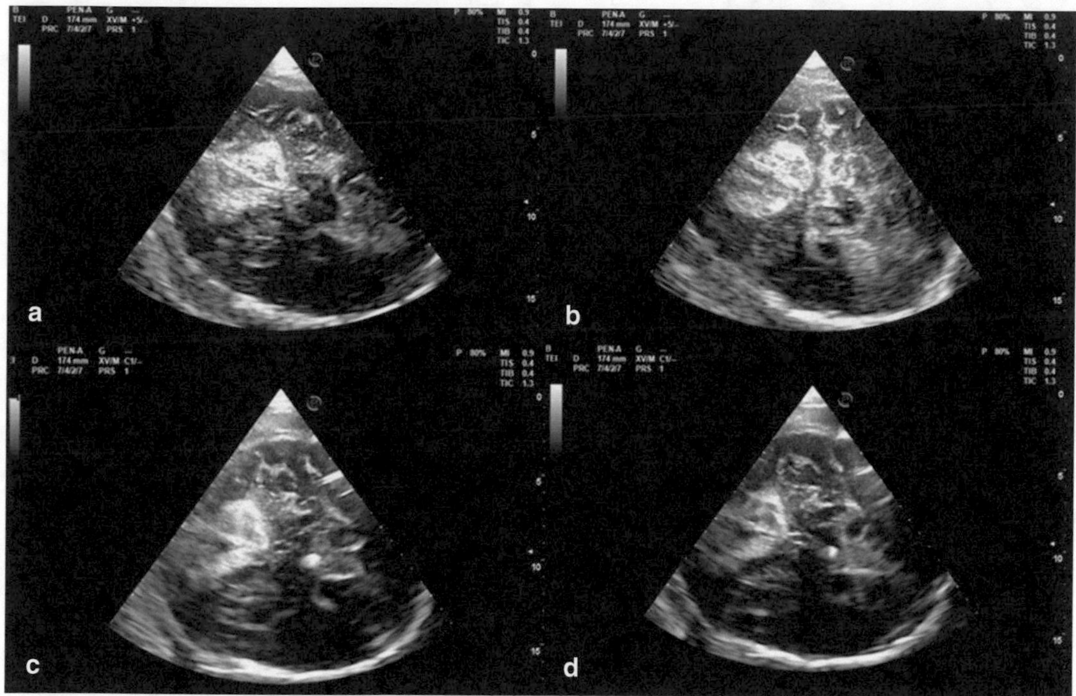

Fig. 29.4 (a–d) Cerebral ultrasound view of a decompressed brain

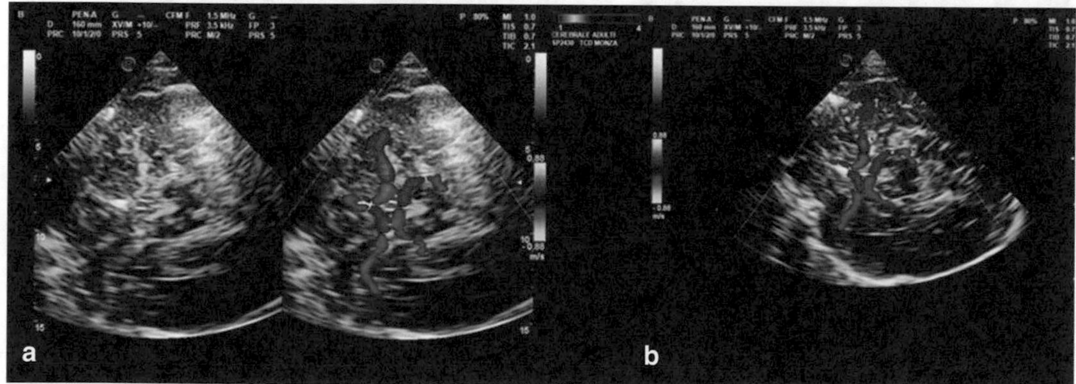

Fig. 29.5 (a, b) Cerebral ultrasound view and color Doppler of vessels in a decompressed brain

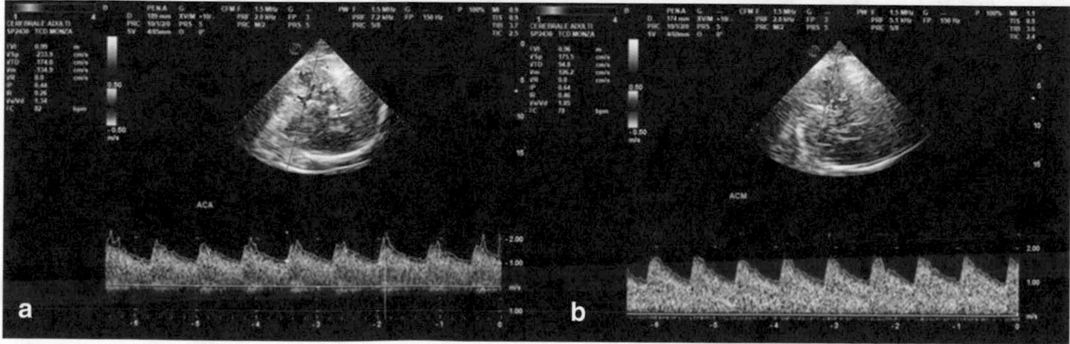

Fig. 29.6 (a–b) Increased blood flow velocity detected with TCCD in both ACA and MCA

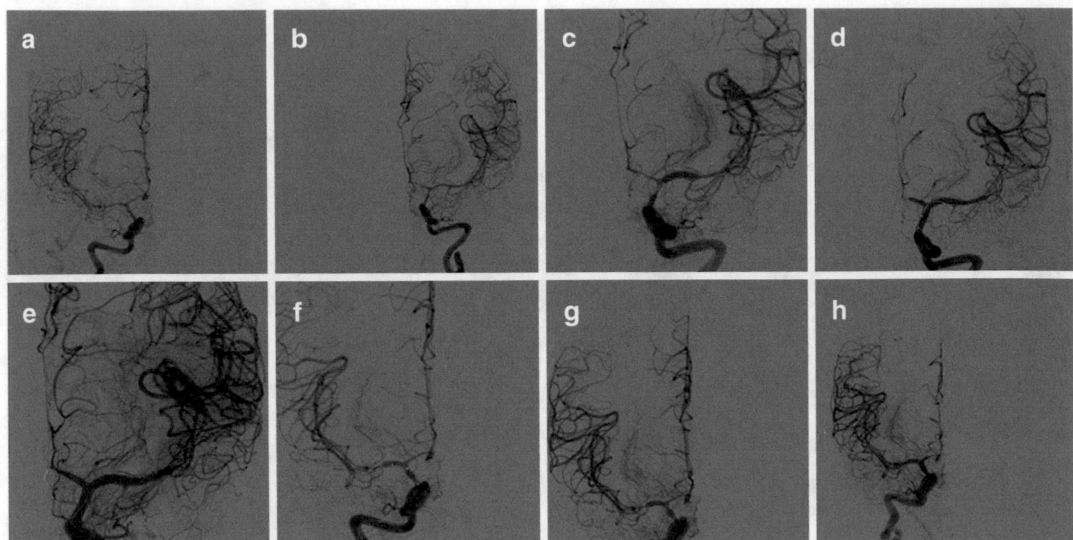

Fig. 29.7 (**a**–**h**) DSA image frames during baloon angioplasty (ACA and MCA) procedure

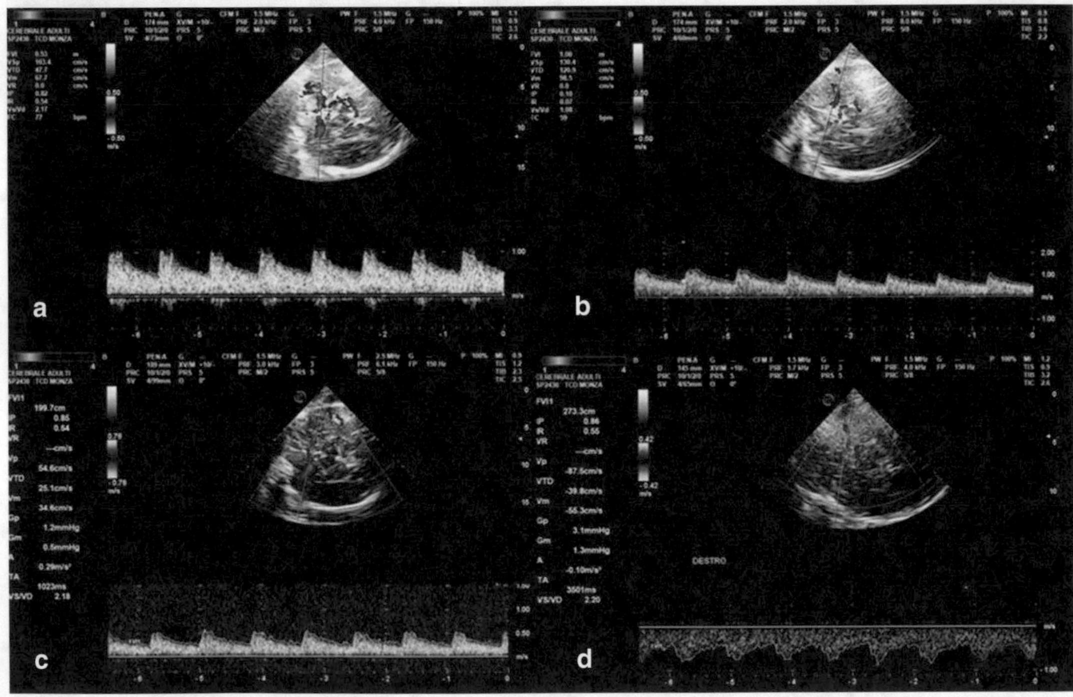

Fig. 29.8 (**a**–**d**) TCCD flow velocities after cerebral angioplastic procedure

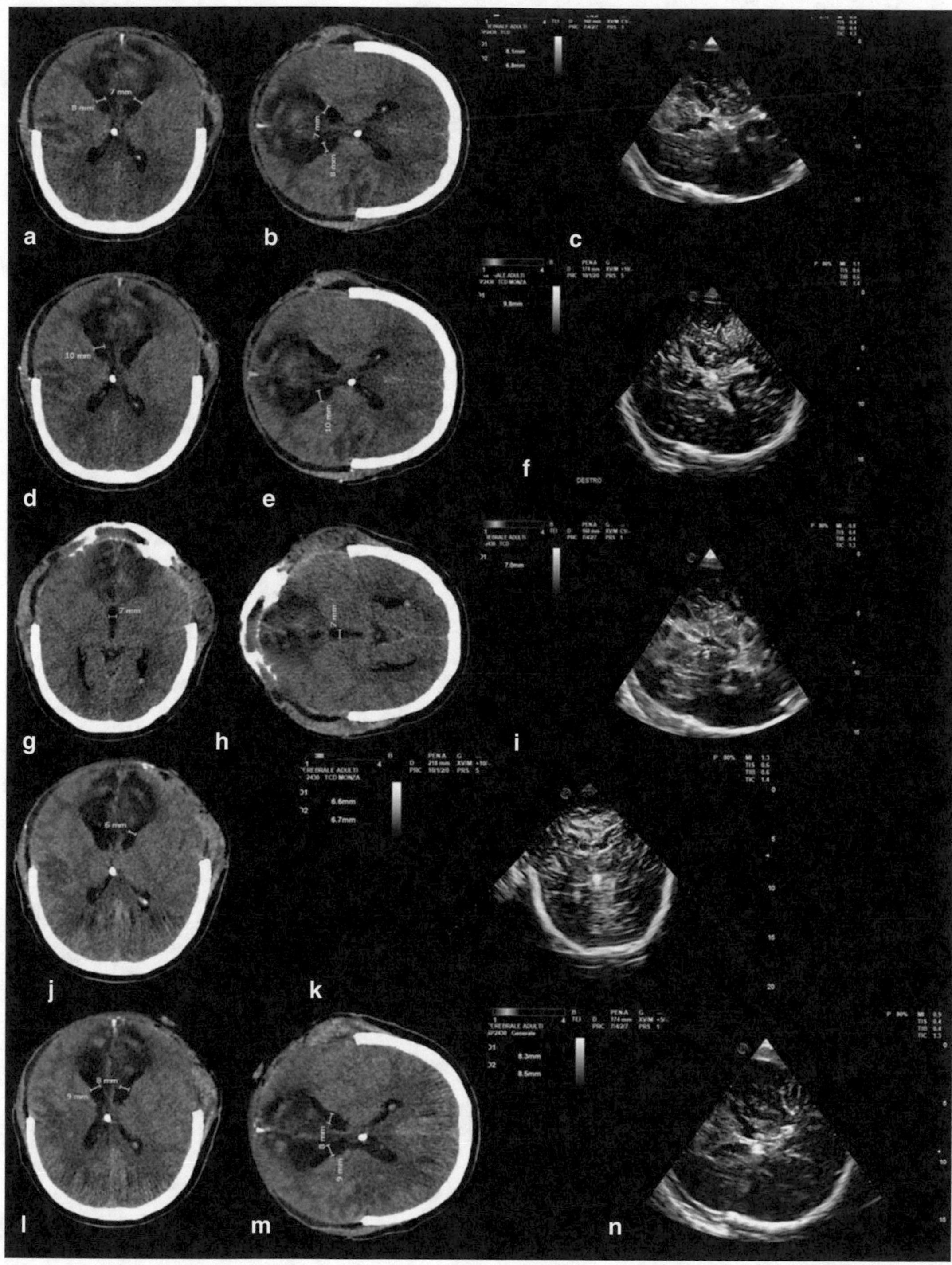

Fig. 29.9 (**a**–**n**) Resolving HCP monitored with the help of brain ultrasound: on the left lateral ventricle size measured on CT head images compared with corresponding ventricles size estimated with brain ultrasound

30 Case 6: Brain Ultrasound for EVD Weaning

Rita Bertuetti, Maurizio Saini, Davide Savo, Francesca Simonassi, Kartika Chandrapatham, and Tarek Senussi

46-Year-old woman was admitted to ICU for right parietal intracranial haematoma associated to massive intraventricular haemorrhage (IVH) secondary to arterioventricular malformation (AVM) rupture (Fig. 30.1a–d). Because of IVH, external ventricular drainage (EVD) was inserted and thereafter the AVM was secured (Fig. 30.2a–d). In the following days resolution of the hydrocephalus and IVH was followed up by means of ultrasound with serial measurements of ventricle size (Figs. 30.3a–c, 30.4a–c, 30.5a–c).

R. Bertuetti (✉)
Department of Anesthesiology, Critical Care Medicine and Emergency, Division of Neurocritical Care, ASST Spedali Civili di Brescia, University Hospital, Brescia, Italy

M. Saini · D. Savo
Department of Emergency, Perioperative Medicine and Intensive Care, Neuroanesthesia and Neurointensive Care Unit, San Gerardo Hospital, ASST-Monza, Monza, Italy

F. Simonassi · K. Chandrapatham
Anesthesia and Intensive Care, Ospedale Policlinico San Martino – IRCCS for Oncology and Neurosciences, Genoa, Italy

T. Senussi
Department of Surgical Sciences and Integrated Diagnostics, University of Genoa, Genoa, Italy

C. Robba, G. Citerio (eds.), *Echography and Doppler of the Brain*,
https://doi.org/10.1007/978-3-030-48202-2_30

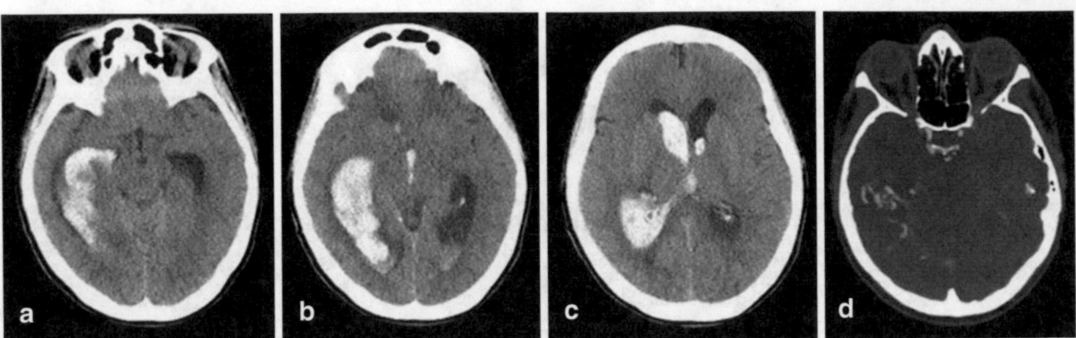

Fig. 30.1 (**a**–**d**) Head CT scan frames showing IVH and angio CT showing right temporo-parietal AVM

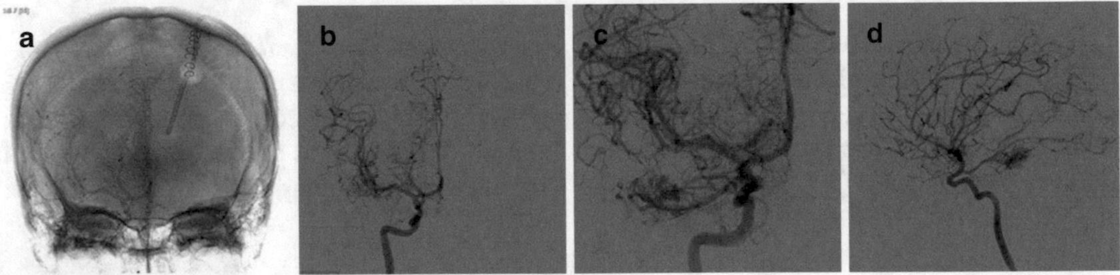

Fig. 30.2 (**a**–**d**) DSA (density subtraction angiography) images during AVM closure procedure

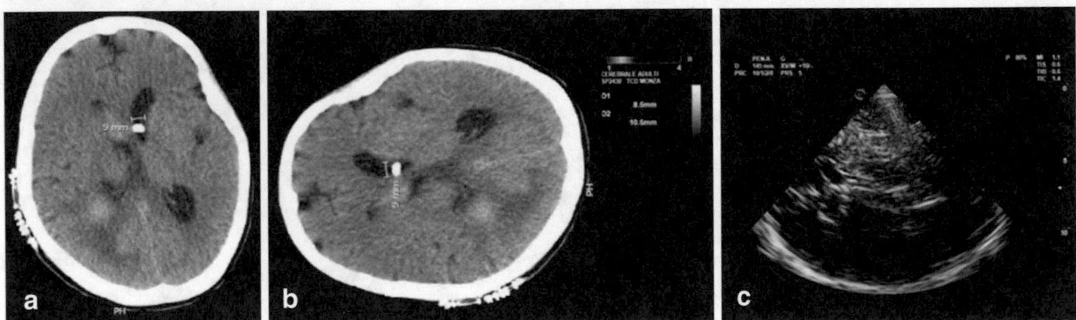

Fig. 30.3 (**a**–**c**) Lateral ventricles size measured on CT head (left and middle panels) and with brain ultrasound (right panel)

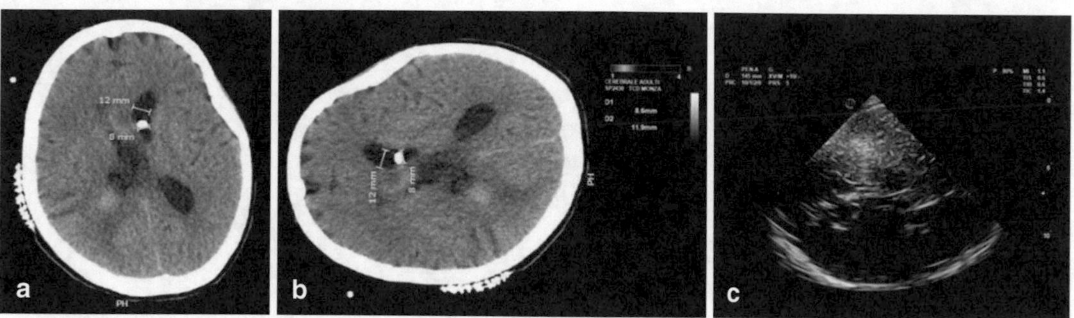

Fig. 30.4 (a–c) Lateral ventricles size measured on CT head (left and middle panels) and with brain ultrasound (right panel)

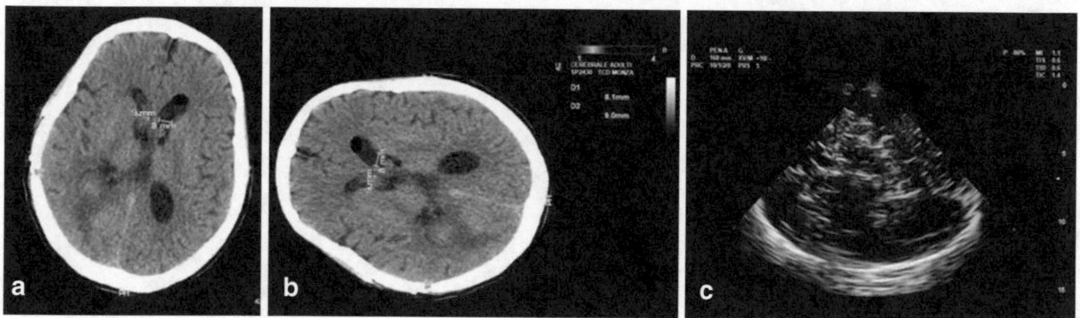

Fig. 30.5 (a–c) Lateral ventricles size measured on CT head (left and middle panels) and with brain ultrasound (right panel)

31 Case 7: Posterior Cranial Fossa Brain Tumor in a Pediatric Patient

Rita Bertuetti, Maurizio Saini, Davide Savo, Francesca Simonassi, Kartika Chandrapatham, and Tarek Senussi

A 2-year-old child, admitted to ICU for hydrocephalus secondary to posterior fossa tumor (Fig. 31.1a–d), was weaned from EVD after surgical resection of the tumor: thanks to the good correlation between brain ultrasound and head CT in the measurement of the ventricle size (Figs. 31.2a–c, 31.3a–c, 31.4a–c and 31.5a–c), clinicians could reduce the number of routine CT scans needed to monitor the resolution of the hydrocephalus.

R. Bertuetti (✉)
Department of Anesthesiology, Critical Care Medicine and Emergency, Division of Neurocritical Care, ASST Spedali Civili di Brescia, University Hospital, Brescia, Italy

M. Saini · D. Savo
Department of Emergency, Perioperative Medicine and Intensive Care, Neuroanesthesia and Neurointensive Care Unit, San Gerardo Hospital, ASST-Monza, Monza, Italy

F. Simonassi · K. Chandrapatham
Anesthesia and Intensive Care, Ospedale Policlinico San Martino – IRCCS for Oncology and Neurosciences, Genoa, Italy

T. Senussi
Department of Surgical Sciences and Integrated Diagnostics, University of Genoa, Genoa, Italy

C. Robba, G. Citerio (eds.), *Echography and Doppler of the Brain*,
https://doi.org/10.1007/978-3-030-48202-2_31

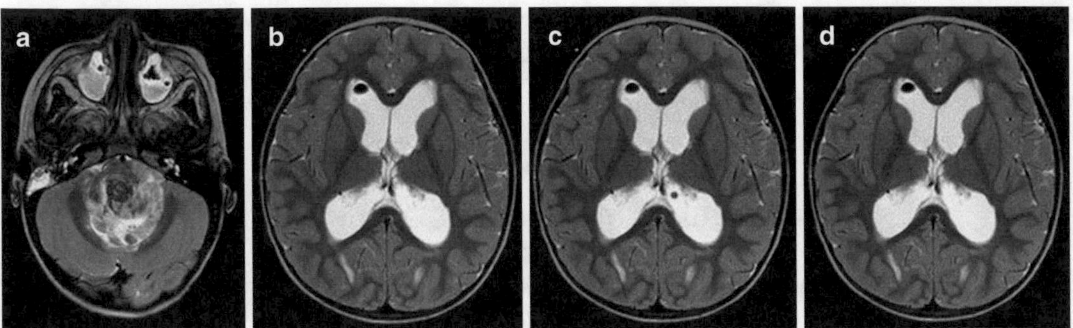

Fig. 31.1 (**a–d**) Pre operative MRI showing posterior fossa tumor and associated obstructive hydrocephalus

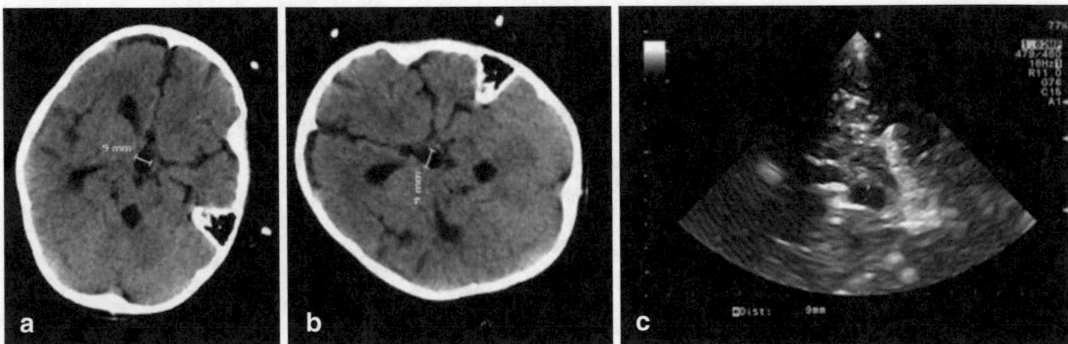

Fig. 31.2 (**a–c**) Ventricles size measured on CT head and on brain ultrasound

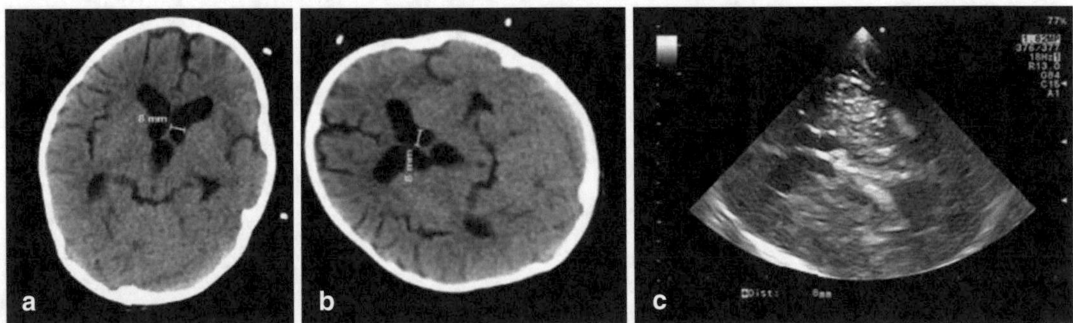

Fig. 31.3 (**a–c**) Ventricles size measured on CT head and on brain ultrasound

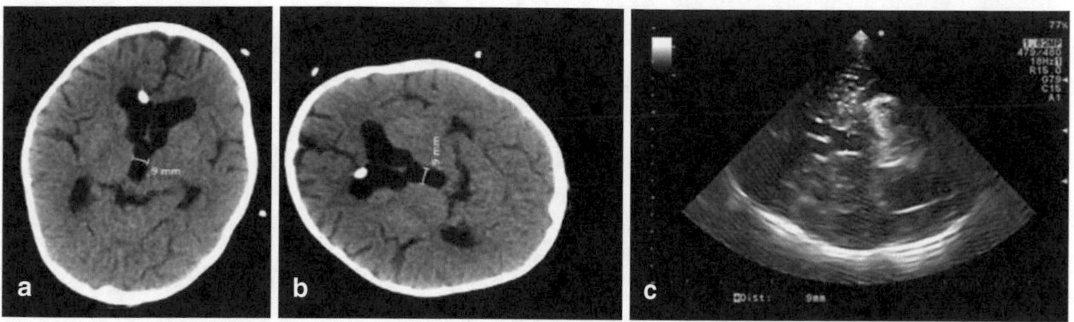

Fig. 31.4 (a–c) Ventricles size measured on CT head and on brain ultrasound

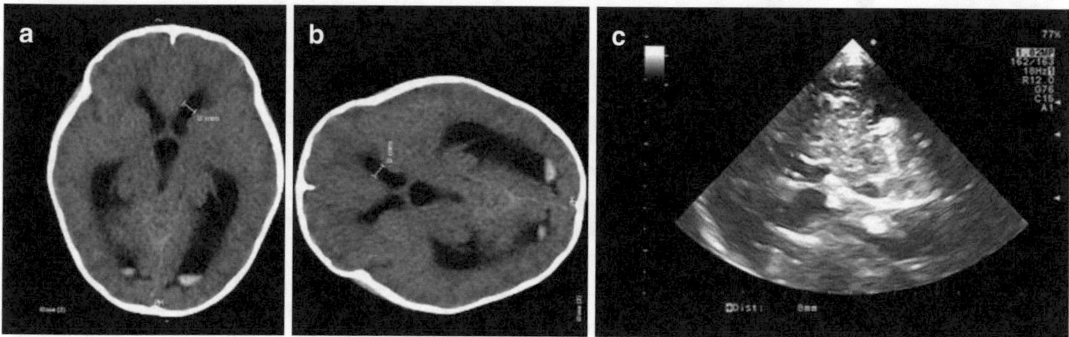

Fig. 31.5 (a–c) Ventricles size measured on CT head and on brain ultrasound

Case 8: Cerebral Circulatory Arrest

32

Rita Bertuetti, Maurizio Saini, Davide Savo, Francesca Simonassi, Kartika Chandrapatham, and Tarek Senussi

49-Year-old lady, rescued at home for loss of consciousness, was found by the ambulance team in cardiac arrest (no flow time of 13 min) with pulseless activity (PEA) rhythm, ACLS (advanced cardiac life support) was started, and ROSC (return of spontaneous circulation) was achieved after 17 min since the event—4 min after the arrival of the rescue team. Once in A&E, since neither the ECG nor the ECHO showed signs of myocardial ischemia; a brain CT angio was performed; this showed aneurysmal subarachnoid hemorrhage (aSAH) Fisher 3 grade, aneurysm of the internal carotid artery, sulcal and basal cistern effacement, and signs of cerebral hypoperfusion. The patient was then admitted to ICU, where a neurological evaluation was attempted after stopping sedation: GCS 3 with dilated pupils; simultanously, TCCD showed oscillatory reverse flow consistent with cerebral circulatory arrest (Fig. 32.1).

Since the clinical course (prolonged no-flow time, poor neurology), the brain CT showing brain swelling, and the TCCD proving cerebral circulatory arrest the patient was deemed unsalvageable. After few hours later the medical board for the diagnosis of brain death was summoned, and after the 6-h observation time according to the Italian law, organ donation was performed.

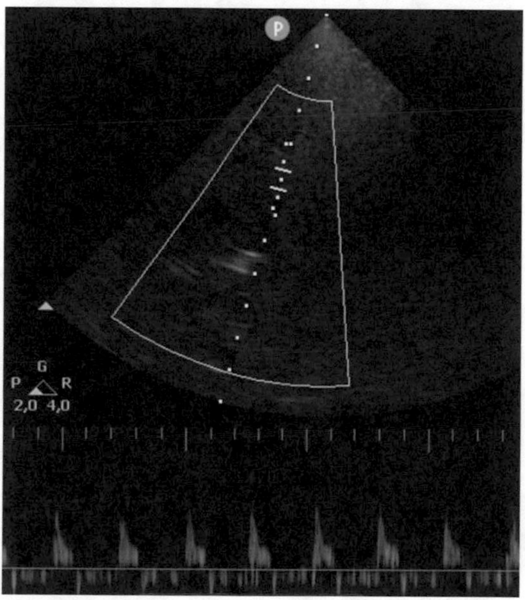

Fig. 32.1 Reverse oscillatory flow at MCA TCCD insonation

R. Bertuetti (✉)
Department of Anesthesiology, Critical Care Medicine and Emergency, Division of Neurocritical Care, ASST Spedali Civili di Brescia, University Hospital, Brescia, Italy

M. Saini · D. Savo
Department of Emergency, Perioperative Medicine and Intensive Care, Neuroanesthesia and Neurointensive Care Unit, San Gerardo Hospital, ASST-Monza, Monza, Italy

F. Simonassi · K. Chandrapatham
Anesthesia and Intensive Care, Ospedale Policlinico San Martino – IRCCS for Oncology and Neurosciences, Genoa, Italy

T. Senussi
Department of Surgical Sciences and Integrated Diagnostics, University of Genoa, Genoa, Italy

C. Robba, G. Citerio (eds.), *Echography and Doppler of the Brain*,
https://doi.org/10.1007/978-3-030-48202-2_32

33 Case 9: Intracranial Hypertension and Hydrocephalus

Rita Bertuetti, Nicola Zugni, Maurizio Saini, Davide Savo, Francesca Simonassi, Kartika Chandrapatham, and Tarek Senussi

Fifty-nine-Year-old lady with a history of poorly controlled arterial hypertension was taken to A&E for sudden intense headache. Upon arrival at the hospital she was in the state of unconsciousness (GCS 3) associated with left anisocoria and arterial hypertension. She was then quickly sedated and intubated for airway protection and was taken to radiology for a head CT. Brain CT angio showed subarachnoid haemorrhage Fisher 4 grade with intraparenchymal haematoma from rupture of a bilobate aneurysm of the left middle cerebral artery (MCA) and initial hydrocephalus sings. The patient was then admitted to ICU where a TCCD was performed just after her arrival. The brain ultrasound showed:

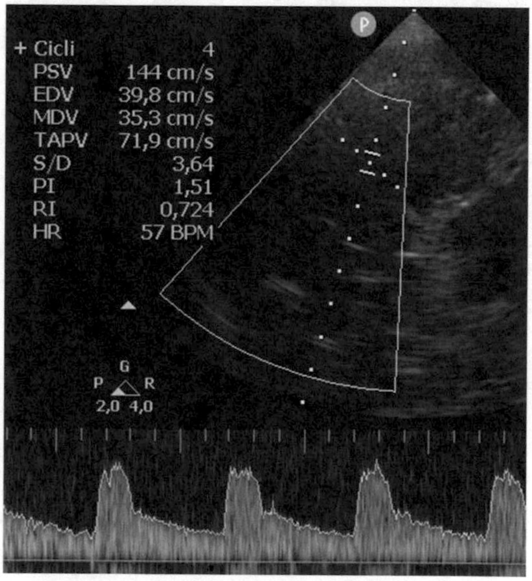

Fig. 33.1 Flow in left MCA

- A right midline shift of 3 mm.
- Estimated ICP with the flow diastolic formula of 21 mmHg and an increased pulsatility index of 1.5 (Fig. 33.1).
- Third ventricle width of 7 mm (Fig. 33.2).

The following day, angiographic coiling of the aneurysm was performed without complications, and sedation was stopped: GCS E4 M6 Vt patient was aphasic with a minor right motor weakness, and the patient was extubated. 24 hours after,

R. Bertuetti (✉) · N. Zugni
Department of Anesthesiology, Critical Care Medicine and Emergency, Division of Neurocritical Care, ASST Spedali Civili di Brescia, University Hospital, Brescia, Italy

M. Saini · D. Savo
Department of Emergency, Perioperative Medicine and Intensive Care, Neuroanesthesia and Neurointensive Care Unit, San Gerardo Hospital, ASST-Monza, Monza, Italy

F. Simonassi · K. Chandrapatham
Anesthesia and Intensive Care, Ospedale Policlinico San Martino – IRCCS for Oncology and Neurosciences, Genoa, Italy

T. Senussi
Department of Surgical Sciences and Integrated Diagnostics, University of Genoa, Genoa, Italy

C. Robba, G. Citerio (eds.), *Echography and Doppler of the Brain*,
https://doi.org/10.1007/978-3-030-48202-2_33

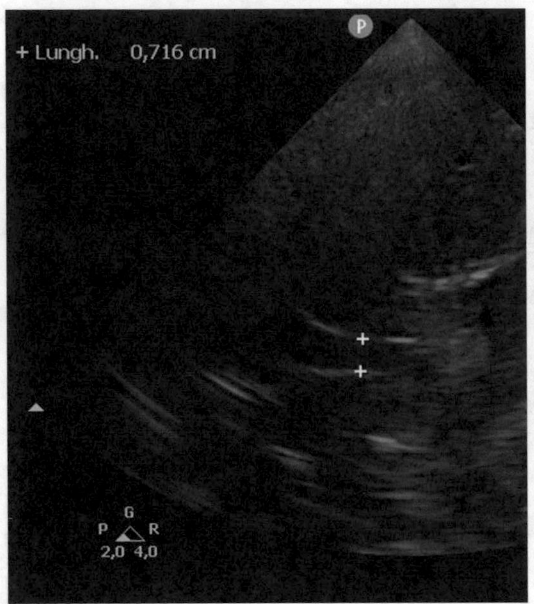

Fig. 33.2 Third ventricle 7 mm wide before the lumbar puncture

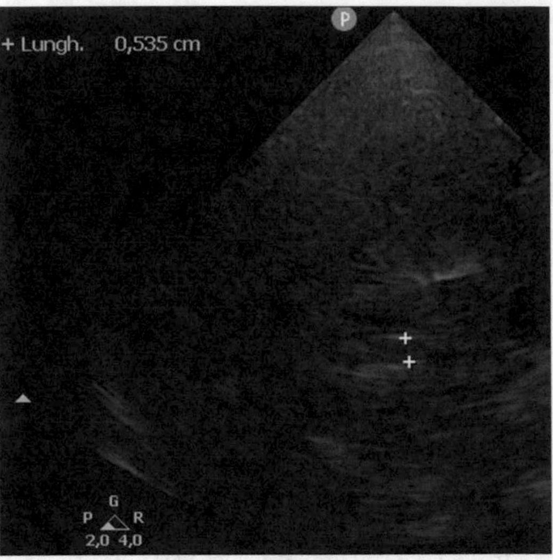

Fig. 33.3 Third ventricle 5 mm wide after the lumbar puncture

GCS dropped to E4 M5 V2; a new brain CT showed increased hydrocephalus with a patent fourth ventricle, the reason why a lumbar puncture was carried out and 20 ml of haematic CSF (cerebrospinal fluid) was subtracted. After the procedure neurological status improved and brain ultrasound showed a narrowed third ventricle (5 mm width) (Fig. 33.3).

34 Case 10: Intracranial Hypertension and Decompressive Craniectomy

Rita Bertuetti, Nicola Zugni, Maurizio Saini, Davide Savo, Francesca Simonassi, Kartika Chandrapatham, and Tarek Senussi

Thirty-five-Year-old young lady, found at the bottom of a stair flight at home, transported by ambulance to the emergency department of a peripheral hospital where the first neurological evaluation is performed: GCS: E4 M5 V2 pupils equal and reactive to light, and blood discharge from the right ear meatus. The anaesthetist decided at this point to intubate the patient before taking the patient to have total body CT scan. Brain CT showed post-traumatic subarachnoid haemorrhage, left subdural haematoma, multiple contusive lesions, temporal bone and petrous bridge bilateral fracture, and left-to-right 5 mm midline shift (Fig. 34.1). After the scan the patient was transferred to a tertiary hospital.

After admission in the ICU of a tertiary hospital, sedation was stopped and a new neurological evaluation revealed a GCS of E3 M6 Vt with upper right limb weakness. After few hours right over left anisocoria was noted and brain ultrasound was then performed: TCCD revealed increased PI in the left MCA with an estimated ICP of 33 mmHg on the left and 22 mmHg on the right; ultrasound measurement of ONSDs showed significantly enlarged ONSD on the right (Fig. 34.2a–d). Invasive ICP monitoring was then positioned, sedation was escalated and boluses of hypertonic saline 5% were injected in order to keep ICP below 20–25 mmHg (Fig. 34.3a, b). Despite optimisation of medical treatment, ICP subsequently spiked above threshold values in the following hours; a new brain CT showed increase of both the haemorrhagic component of the contusions and the midline shift was undertaken. On such a basis, the neurosurgeon on call decided to take the patient to the operating room for decompressive craniectomy (DC). After DC flow velocities in the MCAs and ONSD improved proving normalisation of ICP and CPP. During the following days she developed post-surgical

R. Bertuetti (✉) · N. Zugni
Department of Anesthesiology, Critical Care Medicine and Emergency, Division of Neurocritical Care, ASST Spedali Civili di Brescia, University Hospital, Brescia, Italy

M. Saini · D. Savo
Department of Emergency, Perioperative Medicine and Intensive Care, Neuroanesthesia and Neurointensive Care Unit, San Gerardo Hospital, ASST-Monza, Monza, Italy

F. Simonassi · K. Chandrapatham
Anesthesia and Intensive Care, Ospedale Policlinico San Martino - IRCCS for Oncology and Neurosciences, Genoa, Italy

T. Senussi
Department of Surgical Sciences and Integrated Diagnostics, University of Genoa, Genoa, Italy

C. Robba, G. Citerio (eds.), *Echography and Doppler of the Brain*,
https://doi.org/10.1007/978-3-030-48202-2_34

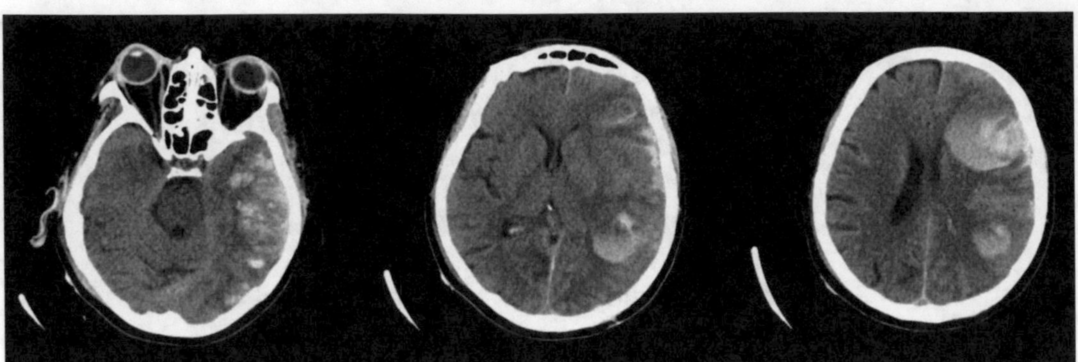

Fig. 34.1 Brain CT scan at admission

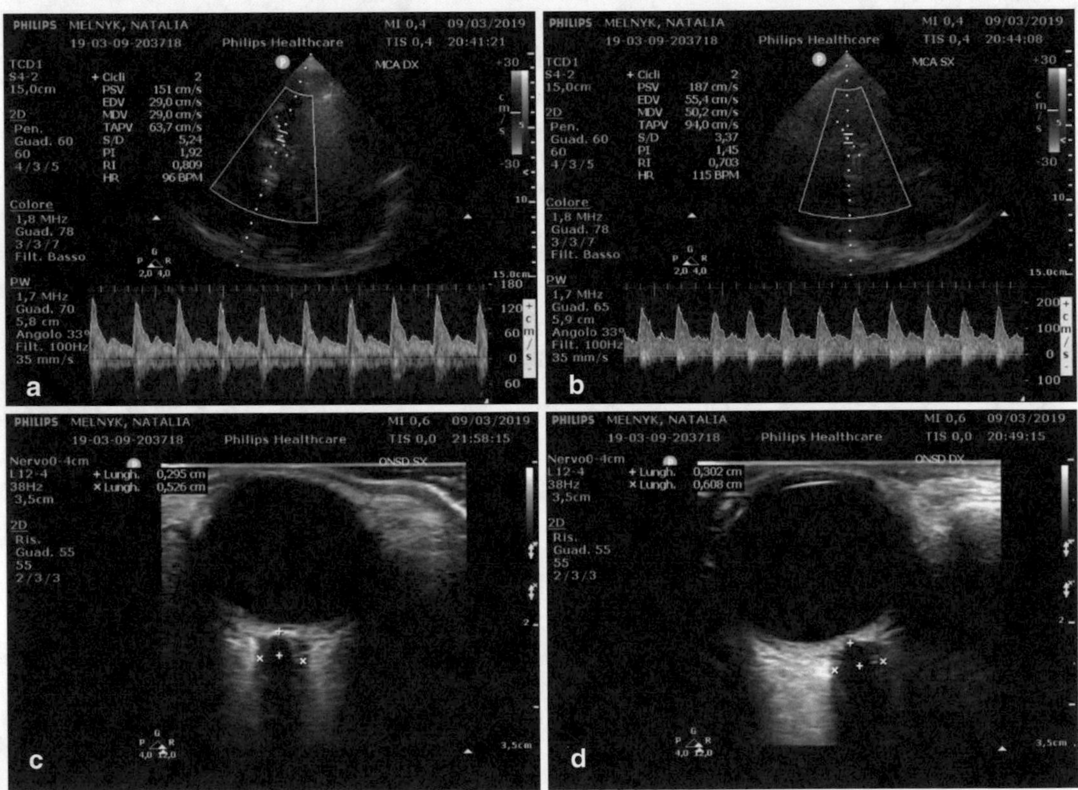

Fig. 34.2 (**a–d**) Panels **a** and **b** showing left MCA flow velocity and ONSD, panels **c** and **d** showing right MCA and ONSD before insertion of the invasive ICP monitoring system

infection complicated by convulsive episodes treated with antibiotics (vancomycin and cefepime) and levetiracetam. On day 7 in ICU she was tracheostomised and quickly weaned from the ventilator.

Her neurological status gradually improved becoming awake with fluctuating levels of attention, intermittently being able to obey commands as for aphasia; after 11 days in ICU, the patient was moved to the neurosurgical ward.

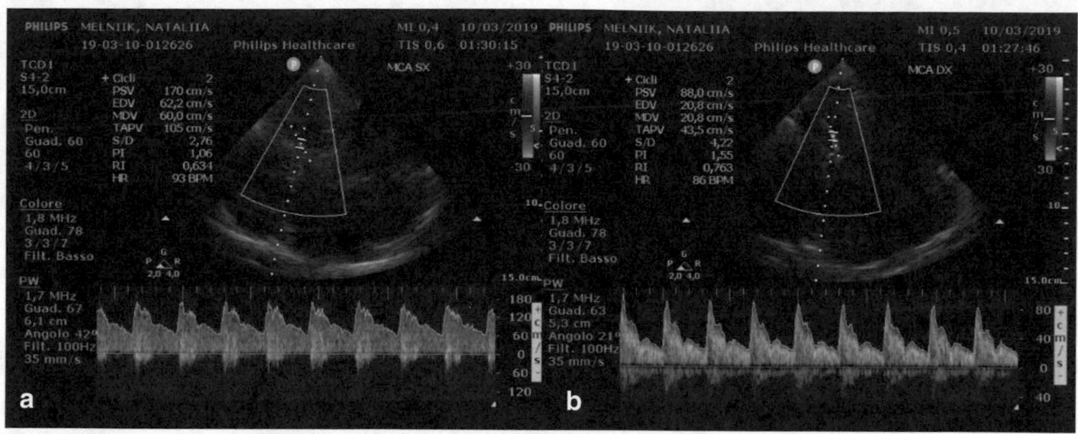

Fig. 34.3 TCCD after DC points out complete normalization of flow in left MCA (left panel), while in right MCA (right panel) PI, despite a decreasing trend, is still above normal limit (PI = 1.55)

Case 11: Hydrocephalus with Ventricular Vegetations

35

Rita Bertuetti, Maurizio Saini, Davide Savo, Francesca Simonassi, Kartika Chandrapatham, and Tarek Senussi

A 19-year-old man was admitted to ICU for polytrauma secondary to a car accident. He reported a severe traumatic brain injury with bilateral interhemispheric and periencephalic hemorrhagic soffusion and frontal contusions. Three days after admission he underwent a right temporoparietal decompressive craniectomy and external ventricular drainage (EVD) placement for uncontrolled intracranial hypertension. In the following months the patients developed multiple hygromas and concomitant Klebsiella pneumonia carbapenemasi producer infection (due to gastrointestinal tract colonization) treated with EVD and antibiotic therapy, respectively. Tracheostomy was performed. Three months after trauma, cranioplasty with autologous bone was performed. During the following weeks, the patient showed a neurological deterioration: an increase of brain ventricle volumes and a hydroaerial level with alteration of cerebrospinal fluid (CFS) signal were observed on CT scan. Similarly brain ultrasound showed remarkably enlarged ventricles (Fig. 35.1). High-quality images obtained with brain ultrasound allowed us to monitor the evolution of hydrocephalus without performing multiple CTs (also given the patient's unstable clinical conditions) (Figs. 35.2a, b and 35.3), but also allowed us to identify two different intraventricular neoformations (Figs. 35.2b and 35.4) consistent with infected vegetations (Fig. 35.3).

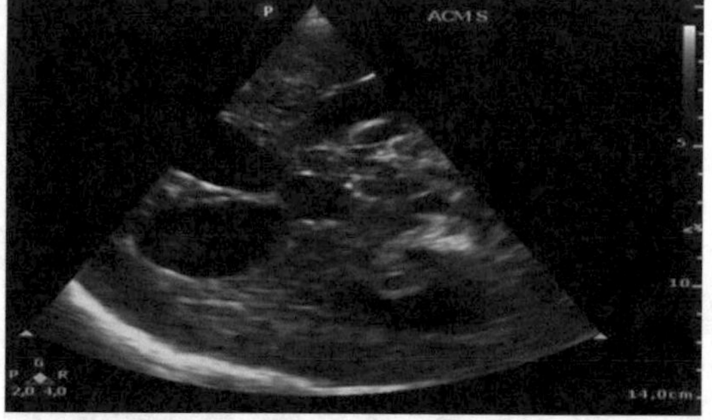

Fig. 35.1 Brain ultrasound (transtemporal window) shows enlarged lateral ventricles, on the top right, in the occipital horn of the ventricle, presence of neoformation can be appreciated

After such findings, a lumbar puncture confirming the presence of turbid CFS was performed

R. Bertuetti (✉)
Department of Anesthesiology, Critical Care Medicine and Emergency, Division of Neurocritical Care, ASST Spedali Civili di Brescia, University Hospital, Brescia, Italy

M. Saini · D. Savo
Department of Emergency, Perioperative Medicine and Intensive Care, Neuroanesthesia and Neurointensive Care Unit, San Gerardo Hospital, ASST-Monza, Monza, Italy

F. Simonassi · K. Chandrapatham
Anesthesia and Intensive Care, Ospedale Policlinico San Martino - IRCCS for Oncology and Neurosciences, Genoa, Italy

T. Senussi
Department of Surgical Sciences and Integrated Diagnostics, University of Genoa, Genoa, Italy

C. Robba, G. Citerio (eds.), *Echography and Doppler of the Brain*,
https://doi.org/10.1007/978-3-030-48202-2_35

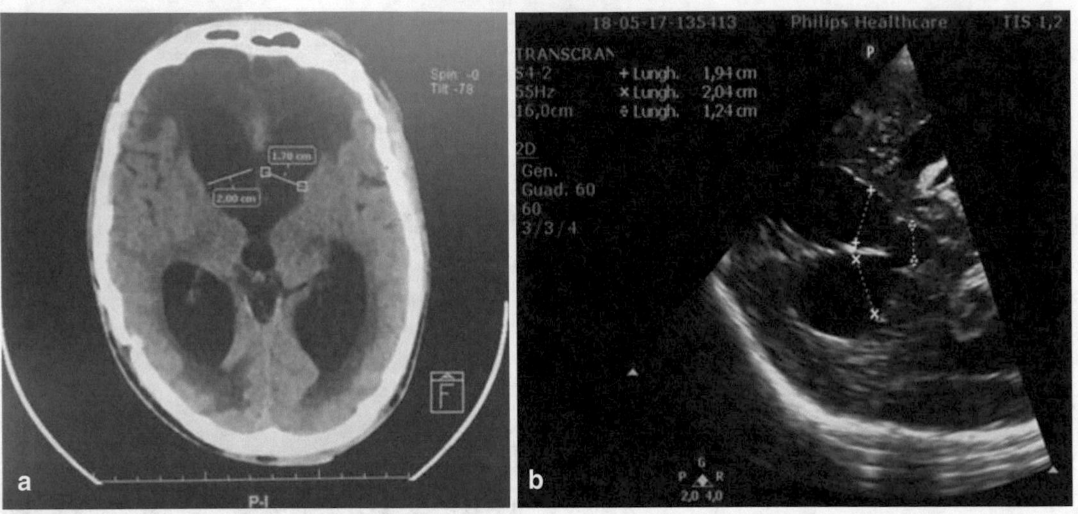

Fig. 35.2 (**a**, **b**) In panel (**a**), on the left, measurement of ventricles size on a TC head image frame. In panel (**b**), on the right, meaurement of ventricle width through using brain ultrasound

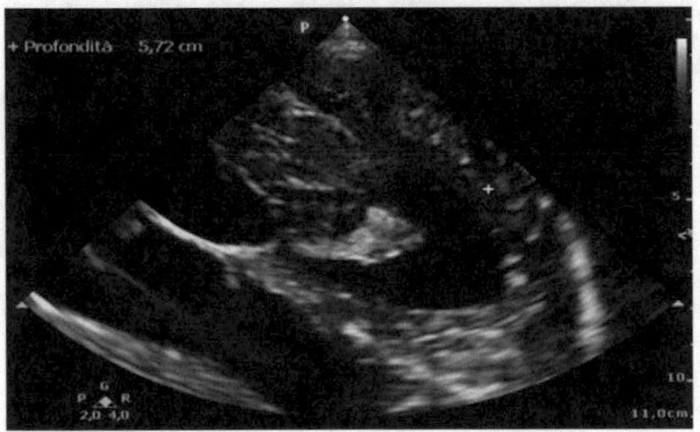

Fig. 35.3 Infectious vegetation in the occipital horn of the left ventricles

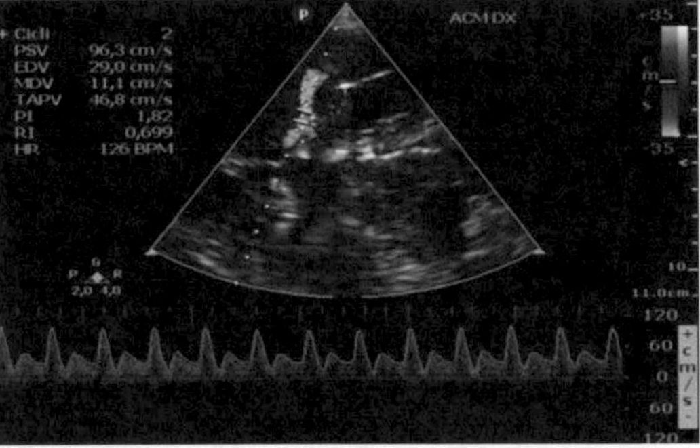

Fig. 35.5 TCCD of right MCA: evaluation of cerebral blood flow and estimation of intracranial pressure in the follow up of hydrocephalus progression. The spectrogram shows increased PI and a diastolic flow velocity at lower limits

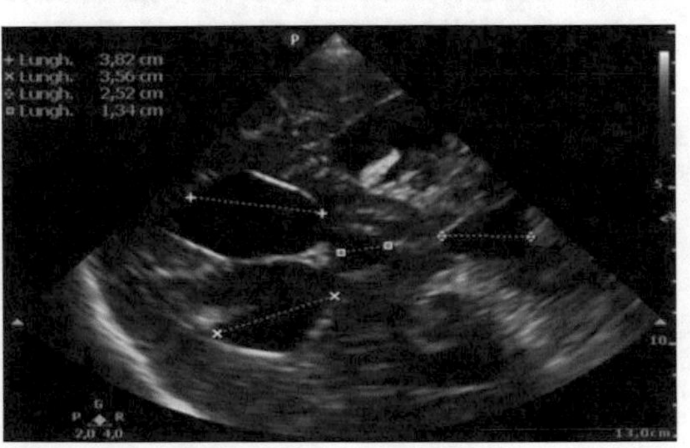

Fig. 35.4 Measurement of the lateral ventricles and third ventricle size through the use of brain ultrasound

and antibiotic therapy was then restored and a new EVD catheter was replaced. Fig. 35.5 shows blood flow velocities evaluated with TCCD in the right middle cerebral artery during the phase of intracranial hypertension secondary to hydrocephalus. Unfortunately, given the serious neurological and infective situation, the patient developed several uncontrolled intracranial hypertension episodes associated with neurovegetative disorders; he died after 6 months from the initial injury.

Case 12: Intracranial Hypertension after Ischemic Stroke

36

Rita Bertuetti, Maurizio Saini, Davide Savo, Francesca Simonassi, Kartika Chandrapatham, and Tarek Senussi

A 40-year-old patient admitted to a trauma center hospital after a workplace accident was diagnosed with a neck injury caused by direct impact with a grinder and complicated with right internal carotid artery laceration. The Glasgow Come Scale at the admission was 13/15. Urgent surgical intervention was needed to repair the damaged vessel and subsequently the patient was admitted to intensive care unit. The day after the trauma, because of neurological deterioration, the patient was intubated and a brain CT was undertaken: it showed a large area of ischemia at the level of the right frontal-temporal-parietal areas with disappearance of the interhemispheric grooves and midline shift. On the basis of brain CT findings decision was taken to insert an intracranial pressure (ICP) probe to monitor the evolving intracranial hypertension. The invasive monitoring system immediately confirmed a condition of intracranial hypertension (ICP = 34 mmHg); alongside TCD sessions were performed in order to evaluate cerebral blood flow (Fig. 36.1). Despite treatment escalation to deep sedation and systemic blood pressure support with noradrenaline, intracranial hypertension worsened causing severe hypoperfusion as showed by a significant reduction in diastolic flow (almost to zero) at the TCCD. Figures 36.2 and 36.3 show the flow in right middle cerebral artery at ICP of 50 mmHg and 57 mmHg, respectively. Mannitol and hypertonic solution boluses were started and support with vasoconstrictors was increased. The efficacy of the treatment was monitored with TCCD and a clear improvement in cranial hypertensive status and cerebral perfusion was observed. Figure 36.4 shows increasing of the diastolic flow with a clear

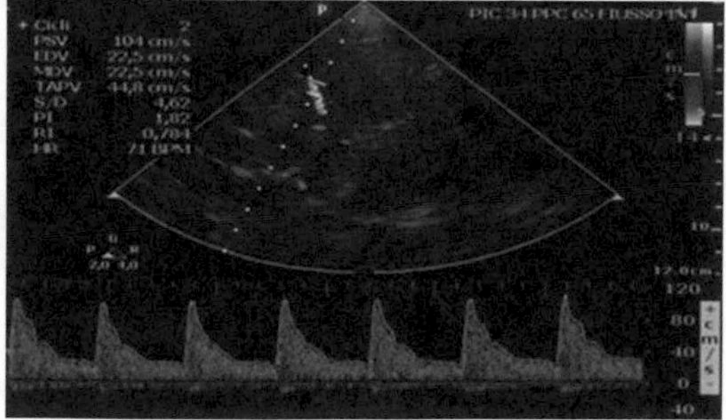

Fig. 36.1 TCCD of right MCA performed in order to assess cerebral blood flow

R. Bertuetti (✉)
Department of Anesthesiology, Critical Care Medicine and Emergency, Division of Neurocritical Care, ASST Spedali Civili di Brescia, University Hospital, Brescia, Italy

M. Saini · D. Savo
Department of Emergency, Perioperative Medicine and Intensive Care, Neuroanesthesia and Neurointensive Care Unit, San Gerardo Hospital, ASST-Monza, Monza, Italy

F. Simonassi · K. Chandrapatham
Anesthesia and Intensive Care, Ospedale Policlinico San Martino – IRCCS for Oncology and Neurosciences, Genoa, Italy

T. Senussi
Department of Surgical Sciences and Integrated Diagnostics, University of Genoa, Genoa, Italy

C. Robba, G. Citerio (eds.), *Echography and Doppler of the Brain*, https://doi.org/10.1007/978-3-030-48202-2_36

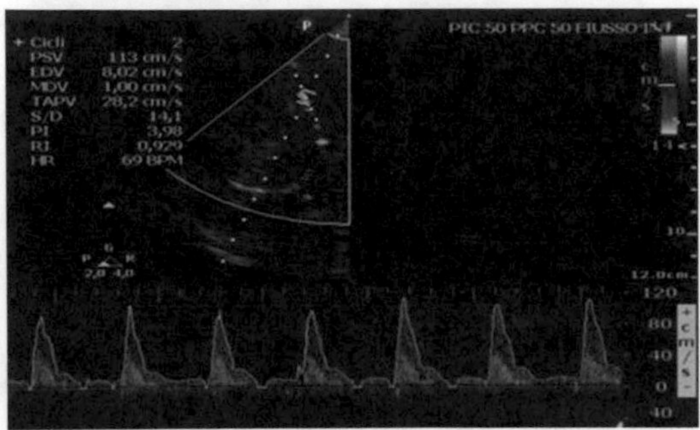

Fig. 36.2 TCCD of right MCA shows almost absent diastolic flow velocity at ICP of 50 mmHg

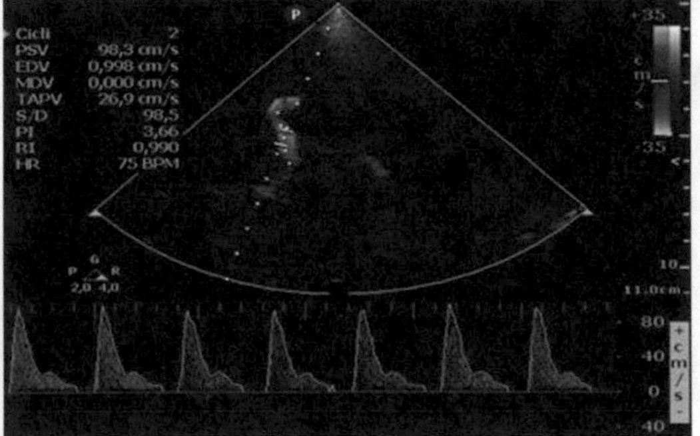

Fig. 36.3 TCCD of right MCA shows almost absent diastolic flow velocity at ICP of 57 mmHg

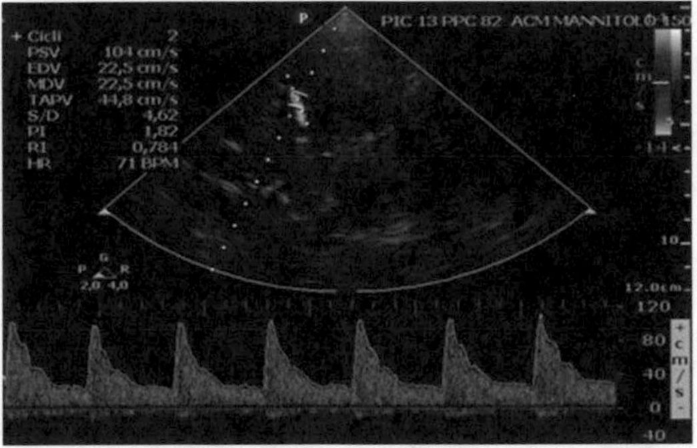

Fig. 36.4 TCCD of right MCA after mannitol bolus and initiation of vasopressors

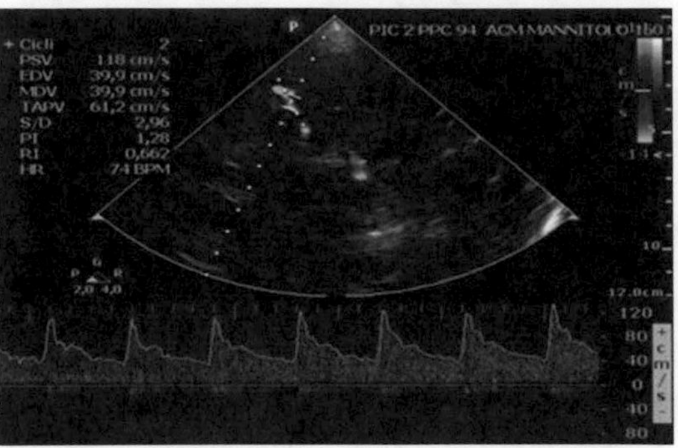

Fig. 36.5 TCCD of righr MCA shows further imprvement of flow after administration of a bolus of hypertonic saline

reduction of the pulsatility index (ICP values = 13 mmHg) after administration of mannitol, and Fig. 36.5 shows a further improvement of the diastolic and systolic flow after administration of a hypertonic solution (values of ICP = 2 mmHg). Despite the medical therapy, in the following days the patient had further intracranial hypertensive crises so, in agreement with the neurosurgeons, it was decided to proceed with a decompressive craniectomy. Subsequently to the decompression, ICP values remained well controlled and the patient was extubated after 4 days and transferred a week later to a neurorehabilitation center due to the neurological sequelae reported (upper and lower left limb motor deficits and partial expressive aphasia). After 1 month cranioplasty with autologous bone was performed.

Printed in the United States
by Baker & Taylor Publisher Services